CH 5,7

COGNITION AND PERCEPTION IN THE STROKE PATIENT

A Guide to Functional Outcomes in Occupational Therapy

THE REHABILITATION INSTITUTE OF CHICAGO
PUBLICATION SERIES
Don A. Olson, PhD, Series Coordinator

Spinal Cord Injury: A Guide to Functional Outcomes in Physical Therapy Management

Lower Extremity Amputation: A Guide to Functional Outcomes in Physical Therapy Management, Second Edition

Stroke/Head Injury: A Guide to Functional Outcomes in Physical Therapy Management

Clinical Management of Right Hemisphere Dysfunction

Clinical Evaluation of Dysphasia

Spinal Cord Injury: A Guide to Functional Outcomes in Occupational Therapy

Spinal Cord Injury: A Guide to Rehabilitation Nursing

Head Injury: A Guide to Functional Outcomes in Occupational Therapy Management

Speech/Language Treatment of the Aphasias: An Integrated Clinical Approach

Speech/Language Treatment of the Aphasias: Treatment Materials for Auditory Comprehension and Reading Comprehension

Speech/Language Treatment of the Aphasias: Treatment Materials for Oral Expression and Written Expression

Rehabilitation Nursing Procedures Manual

Psychological Management of Traumatic Brain Injuries in Children and Adolescents

Medical Management of Long-Term Disability

Psychological Aspects of Geriatric Rehabilitation

Clinical Management of Communication Problems in Adults with Traumatic Brain Injury

Cognition and Perception in the Stroke Patient: A Guide to Functional Outcomes in Occupational Therapy

Rehabilitation
Institute of
Chicago

COGNITION
AND
PERCEPTION
IN THE
STROKE PATIENT

A Guide to
Functional
Outcomes in
Occupational
Therapy

Kathleen Okkema, MBA, OTR/L
Formerly, Supervisor in Occupational Therapy
Rehabilitation Institute of Chicago
Associate Therapist
Rausch and Associates
Chicago, Illinois

AN ASPEN PUBLICATION®
Aspen Publishers, Inc.
Gaithersburg, Maryland
1993

Library of Congress Cataloging-in-Publication Data
Okkema, Kathleen.
Cognition and perception in the stroke patient : a guide to
functional outcomes in occupational therapy / Kathleen Okkema.
p.   cm. — (The Rehabilitation Institute of Chicago
publication series)
Includes bibliographical references and index.
ISBN: 0-8342-0362-6
1. Cerebrovascular disease—Patients—Rehabilitation.
2. Cognition disorders—Patients—Rehabilitation. 3. Occupational
therapy. 4. Perception, Disorders of—Patients—Rehabilitation.
I. Title. II. Series.
[DNLM: 1. Cerebrovascular Disorders—rehabilitation.
2. Cognition. 3. Occupational Therapy. 4. Perception. WL 355
0415c]
RC388.5.O44 1993
616.8'106515—dc20
DNLM/DLC
for Library of Congress
92-48191
CIP

Aspen Publishers, Inc. grants permission for photocopying for limited
personal or internal use. This consent does not extend to other kinds of
copying, such as copying for general distribution, for advertising or
promotional purposes, for creating new collective works, or for resale. For
information, address Aspen Publishers, Inc., Permissions Department,
200 Orchard Ridge Drive, Suite 200, Gaithersburg, Maryland 20878.

The author has made every effort to ensure the accuracy of the information
herein. However, appropriate information sources should be consulted, especially for new or unfamiliar procedures. It is the responsibility of every practitioner to evaluate the appropriateness of a particular opinion in the context of
actual clinical situations and with due consideration to new developments. The
author, editors, and the publisher cannot be held responsible for any typographi-
cal or other errors found in this book.

Editorial Resources: Ruth Bloom

Library of Congress Catalog Card Number: 92-48191
ISBN: 0-8342-0362-6

Printed in the United States of America

1 2 3 4 5

Table of Contents

Series Preface ix

Preface xi

Guide to the Use of This Book xiii

Acknowledgments xv

PART I—COGNITIVE AND PERCEPTUAL EVALUATION   1

Chapter   1—Evaluation of Cognition and Perception: Overview of
                 Occupational Therapy Practice   3
            Development of the Occupational Therapy Cognitive
                 Protocol: Review of the Literature   3
            Assessments Developed by Occupational Therapists   4
            Thoughts on Formal Testing   6
            The RIC Occupational Therapy Cognitive and
                 Perceptual Evaluation Protocol   6

Chapter   2—Evaluation: General Methods and Philosophy   9
            Purpose of Evaluation   9
            Chart Review   9
            Interview 10
            Activity Analysis 10
            Formal Testing 11

Chapter   3—Factors Influencing Cognitive and Perceptual Evaluation 13
            Psychosocial Factors 13
            Primary Senses 15
            Expressive Language Deficits 19
            Motor Function 20

Chapter 4—Cognitive and Perceptive Techniques **23**

Cognitive and Perceptual Evaluation Overview 23

Evaluations for Cognition 23

Evaluations for Visual Perception 36

Evaluations for Visual Analysis and Synthesis 43

Evaluations for Body Awareness 50

Evaluations for Motor Planning 54

PART II—GOAL WRITING AND TREATMENT PLANNING **59**

Chapter 5—General Considerations for Goal Writing and Treatment Planning **61**

Evaluating Skill Deficits 61

Analyzing the Impact of Component Skill Deficits on Function 62

Setting Realistic Functional and Component Skill Goals 63

Planning Treatment To Address Mutual Goals 65

Planning Treatment 66

Evaluating the Effectiveness of Treatment 67

Chapter 6—Frames of Reference and General Principles for
       Cognitive and Perceptual Treatment **69**

Consideration of Various Frames of Reference 69

General Approaches to Treatment 73

Educating the Adult Learner 82

Adapting the Environment 84

Chapter 7—Cognitive and Perceptual Treatment Techniques **85**

Cognitive Treatment Ideas 85

Perceptual Treatment Ideas 95

Conclusion 115

Chapter 8—Driver Rehabilitation after Stroke **117**
Roseann Cumbo-Misheck

Referral Process 117

Clinical Evaluation 118

Behind-the-Wheel Evaluation 119

Driver Training 119

Poor Clinical or Driving Performance 122

Evaluation of Deficits 123

Treatment Suggestions 128

Conclusion 130

Appendix 8-A—List of Vendors 131

Chapter 9—Case Example Illustrating Evaluation and Treatment Principles **133**

Medical and Social History 133

Initial Evaluation 133

Goals 134

Treatment 135

Outcome 137

PART III—EVALUATION AND TREATMENT GUIDES 139

Chapter 10—Cognitive Evaluation Guide 141
    Arousal 141
    Attention 143
    Orientation 148
    Topographical Orientation 149
    Memory 149
    Problem Solving 151

Chapter 11—Perceptual Evaluation Guide 155
    Visual Perception 155
    Visual Analysis and Synthesis 159
    Visual Construction 163
    Body Awareness 166
    Body Awareness Tests 167
    Motor Planning 172

Chapter 12—Goal Writing and Treatment Ideas 175
    Cognitive Goals and Treatment 175
    Perceptual Goals and Treatment 179
    Group Goals 184
    Group Treatment 184

Bibliography 191

Index 199

Series Preface

Key words in today's rehabilitation vocabulary are "functional outcomes." The physician, nurse, and therapist are being judged on the outcomes produced in the therapy setting. Research in nursing, allied health, and medicine are focusing on demonstration of functional outcomes in all of our patient activities. Occupational therapists have been leaders in this area primarily because all of their therapeutic activities are directed at that end result—functional outcomes to maximize the patients' quality of life.

The need to document the patients' severity of disability and the outcomes of our rehabilitation have been long-standing. We continue to seek a uniform language among professionals to describe functional outcome and change across disciplines. It is our goal to document and establish measures against which patients' progress can be assessed. We continue to seek comprehensive approaches to our patients to reintegrate them into the community and maximize their quality of life.

The Procedural Manuals developed by the Rehabilitation Institute of Chicago are directed to accomplish the above goals, but also to share the expertise of our staff with our colleagues throughout the world. Twenty Procedural Manuals make up this cooperative program that has been developed between Aspen Publishers, Inc., and the Rehabilitation Institute of Chicago. This new manual, *Cognition and Perception in the Stroke Patient: A Functional Guide to Outcomes in Occupational Therapy* is our latest effort to share in an organized fashion our approaches to better management and care of our patients.

As rehabilitation professionals we continue to try to meet the challenges of providing maximum services for the people we work with. In order to meet this challenge we need to continue to expand our knowledge, our experiences, our teamwork, our ability to collaborate, to coordinate, and to plan. This manual is but one tool to assist you in meeting the common goals you share with your colleagues and the patients you work with in your facility.

Rehabilitation medicine relies on an interdisciplinary approach to patient care. The way the treatment staff works together as a team, and the approach they adopt, will determine the success or failure of the outcome of their treatment. We all want our patients to recover to their maximum potential and to learn skills that will offer them independence in their home communities. The procedures set forth in this series are directed at improving our individual approaches, our team approaches, but more importantly, the outcomes possible with our patients.

Don A. Olson, PhD
Coordinator
Rehabilitation Institute of Chicago
Publication Series
Director, Education and Training Center
Associate Professor
Departments of Physical Medicine and
Rehabilitation and Neurology
Northwestern University Medical School

Cognition and Perception in the Stroke Patient: A Functional Guide to Outcomes in Occupational Therapy provides both theoretical and practical information for the evaluation and treatment of cognitive and perceptual problems experienced by stroke patients. The text is based on standards for cognitive and perceptual evaluation that were developed for use by occupational therapists treating stroke patients at the Rehabilitation Institute of Chicago (RIC). The stroke patients who receive treatment at RIC show a wide range of abilities. Some have had severe strokes, making them dependent on others for all aspects of care. Others demonstrate mild deficits that interfere only with high-level skills such as work, leisure, or social activities. Thus, our department required a wide range of evaluation and treatment activities in order to meet individual patients' needs.

To help the therapist define and treat various cognitive and perceptual deficits, they are listed in a hierarchical order throughout the book. In reality, the patient will show problems in a variety of component skills. One deficit will influence another and make analysis of the major factors that limit function complex. It is hoped that by looking at the problem areas discretely, the occupational therapist will be able to define difficulties accurately. He or she must then determine how one problem affects another, and must plan treatment that will address a variety of limiting factors in a manner that is relevant for each patient.

Throughout the book, the importance of functional observations and treatment techniques is emphasized. It is believed that the most benefit can be provided to our patients by carefully observing them during meaningful activities. Analysis of their performance, followed by specific testing when necessary to clarify observations, will ensure a relevant and accurate assessment. The text also emphasizes the importance of involving the patient, the family, and other caregivers in the treatment process. It is hoped that therapists will strive to understand the cultural, social, and emotional factors that contribute to performance. By considering all of these factors, the therapist can provide an effective treatment plan.

Many types of evaluation and treatment activities are included because it is believed that each patient will benefit from a unique combination of tasks. The skilled therapist should be familiar with a wide range of techniques and should use those that best suit the patient's needs. The methods and techniques described have been useful with various patients at RIC. It must be emphasized that each patient receives only a few of the many evaluation procedures described. The evaluations that are chosen reflect the skills and goals of that patient. In other settings, where the goals of treatment or the types of patients differ, the information should be used selectively to meet those needs.

This book was written to provide structured information for students or new therapists as well as more theoretical information that can assist the experienced therapist to solve evaluation and treatment problems related to cognition and perception. The information can also help therapists establish department protocols for evaluation, goal writing, and treatment in the areas of cognition and perception.

Guide to the Use of This Book

This manual was written to help occupational therapists effectively evaluate and treat cognitive and perceptual deficits in patients who have had a cerebrovascular accident. The book is intended to be used as a working tool in the clinic as well as a reference book for planning treatment. Theoretical concepts discussed in the literature and practical considerations gained through experience are combined to provide evaluation and treatment suggestions that are both academically sound and clinically useful. Although more than one frame of reference is used, it is hoped that the functional foundation of occupational therapy is clearly reflected throughout the book. The subject matter of this book is complex; however, efforts were made to present the information in a clear and logical manner. The manual is not intended to be used as a "cookbook." The therapist must always be aware of a patient's subtle variations in performance and use good clinical judgment in selecting evaluations, interpreting evaluation results, setting goals, and planning treatment.

The book is divided into three parts with several units in each. Part I provides in-depth information about cognitive and perceptual evaluation. Background information about the testing sequence and rationales for the tests selected are given. In addition, information is given about how other areas, such as poor vision, may influence cognitive and perceptual evaluation.

Part II describes the goal writing and treatment planning process. General information about setting goals and planning treatment is provided. Current frames of reference are described and rationales are given for the treatment approaches used by the occupational therapy department at the Rehabilitation Institute of Chicago.

Included in this section are suggestions for remediation as well as compensation.

Part III is the evaluation and treatment guide. This part of the manual is designed to be used in the clinic and provides protocols and scoring methods. Although the guide is arranged in an easy-to-use format, the therapist should be familiar with the background information and rationales for evaluation protocols before using it. The protocols provided are meant to be used in a selective way based on each patient's performance in self-care tasks, activities related to their prior roles, and activities performed in the clinic. Good observational skills and a holistic approach to the patient's care is necessary for effective use of the evaluation protocols. Part III also contains goals and treatment suggestions to help attain each goal. Information is arranged in a chart format to simplify its use in the clinical setting. These goals and treatment ideas are suggestions that are designed to be modified to meet each patient's needs. Information pertaining to group goals and treatment is provided in this part. The charts summarize information and provide specific ideas to complement the more theoretical information presented in Part II.

This manual is intended to assist the therapist in understanding each patient's cognitive and perceptual deficits. By increasing understanding, it is believed that the therapist will write realistic goals, help the patient and caregivers to understand the impact of these deficits on function, and provide optimal treatment. It is hoped that the book will stimulate further exploration of cognitive and perceptual deficits, encourage the therapist to routinely evaluate treatment effectiveness, and positively affect the care of stroke patients.

Acknowledgments

This book was made possible because of the support of many people both at the Rehabilitation Institute of Chicago and outside of the Institute. We are especially indebted to the Buchanan Family Foundation which provided financial support that allowed the authors to prepare for the writing of the book, investigate and research testing methods, and develop occupational therapy standards for the evaluation of cognition and perception for our stroke patients.

Many people aided in the development of the book and I would like to express my appreciation for their dedication, knowledge, and assistance with this project. Special thanks and appreciation go to the following people:

Carolyn Weber, MS, OTR/L

Shari Intagliata, MS, MPA

Kathy Culler, MS

Marlene Morgan, MOT,

Gerri Gibson

Oscar Izquierdo

and to the Stroke Survivors who have taught me so much about evaluation and treatment.

Also, to my husband Jim and my son Tim, who provided ongoing encouragement to help me maintain the balance between work, rest and play.

Contributor

Roseann Cumbo-Misheck, OT
Clinical Specialist
Department of Occupational Therapy
Rehabilitation Institute of Chicago

Part I

Cognitive and Perceptual Evaluation

Evaluation of Cognition and Perception: Overview of Occupational Therapy Practice

DEVELOPMENT OF THE OCCUPATIONAL THERAPY COGNITIVE PROTOCOL: REVIEW OF THE LITERATURE

It cannot be disputed that occupational therapists (OTs) require information about cognitive and perceptual function in order to treat their patients effectively. Cognitive and perceptual skills affect all aspects of self-care and can have a significant impact on the patient's ability to profit from treatment (Anderson et al. 1974; Dombovy et al. 1986; Feigenson et al. 1977; Jongbloed 1986). The need for evaluation methods useful to OTs is evident.

After review of a large body of literature, the Rehabilitation Institute of Chicago (RIC) cognitive and perceptual evaluation was developed. The goal was to create an accurate, flexible, time-efficient, easily used test battery that combines functional observations with formal tests. The protocol recommends beginning the evaluation with observations of self-care skills. Tests can then be selected to clarify deficits further. The tests are presented in a hierarchical manner from most basic to most complex. Thus a simple test may be used to help define deficits in a patient with more involved problems, and a difficult test may be used to detect subtle problems in a patient with high-level skills. In developing this protocol several years ago, there were few occupational therapy tests available for testing patients who had had a cerebrovascular accident (CVA). Since that time several occupational therapy batteries

have become available. These may be useful for departments that do not have a protocol established. Most of them, however, do not cover the wide range of cognitive and perceptual deficits found in patients who have had a CVA; do not integrate functional observations into their protocols; have varying degrees of psychometric strength; and, in order to be reliable, many must be given as a complete battery, thus eliminating the flexibility to choose specific tests based on the patient's presentation.

A review of occupational therapy approaches to cognitive and perceptual evaluation follows. It is clear that the best method of gathering cognitive and perceptual information remains open to debate. There are some who believe that cognition and perception (Morse 1986; Arnadottir 1990; Fisher 1992) can best be evaluated through functional observations made during self-care activities. It is by these observations that OTs make a unique contribution to the treatment team. The daily living skill evaluation takes place in realistic settings rather than the sterile environment found in a testing situation. The complexity and decision-making requirements that standard tests seek to simulate can be found in many daily living tasks. The problem with this functional method is that it is sometimes difficult to delineate clearly a cognitive or perceptual deficit through observation alone. Because a patient who has difficulty buttoning a shirt may have motor loss, visual spatial deficits, motor-planning problems, or decreased attention, observation often must be supplemented with more discrete tests or a series of observations. As Mosey (1986, 9) states in *Psychosocial Components of Occupational Therapy*, "At times it is necessary to divide to understand." Without a clear picture of the deficits interfering with function, our effectiveness and professionalism can be questioned.

ASSESSMENTS DEVELOPED BY OCCUPATIONAL THERAPISTS

To define deficits more clearly, some OTs have developed standardized tests designed to look at cognitive and perceptual skills. Occupational therapy is in a preliminary phase of test development, and further efforts toward standardization are needed to provide useful tests for the CVA population. A review of some of these evaluations follows.

The Loewenstein Occupational Therapy Cognitive Assessment (Katz et al. 1989) has been tested with 28 patients with CVA, 20 patients with craniocerebral injury, and 55 normal adults. It evaluates orientation, perception, visuomotor organization, and thinking operations through a series of 20 subtests. Inter-rater reliability, internal consistency, limited criterion validity, and construct validity were established. The test was not available in the United States when the RIC protocol was developed. Although some useful statistical analysis has taken place, this test does not include a clear attempt to use functional observations as a basis for evaluation.

The Allen Cognitive Level Test (ACL), a leatherlacing activity, is being used in clinics with adult brain-injured patients (Smith 1990); however, there is no specific information about what skills it tests in these patients. Although there is a body of literature to support its use with adult psychiatric patients (Allen 1985; David and Riley 1990; Mayer 1988), little has been published about its usefulness with brain-injured adults. It is described as a cognitive test; however, in a study of 71 psychiatric patients, David and Riley (1990) found a relationship between the ACL and the Symbol Digit Modalities Test, a test of visuomotor speed and attention. These authors suggest that the ACL measures novel perceptual motor learning and speculate that the test may be sensitive to neurological dysfunction. They recommend further investigation with neurologically involved patients. Mayer (1988) studied 40 adult psychiatric patients and found that the ACL test was related to fluid perceptual-integrative skills of perceptual organization and distractibility as measured by the Wechsler Adult Intelligence Scale-Revised (WAIS-R). Some of the WAIS-R subtests that

are used to measure perceptual organization include Block Design and Object Assembly, while distractibility is correlated with performance on the Digit Symbol test and the Digit Backwards test. In summary, this test may be useful as a tool for observing a patient's ability to follow instructions to attend to a task and to perform a visual construction task. It does not evaluate memory; distinguish various learning modalities such as visual, tactile/kinesthetic, or auditory learning; allow analysis of specific factors that contribute to performance; or provide alternatives for analyzing the components of a visual construction task. In addition, unilateral performance of the test by clamping the work in a vice is awkward and may be rejected by patients. Finally, the language skills required may be too advanced for many CVA patients.

The Saint Mary's CVA Evaluation has been studied with 100 CVA patients for construct validity; however, it was not given to a control group, and reliability information was not reported. This battery looks at self-care, left-side function, recovery stage, perception, and strength (Harlowe and Van Deusen 1984; Van Deusen-Fox and Harlowe 1984; Van Deusen and Harlowe 1987). Although this test battery includes self-care evaluations to define perceptual deficits, the procedures were not clearly described. Furthermore, when analyzing the bilateral awareness scale, the authors concluded that functional observations are not as sensitive as more rigorous test procedures in separating unilateral neglect from other perceptual problems (Van Deusen and Harlowe 1987).

The Test of Orientation for Rehabilitation Patients (TORP) has been evaluated for content validity and inter-rater reliability (Dietz et al. 1990). It is designed to evaluate five domains: person and personal situation, place, time, schedule, and temporal continuity. Many of these items are also addressed in the RIC evaluation protocol in a less formal manner. The authors state that 25 minutes are required to prepare to administer each test. Evaluation time using the TORP can range from 5 to 30 minutes. When a standard test is desired, the RIC protocol recommends Benton's test of temporal orientation, a fast, easily administered evaluation (Benton 1983d).

Tan and Zemke (1991) established adult norms for the Motor-Free Visual Perception Test (Colarusso and Hamill 1972). Previously, norms were limited to children. This test battery evaluates a range of visual perceptual skills and is administered by the Communicative Disorders Department at RIC. Based on evaluation of 104 older adults, aged 60 to 89, Tan and Zemke found lower scores and slower response times with increasing age.

The Ontario Society of Occupational Therapists Perceptual Evaluation was developed to provide a standardized, quantifiable, and valid assessment procedure for evaluating perceptual deficits in patients with acquired brain damage (Boys et al. 1988). Patients with cerebral trauma and aphasia were excluded. The 28 tests included in the battery measure sensory function, scanning and spatial neglect, apraxia, body awareness, spatial relations, and visual agnosia. After administering the test battery to 80 experimental and 70 control subjects, Boys et al. concluded that the test was able to differentiate normal from impaired subjects and that most sections of the test demonstrated construct validity. The authors state that the test provides considerations for self-care evaluation, but this information was not described. The time required to administer the test was not indicated, but because of the number of items, it appears to be lengthy.

The Rivermead Perceptual Assessment Battery is composed of 16 subtests that can be administered in less than an hour and is designed to measure visual perception. It provides normative data for adults under age 69 years and evidence of reliability and validity (Whiting et al. 1985). The Rivermead Behavioral Inattention Test is described as a test that provides an objective method of evaluating daily skills for unilateral neglect. It was given to 28 CVA patients and 14 neurologically intact persons. The test was found to be reliable and valid; however, a significantly longer time was required to administer this test than other tests of neglect such as letter cancellation and design copying (Wilson et al. 1987). This test represents an attempt to combine functional activities with cognitive and perceptual testing; however, many of the functional tasks are actually simulations leading to some of the same relevance problems encountered with psychological tests. A Rivermead Memory Test is also available.

The Chessington Occupational Therapy Neurological Assessment Battery is composed of 12 tests measuring visual perception, constructional ability, sensory motor ability, and ability to follow instructions. Product information indicates that the test provides normative information and is valid in measuring these factors in stroke patients. The test is cumbersome and costly, largely because of the types of test activities included (Nottingham Rehab Catalogue 1990).

The Cambridge Apraxia Battery (Fraser and Turton 1986) is a battery consisting of 8 subtests designed to be administered in 30 to 45 minutes. It was standardized on 60 men and women ages 20–79. Inter-rater reliability was established between two raters evaluating four normal subjects. Although statistical analysis was not provided, the authors believed that inter-rater reli-

ability was acceptable. Subtests such as manual form perception, a finger maze, awareness of double tactile stimuli, ability to imitate postures, and ability to pantomime object use were included. Three underlying performance factors were identified: attention, spatial imagery, and registration of sensory input. Suggestions for interpreting results were provided. The subtests described were very similar to those developed by Chapparo and Ranka (1980) and used in the RIC OT department. It was our experience that giving a battery of tests was often time consuming and not necessary. Our goal was to choose tests that were short, valid and reliable, and that could be given individually based on the patient's presentation.

Soderback (1988a), a Swedish OT, describes the Intellectual Housework Assessment used for the evaluation of brain-damaged adults. This Swedish assessment uses observation of the activities of preparing potato soup and rolls or making cheese pasties and stock to evaluate eight factors relevant to performance. The factors are perceptual, spatial, verbal, numerical, praxis, memory, logical, and attentional. For each factor, critical points in task performance are identified. For instance, some of the observations that would suggest adequate attention include noticing the time, turning off appliances, and ensuring that food does not overcook while the table is set. Soderback presents two versions of the test to allow valid retesting after a short period of time. Analysis of the test demonstrates inter-rater reliability, concurrent validity, and construct validity; however, a high degree of correlation exists between various subtests. Soderback states that the evaluation can be used as a "proficiency test" and that it provides unique information to the rehabilitation team. The evaluation would not be appropriate for testing patients who are at a lower level of function.

Arnadottir (1990), in her book *The Brain and Behavior: Assessing Cortical Dysfunction through Activities of Daily Living*, describes a standardized test for OTs that combines functional observations of basic self-care skills with cognitive and perceptual assessment. Although this test focuses most specifically on perception, Arnadottir does provide a checklist with which to delineate whether memory, insight, judgment, confusion, alertness, attention, organization, and sequencing are present or absent. Her approach to standardizing observations of cognitive and perceptual deficits during basic self-care tasks seems promising, since it capitalizes on the OT's unique role on the treatment team while allowing the therapist to quantify observations and draw systematic conclusions. Arnadottir indicates that delineating deficits during functional observations is often difficult, and alludes to the benefit of using other test methods to clarify problems areas; however, she does not provide specific guidelines for using these tests. In addition, she states that analysis of high-level activities of daily living (ADL) would be beneficial.

The Assessment of Motor and Process Skills (AMPS) is described by Fisher et al. (1992) as an evaluation that allows simultaneous evaluation of 15 motor and 20 process skills during a two- or three-step advanced daily living task. The patient is allowed to choose two to three relevant and familiar meal preparation, home maintenance, or laundry tasks that will serve as the basis for the evaluation. Rigorous testing is being applied to ensure that this test is psychometrically sound, clinically relevant, and free of cultural bias. When released for general use, it promises to provide a functional, yet sensitive, test to analyze performance strengths and weaknesses.

THOUGHTS ON FORMAL TESTING

Although there are some OTs who believe that formal cognitive and perceptual testing should be done only by a psychologist to avoid duplication of services, to ensure that the patient does not benefit from the practice effect if a test is given twice, and to take advantage of the highly trained psychologist's expertise in interpreting test results (Morse 1986), there are many OTs who believe that it is acceptable to borrow well-constructed evaluations from other disciplines to test for deficits that may affect function (Siev et al. 1986; Farver and Farver 1982; Van Deusen and Harlowe 1987; Kaplan and Hier 1982; Titus et al. 1991).

The content of many of the occupational therapy cognitive batteries previously described actually appear to be shortened or modified versions of tests borrowed from psychology. However, generally they lack the research that strengthens most well-established psychological tests. When developing standardized tests, OTs must be careful to apply high standards of scientific scrutiny to ensure that these batteries really measure the skills intended. When long standardized tests are shortened and modified to meet OTs' practical objectives, it must be realized that the qualities of sensitivity, reliability, and validity that were carefully established may be lost. Finally, caution must be used in describing these tests as unique occupational therapy batteries because their content may not reflect the philosophy of occupation.

It is believed that the development of standardized occupational therapy evaluations is a positive step in the growth of the profession. However, the use of tests already devised by other highly skilled professionals can allow OTs to focus more energy on refining ADL evaluations and on determining the functional implications of particular deficits. Work such as that of Arnadottir (1990), Fisher (1992), and Soderback (1988a) seems very promising in further establishing the unique role of occupational therapy.

The Russian neuropsychologist, Luria ([1962] 1980), describes many brief tests suitable for bedside evaluation. Although these are not standardized tests, Luria emphasizes their use as a means of making systematic observations. He states that these simple tests are designed for patients with known brain damage and are activities that can be performed easily by an unimpaired person. Their purpose is not so much to describe quantitative information as qualitative information. Patients who are functioning at a higher level, however, may require more sensitive tests to differentiate normal from abnormal performance.

It is believed that "tests" similar to those described by Luria ([1962] 1980) may be used effectively as a method of examining various types of behavior in a systematic way. When observation of complex ADL tasks is confusing because of the great number of variables, systematic analysis of specific tasks can clarify problem areas. A simple clinical tool may be faster and more specific than continuing to observe complex ADL tasks. For advanced patients who do not show deficits in basic ADL tasks, standardized tests can help detect subtle problems. With these patients it is important to use tests that clearly establish normal performance so that challenge appropriate to their age and educational level can be provided.

THE RIC OCCUPATIONAL THERAPY COGNITIVE AND PERCEPTUAL EVALUATION PROTOCOL

Review of the literature, consideration of the needs of our staff, reflection on the needs of our patients, and discussion with other disciplines resulted in the RIC occupational therapy cognitive assessment protocol that provides

- a means of observing component skill deficits in function
- a method of testing deficits that are not clearly defined through functional observation
- a flexible format that can be used with patients with either high-level function or low-level function
- time efficiency
- established procedures to facilitate communication and consistency between therapists

The recommended evaluation process includes observation of deficits during self-care evaluation and selective testing to clarify the patient's deficits for goal setting, treatment planning, and caregiver teaching.

As described in Chapter 2, chart review is recommended as the first method of gathering data pertinent to cognition and perception. Next, functional observations are combined with activity analysis to identify deficits that relate specifically to each patient's roles, habits, and interests. The interplay between various cognitive strengths and weaknesses can be analyzed to make practical recommendations for treatment and suggestions for carry-over by the patient, caregiver, or team. When the information from these observations is clear, no further testing is required.

Because of the complex interaction of various cognitive and perceptual deficits in activity, it is likely that some questions about the nature of a patient's deficit may remain after functional observations have been completed. Literature on clinical problem solving indicates that the problem-solving skills of an entry-level practitioner are different from those of an experienced practitioner (Balla et al. 1990; Fleming 1991a, 1991b). Although an experienced practitioner may readily make pertinent observations of function and then use these observations coupled with scientific knowledge to identify a problem, the newer practitioner may have difficulty. Our experience as a training center for students and as an employer of many recent graduates confirms these findings. The need is evident for evaluation materials that help to clarify nebulous problems and allow the newer OT to refine observational skills. The use of specific evaluations can facilitate the development of clinical problem-solving expertise by helping the clinician link test results to patient performance problems.

Despite more sophisticated problem-solving skills, experienced staff may also need additional information to clarify their observations (Fleming 1991a). When a patient presents complex or overlapping deficits, or when the pattern of deficits is unfamiliar, the experienced clinician may seek more data. This may be done by observing the patient in additional functional tasks that emphasize the areas in question, by using evaluations designed to test the problem areas, or by consulting with another discipline that has performed objective tests. For the experienced therapist, then, it is also valuable to have evaluation tools that can be used to clarify more difficult or subtle deficits.

When using self-care observations for an initial evaluation, occasionally it can be difficult to provide challenges appropriate to the patient's level of function. This difficulty is evident with both high-level and low-

level patients. The first two or three days of contact with a CVA patient in a rehabilitation setting usually are devoted to rapport building; evaluation of basic self-care skills; and initial assessment of psychosocial, motor, and cognitive and perceptual deficits. In an acute care or long-term care facility, even less time may be available for these initial assessments. Although functional observations of some patients provide useful information in a time-efficient manner, other patients may be better evaluated through formal testing.

Patients who are severely impaired may be unable to participate in many aspects of basic self-care during the initial evaluation phase. Since these patients also have difficulty participating in formal testing, a series of structured observations of simple therapeutic activities (such as following one- or two-step motor commands; identifying objects; and engaging in oral/facial hygiene, mobility, or feeding) may provide the best information.

A very-high-level patient may display no difficulty with basic self-care or even homemaking tasks observed during the first few days of treatment; however, the therapist should be cautious in deciding that no deficits are present. In order to set realistic goals and anticipate function in a less structured setting, the high-level patient must be challenged by more complex and abstract tasks. Because of clinic realities and patient priorities, it may be difficult to arrange such high-level functional tasks during the initial evaluation phase. These more subtle deficits may be quickly evaluated through carefully selected advanced standardized or nonstandardized tests. Then, as therapy continues, the effects of these deficits can be validated in high-level community, homemaking, or work tasks.

To allow flexibility and promote clear problem delineation, the RIC occupational therapy cognitive and perceptual assessment includes standardized and nonstandardized tests as well as functional observations to help the therapist

- identify accurately the skill deficits observed in function
- evaluate whether high-level responses are within normal ranges
- provide cognitive challenges that can be used early in the hospital stay to observe advanced cognitive and perceptual skills

Although the original intent was to select only standardized tests for this protocol, it became evident that standardized tests are not appropriate for many of the patients, are time-consuming, and do not always provide more information than do nonstandardized activities. Varieties of standardized and nonstandardized tests that had been supported by occupational therapy literature or neuropsychological literature were therefore chosen. These tests are meant to be used selectively to isolate problem areas that cannot be defined clearly through functional observations. It is never recommended that all of the tests be given to one patient. Instead, the therapist should use judgment based on knowledge of the patient and the test materials to select several assessments that relate to problem areas observed functionally. The strengths and limitations of each test should be considered when choosing evaluation tools. A wide range of tests is available, so that the chosen test may best correspond to the patient's level of function. The standardized tests that are recommended have well-developed norms and are supported by validity and reliability data. They therefore allow the therapist to detect subtle deficits, since scores can be compared with norms for the person's age, sex, and, in some cases, educational level. These standardized tests are also appropriate for research.

The RIC occupational therapy cognitive and perceptual protocol is unique in combining both functional observations and specific tests to aid in problem definition, goal setting, and treatment planning. Guidelines suggested by Abreu and Toglia (1987) to make qualitative as well as quantitative observations of function can be used during the evaluation process. The functional observations and tests that we have chosen are arranged in a hierarchical manner, allowing the therapist to choose tests that will challenge the patient without overwhelming him or her. The OT can observe performance while analyzing the strategies and the conditions that enhance effectiveness. Directions for nonstandardized tests and functional tasks can be modified to observe the patient's ability to learn from instruction. If the suggested instructions are not effective in eliciting good performance, the therapist can change the instructions or provide cues. These must be noted in the interpretation of performance so that another rater can duplicate the test if needed. Directions for standardized tests cannot be altered, since the norms are based on the use of specific instructions. Some of the standardized tests, however, especially those by Benton (1983a) and Benton et al. (1979, 1983) allow for some repetition and teaching prior to beginning the test. When teaching prior to the test is used, the type of information that is most helpful to the patient should be noted.

In summary, it is felt that there is a place for both functional observations and formal testing in the OT's evaluation of cognition and perception. Although observation of functional activities usually should be the first choice for evaluation, there are many instances when these observations do not provide all of the information needed to identify specific component skill deficits. The therapist should then have access to other well-developed tools that can assist in assessment and identification of problems related to occupational performance.

Chapter 2

Evaluation: General Methods and Philosophy

PURPOSE OF EVALUATION

Evaluation of the cognitive and perceptual status of a patient who has had a cerebrovascular accident (CVA) is important to better comprehend functional level, to set realistic goals, to help remediate or compensate for deficits, and to assist the patient and family in understanding the consequences of these problems. Various evaluation methods may be used, depending on the knowledge of the therapist and the patient's current functional level and anticipated roles. It is important, therefore, for the therapist to consider his or her strengths and weaknesses in the areas of cognitive and perceptual evaluation and to clarify for the client how the information will be used to assist recovery or adaptation to disability. This chapter provides a framework for using the more detailed information found in the following chapters.

Evaluations must be performed with a clear purpose. They should provide information that will help direct treatment, improve function, or facilitate adaptation to disability and should relate to the daily living skills that the therapist is planning to address in treatment. For instance, it may not be important to evaluate high-level visual analysis and synthesis skills when a patient's functional activity will be limited to performing oral/facial hygiene and self-feeding in a nursing home environment. When a person is planning to return to work or perform home management tasks, however, this type of evaluation may provide useful information.

The evaluation sequence proposed in this book involves, first, gathering information about the patient's current status, past roles, and anticipated functional level. This information is collected through chart review, interview with the patient and/or family, and observation. Next, activity analysis is used to evaluate relevant areas of function and to define the components that are difficult for the patient. Having formed a preliminary idea about the nature of the problem, the therapist can then use formal testing to validate his or her ideas, demonstrate problems to the patient and family, and establish a baseline for treatment. In this way, evaluation is focused on relevant activities, is not unnecessarily long, and provides the information needed to address treatment in a comprehensive manner.

CHART REVIEW

The first step in the evaluation process is to review the patient's medical record. The therapist can gather information about the patient's medical history, precautions, current medications, site of lesion, previous functional status, and possible discharge destination. This information is important to help the therapist visualize the patient and plan the initial evaluation session. For instance, the therapist will plan to evaluate responses to basic sensory modalities and perform evaluations that require less active participation if the chart indicates a severe stroke with numerous medical complications. When chart data describe a more functional patient, the therapist will prepare evaluations that provide a higher degree of challenge. Information in the medical record about previous functional status will also help guide the evaluation process. For example, if a patient is hospitalized for a second stroke, it is important to determine the level of independence regained prior to the current admission. The therapist can then plan evaluations that take into account any prior limitations and that relate to expected functional outcomes.

Chart information is also important to verify the patient's responses to orientation questions such as address, birth date, or the names of family members; this can help in assessing remote memory. The chart may describe the patient's educational level. On the basis of this information, the therapist can more accurately interpret the results of language-based tests and evaluations requiring more abstract or academic problem-solving skills. In addition, the therapist may be required to know the patient's educational status in order to use the norms for scoring a standardized test. Awareness of previous work, family, and leisure roles can help in the selection of evaluation activities that are meaningful to the patient. To use test information correctly, the therapist must be aware of the many medical and psychosocial factors that influence performance and must consider these factors in test selection and interpretation. Thorough chart review is one method of gathering preliminary medical and psychosocial information relevant to the evaluation process.

In summary, chart review is important to provide the following data:

- medical information
  1. past medical history
  2. current deficits: site of lesion, extent of motor and cognitive involvement
  3. medications
  4. precautions
- psychosocial information
  1. family configuration
  2. prior living situation
  3. expected discharge destination
  4. previous educational level
  5. prior work, family, and leisure roles

INTERVIEW

Although it is helpful in the preliminary phase of the evaluation process, chart review does not usually provide the depth of information needed by the occupational therapist (OT) to thoroughly address values, interests, roles, and habits. Interviewing the patient and/ or the family is critical to gathering additional information that will help the OT select relevant evaluation tasks and interpret the results. Failure to perform this step leads to irrelevant evaluation or treatment methods and misunderstandings about the purpose of occupational therapy intervention. An interview may be an informal discussion of the patient's previous life style and current goals or can be structured through the use of tools such as the Occupational Functioning Screening Tool described by Hawkins Watts et al. (1986). A clearly focused informal interview conducted during the first several days of occupational therapy generally is sufficient to direct evaluation and treatment. The therapist should obtain information about the patient's previous daily routine, the roles and activities that were most meaningful, how well those roles were performed in the past, and which roles and activities the patient and family see as priorities to address in treatment. Questions that may be asked include the following:

- How did you (or your relative) spend a typical weekday and weekend morning, afternoon, and evening?
- Which of these activities are most important to you?
- What activities do you enjoy most? (What do you do for fun?)
- On what occupational therapy activities would you like to work?
- Why do you want to work on these activities?

These questions should be expanded upon and reworded as needed to obtain information about previous roles, habits, and values. The answers should be used to select meaningful activities and to decide which formal tests relate best to the patient's goals.

ACTIVITY ANALYSIS

Activity analysis is a tool that OTs can use efficiently to provide valuable information to the patient, the family, and the treatment team. Our expertise in analyzing task components and the effects of deficits on function are unique and should be the basis of the occupational therapy evaluation. Skillful use of activity analysis allows us to identify performance components, such as motor skill, cognitive abilities, or perceptual performance in almost any situation. Mosey (1986), in her book *Psychosocial Components of Occupational Therapy*, describes two types of activity analysis. Generic activity analysis involves studying all possible characteristics of task performance. She provides a two-page sample outline describing a multitude of factors that can be considered. She also describes a restricted approach to activity analysis in which certain characteristics are studied to meet specific needs. This is the approach that will be used to identify cognitive and perceptual motor factors that are inherent in functional and clinical activities.

Observation of the patient's interaction with his or her family, another patient, or with us can provide some information about initiative, self-concept, awareness of the environment, orientation, and cognitive status. The way in which he or she responds to structured physical assessments and interview techniques can also provide data useful to the cognitive and perceptual evaluation. When a patient is observed in functional tasks, however, the OT's activity analysis skills are called into full play. Because the interaction of various psychosocial, cognitive, and perceptual/motor components is so complex, the therapist must carefully observe performance patterns to decide which deficits most interfere with performance (see also Chapter 6).

Even a basic task such as face washing involves cognitive and perceptual motor skills such as initiation, attention, body awareness, and motor planning. A complex activity such as meal preparation requires many cognitive and perceptual skills ranging from attention and initiation to problem solving and visual analysis. From functional observations the OT will form a hypothesis about the major causes of performance difficulty. When needed to clarify observations, appropriate evaluations can then be selected to test this hypothesis.

FORMAL TESTING

Formal tests are used to clarify problem areas, to provide a baseline for treatment, and to demonstrate subtle or abstract deficits to patients and caretakers in a concrete manner. In all cases, the therapist should have a clear rationale for performing a test. Without careful consideration, tests may be an unnecessary expense and a poor use of the patient's therapy time. Properly used, however, tests can facilitate goal setting, treatment planning, and understanding of the patient's problems. In most cases, tests for cognition and perception can best be used after working with the patient for several days. During this initial period the OT can collect data by using the approaches described above. When rapport has been established and the therapist has preliminary ideas about the patient's cognitive and perceptual problems, selected tests can be performed to define deficits more clearly. Although performing these tests too early may compromise rapport and the results may be unfocused, waiting too long will limit their usefulness in goal setting and treatment planning. Optimal

timing will vary for each patient. If the therapist is conscious of the rationale for performing each test and has effectively used the information gathered from chart review, interview, and activity analysis, formal testing may be justified at various points in the treatment process.

For example, early in a patient's stay, observation may indicate severe attentional deficits that respond well to a quiet environment. The family plans to take the patient home with 24-hour attendant care. Both the patient and the family feel that independent feeding in a quiet environment is an appropriate goal and do not want to address other self-care areas. The therapist may decide not to perform further cognitive or perceptual testing, since the information gathered through other methods has provided enough data to ensure competent treatment of the patient. As time progresses, however, the patient's status may improve. Both the patient and the family may then feel that other self-care goals should be addressed, and they hope to require assistance at home only for bathing. Because of this change in circumstances, further evaluation of selected cognitive and perceptual components can be justified to clarify deficits that may affect performance and to provide patient and family education that will assist in a smooth transition to home.

To use tests well, the therapist must be aware of evaluation procedures, scoring methods, and factors influencing interpretation. Familiarity with the strengths and limitations of each evaluation is also important for making a good choice of tests. Standardized tests have limitations because they are usually administered in sterile clinical environments, are lengthy, cannot be modified to suit the patient, and generally do not have research available to support correlations with function. On the other hand, they do allow the therapist to better isolate deficit areas and compare the patient's performance with that of age- and sex-controlled norms. In addition, the use of respected standardized tests can provide factual support for our observations and should be used whenever research is being conducted.

When interpreting test results it is important to consider

- demographic factors such as age, sex, education, previous roles, and personality
- neurological factors such as lesion size, time since onset, and location of the CVA
- psychometric factors related to test-taking skills
- functional considerations regarding how the test information will be used to improve daily life (Diller and Gordon 1981)

Age-related changes in the elderly are well documented (Kinsbourne 1974). For diagnostic purposes it is important to know whether performance is within the normal range for the patient's age group. Functionally, however, any deficit, even if it is not abnormal for an elderly patient, may affect learning and performance skills. Consideration of these factors will help ensure that the therapist selects tests that will be useful in improving daily living skills and that the tests are interpreted accurately.

If the patient is being seen by a psychologist or a practitioner of another discipline that uses standardized cognitive and perceptual tests, it is important to avoid duplication and to share evaluation results. This requires communication and collaboration between the disciplines about evaluation plans and results. Failure to communicate may result in invalid testing (for example, if the same test is given twice), needless expense, and frustration for the patient. Ideally, each facility will develop specific protocols describing interdisciplinary test procedures and information exchange.

Nonstandardized tests can also be used in evaluation and re-evaluation protocols within a department. Al-though these tests do not have reliability or validity data and have not been norm-referenced, they can facilitate consistency between therapists when evaluating, treating, and communicating patient status if they are performed in the prescribed manner. Consistency, in turn, can be beneficial in gauging quality of care within the department, since standards are in place against which to judge patient evaluation, treatment, and documentation. In addition, they are often shorter than standardized tests and can be adapted to suit the patient's functional level. Many of the nonstandard tests suggested in this book are supported in the clinical literature; however, they must be interpreted cautiously, since there are no statistical data to support their validity or to establish normal performance.

Although formal tests can help clarify the type of cognitive or perceptual deficits observed in function, their limitations must be understood. When administered correctly and interpreted carefully, these tests can be a useful adjunct to activity analysis, patient interview, and chart review. Used together, these methods can provide helpful information with which to define specific problem areas that interfere with function and to enhance occupational therapy treatment.

Chapter 3

Factors Influencing Cognitive and Perceptual Evaluation

Because the deficits experienced by a stroke survivor are so complex, a variety of factors must be considered in order to perform an efficient and effective evaluation. The interplay of cognitive, perceptual, and motor factors is complex, making identification of specific problem areas difficult. A rational, systematic approach therefore must be used to examine problem areas. If the therapist fails to think seriously about the wide range of elements that affect function, he or she may incorrectly attribute performance errors to particular cognitive or perceptual deficits when, in reality, another problem may be limiting optimal function. Some of the factors that should be considered when evaluating cognitive and perceptual status include the following:

- psychosocial style
- primary visual, auditory, and tactile acuity
- receptive and expressive language skills
- motor skills such as upper extremity use, balance, and postural stability

When cognitive and perceptual skills during functional activities are observed, the interplay of all of these factors becomes especially important.

PSYCHOSOCIAL FACTORS

Concerned with the holistic function of each patient, occupational therapists (OTs) recognize that psychosocial factors have a strong influence on a patient's suc-

cessful return to former roles (Bach-y-Rita 1980; Fune 1990). The Model of Human Occupation (Kielhofner 1985) and other occupational performance models are gaining favor as unifying foundations for the practice of occupational therapy (Arnadottir 1990; Pedretti and Pasquinelli-Estrada 1985; Mosey 1986). These theories consider human desires and motivations that lead to effective role fulfillment.

The Model of Human Occupation (Kielhofner 1985) is useful in understanding the ways in which motivation and performance skills combine to produce successful outcomes. This model proposes that human beings engage in occupational behavior because of an innate desire to explore and master the environment. According to the theory, individuals can effect changes in themselves and their world through ongoing interaction with the environment. Behavior is believed to be guided through three subsystems. The first subsystem, volition, describes the urge or motivation to explore and master the environment. Values, goals, personal standards, belief in oneself, and interests stimulate a person to engage in particular activities. Through the second subsystem, habituation, one develops daily routines. These routines help one to fulfill roles and organize daily activities. Finally, the performance subsystem encompasses the skills needed to interact with the environment. These skills include motor skills, process skills such as problem solving, and interpersonal skills. Skills are shaped and limited by psychological and philosophical beliefs, neurological integrity, cognitive abilities, and musculoskeletal potential. A stroke can affect all levels of the subsystem hierarchy. Performance components, which form the base of the hierarchy, rely on a well-integrated neurological system and physical abilities, while the highest levels of occupational behavior, values, and interests require a good self-concept and the desire to interact with the environment. Awareness of the impact of a stroke on these subsystems helps a therapist choose relevant evaluations and improves his or her interpretation of behavioral observations.

A person who has had a stroke comes to the therapist with previously established goals, standards, habits, and performance skills that are now altered by the cerebrovascular accident (CVA). It is the therapist's job to learn as much as possible about the patient's previous performance patterns and then to determine how the stroke affected them. It is useful to understand the patient's previous interests and ways of coping with new situations in order to choose relevant evaluations and set realistic expectations for therapy.

Because the subskills of motor performance and neurological integrity are often impaired after a stroke, the patient may no longer be able to perform previous habits, roles, and leisure activities in the accustomed manner. This loss of ability to engage in the tasks that previously defined one's place in society may result in depression or role confusion. In addition to psychological stress caused by the loss of function, a stroke often causes cognitive changes that affect motivation and the ability to adjust effectively to the disability. After a CVA, occupational roles frequently are disrupted, and coping skills, learning strategies, and motivation may be impaired as a result of neurological damage. The therapist must use skills, tact, and understanding in order to facilitate patient involvement, assist in identifying strengths, and determine realistic performance goals.

To best evaluate the patient, the therapist must find activities that are relevant, role-appropriate, and interesting, yet are suited to the patient's current motor and neurological skills. The patient's response to the testing situation then must be carefully monitored. Anxiety about test performance or a belief that the tests are degrading or meaningless may affect results negatively. Anxiety, disinterest, insufficient challenge, or excessive challenge may result in a lack of involvement in the activity. Generally a patient who is optimally engaged in a task or test will be focused on it and will not talk excessively or be distracted by irrelevant stimuli. If the patient is not fully participating in an activity, the therapist should determine why involvement is not optimal. On the basis of observations in other situations,

knowledge of the patient, and discussion with the patient or the family, the OT can modify the test activity, try to elicit cooperation through re-explaining its importance, or account for psychosocial factors in the interpretation. Because the skillful therapist can make observations of cognitive and perceptual components during a wide range of tasks, tests or activities can be modified to elicit maximal patient involvement.

Understanding previous roles, interests, and habits is important not only in selecting tests or interpreting performance, but also in assisting the therapist to separate the effects of the CVA from previous patterns of behavior. Information about former occupational performance can be gained through a structured interview; however, is more often accomplished informally during the first few therapy sessions as the therapist works to build rapport and determine the patient's and/or family's goals. When working with a severely aphasic patient, it is especially important to gather information regarding past performance through chart review and discussion with significant others. Since the patient is unable to share goals and interests verbally, effective evaluation and treatment rely on the therapist's gathering as much information as possible. Ideas and activities can be presented that are geared to expected interest areas and then modified according to the patient's response. In this way collaboration and rapport are begun during the evaluation period. Integration of information about the patient's former life style with other evaluation data results in a more accurate assessment and goals that reflect the patient's previous interests as well as his or her current abilities.

Fine (1991) describes the personal threat experienced when a person faces the trauma of a major illness. The loss of physical, cognitive, and perceptual skills; the confinement to an impersonal hospital environment; and the disruption of life roles cause pain and humiliation. The ability to respond positively to such adversity requires cognitive and behavioral coping skills as well as social support. Some of the qualities that Fine (1991) describes as helpful in adapting to trauma are: maintaining hope, finding meaning, accepting challenges, remaining committed, and developing a sense of control. She proposes that by understanding a patient's inner drives, occupational therapists can help "patients refine their adventures, find meaning and purpose in their ordeals, discover there is more to themselves than current circumstance suggests, and transform the dross of their adversity into the gold of their accomplishments" (p. 501). It is evident that psychosocial factors are very important during the evaluation and treatment process. Awareness of the patient's feelings following the trauma of a stroke can help therapists interact compassionately, understand performance, and assist in the recovery process.

PRIMARY SENSES

Before a cognitive and perceptual evaluation is conducted, the patient's visual, tactile, and auditory sensory status should be determined. This information can be gained from the chart, consultation with other disciplines, referral for specific audiometric or ophthalmologic testing, or tests performed by the OT. Impairment of these primary senses may adversely affect performance on perceptual and cognitive testing and may necessitate adaptation of the evaluation process.

Visual Screening

Basic information about the patient's visual status should be available before visual perceptual testing is performed. Important areas to assess include visual fields, visual acuity, visual range of motion (ROM), the ability to perform accurate saccadic eye movement, and the ability to pursue visually a moving object (Exhibit 3-1). These skills are important, since a defect in any one of them will cloud the results of visual perceptual testing. Screening tests using simple hand-held charts and targets can be performed by the OT. When more specific information is needed (for instance, when evaluating vision prior to driving training), a therapist should obtain specialized equipment and training or should refer the patient to an ophthalmologist. Chapter 8 provides additional information about evaluating vision prior to driving training.

Hemianopia

Homonymous hemianopia, an inability to detect stimuli in the right or left half of both visual fields, is

---

Exhibit 3-1 Definitions of Visual Testing Terms

Visual field—The limits that the eye can detect when focused on a fixed location (Normally, a person is able to detect 60 degrees inward, 70 to 75 degrees downward, and 100 to 110 degrees outward [Siev et al. 1986].)
Visual acuity—The ability to detect detail
Visual range of motion—The ability to move the eyes in all directions
Saccades—The ability to smoothly, accurately, and rapidly move the eyes between two fixed points
Pursuit—The ability to follow a moving target with the eyes in a steady and precise way

---

often evident after a CVA. A lesion of the optic tract after the fibers have crossed at the optic chiasm produces the characteristic symptoms of visual loss in the right or left half of both visual fields. In some cases the lesion may affect fibers that carry visual images from the upper or lower quadrant of the eye. A patient with this defect will show a smaller area of right or left, upper or lower visual field loss.

A patient who spontaneously compensates for hemianopia may not show functional difficulties during simple activity of daily living (ADL) tasks. In tasks requiring more complex and rapid visuomotor integration, however, the deficit may be more evident. It is important to perform specific testing when a patient will be driving or performing work or community activities that require a rapid response to visual information. The additional problem of unilateral visual inattention complicates hemianopia and is often present in those who do not compensate. Although it is not necessary to test formally every stroke patient for hemianopia, since there may be no effect on relevant ADL tasks, it is important to observe the patient carefully as new activities are begun and to use formal tests if deficits that interfere with safe, effective skill performance are suspected.

Visual fields may be examined through sophisticated measures such as perimetry testing (see Chapter 8) or through less accurate, but simpler, techniques such as confrontational testing. For confrontational testing, the examiner faces the patient and asks him or her to look forward. A target visual stimulus, such as a finger, a dowel with a painted tip, or a pencil topped with a colorful eraser, is presented in the patient's right or left peripheral field. The patient is asked to respond verbally or through gesture when the stimulus is detected. A gross assessment can be made with both of the patient's eyes open, or a patch can be used to cover first one eye, then the other. By testing each eye separately, the therapist can specify more accurately the location of peripheral limitations.

Moving stimuli, such as wiggling fingers, are detected more easily than static stimuli. For this reason, patients who are suspected of having severe deficits can be tested first by using moving stimuli. The patient is asked to respond verbally or nonverbally when movement is detected. Since a patient conceivably could state that the object or movement was detected even when it was not, a confused or unreliable patient can be tested in another way. One or two objects are gradually moved into the visual field and the patient is asked to indicate how many objects are seen (Figures 3-1 and 3-2). If the patient is guessing, it becomes evident by the random responses that are given. Once hemianopia has

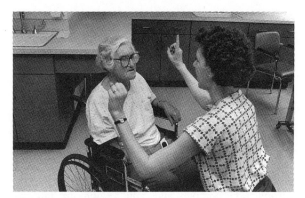

Figure 3-1 Visual fields can be tested by asking the patient how many fingers are visible.

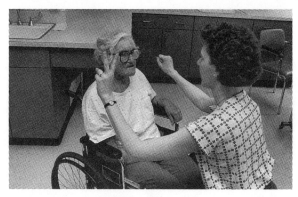

Figure 3-2 Confrontational testing of the visual fields is quickly administered, although it is not as accurate as sophisticated methods such as perimetry.

been detected, further tests can be modified so that visual information is presented in the intact visual field.

Hemianopic testing requires a high degree of cooperation from the patient. Patients with motor impersistence, usually left-side hemiplegics, may not be able to keep their eyes forward during the test. They may easily be distracted or lose interest and concentration on the test. The test should be done in a quiet location at a time when the patient is able to cooperate at an optimal level. Often it is best to wait until rapport has been established if this test is likely to be difficult and confusing for the patient.

Acuity

A patient with diminished acuity may not be able to distinguish lines, letters, or figures used in visual perceptual testing. Functionally, there may be difficulty in distinguishing buttons on a shirt or items in a drawer or a cabinet. Awareness of acuity deficits will allow the therapist to separate them from visual perceptual problems. It is preferable to obtain acuity information from the chart or from an optometrist; however, the patient's or family's report about previous visual limitations may also be helpful. When the treatment focus is on basic ADL, the OT generally will not need to perform specific acuity tests in order to judge the patient's ability to participate in the visual components of the task. Observation of function and discussion with the patient and family frequently provides sufficient information.

In those instances in which more information is needed, especially for driving, pursuit of leisure interests such as reading, or return to work, there are several methods that the therapist can use to screen for acuity. A modified Snellen test, distributed through the Lighthouse for the Blind, uses pictures rather than letters as the stimuli and can therefore be used with aphasic patients (Figure 3-3). Responses can be given verbally or

by pointing to the object that is seen. A functional test that equates various sizes of type to acuity ratings can also be used. For example, the patient can be asked to read the following materials placed 16 inches from the eyes: classified advertisements [20/30], textbooks or magazines [20/60–20/70], or newspaper subheadings [20/80–20/130] (Abreu 1987) (Exhibit 3-2). The numbers in brackets correspond roughly to the acuity level required for reading each type of material. All visual testing should be conducted while the patient is wearing the appropriate corrective lenses. Since our intent is not to test vision but to ensure adequate sight for func-

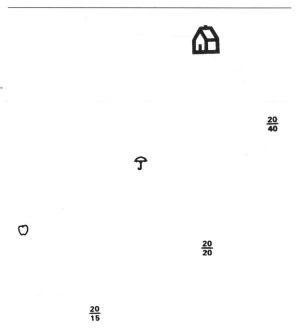

Figure 3-3 This modified Snellen test uses pictures rather than letters for acuity testing. Available from the Lighthouse for the Blind. Courtesy of Lighthouse Low Vision Products, Long Island City, NY 11101.

Exhibit 3-2 Correlation of Various Type Sizes with Visual Acuity

Various sizes of type have been correlated with acuity ratings. The patient is asked to read printed material from a distance of 16 inches.

ENGLISH BULL DOG PUPS
AKC. guaranteed. $500-$600.
Possible delivery. 217-357-3378.
ENGLISH SPRINGER SPAN.
AKC. 8 wks., liver & white.
Excellent pedigree, $200. 532-5485
ENGLISH—Bulldog pups, 10 wks., AKC reg. M & F, shots & wormed. $500. 756-2188
GERM. Shep—rare blk. F, 8 mos., lg. boned, gd. w/kids, hsbrkn., AKC. baby allergic. must sell. $450/ofr. 749-0012.

that she continued her observations for our years. Here she offers a rare glimpse of the beavers' struggle to save their habitat, find food and raise their young despite great natural hardships—and human destruction.

tional tasks, glasses, if normally worn, should be part of the evaluation.

The therapist is cautioned never to report the results in terms of acuity unless specialized, sophisticated testing is used. Rather, the task and the patient's performance should be described. For example, it would be accurate to state that the patient was able to read magazine print from a distance of 16 inches, but it would not be correct to state that acuity was measured at 20/60. These acuity tests, while useful for screening, cannot be expected to substitute for, or be equivalent to, the more sophisticated tests performed by optometrists or specially trained therapists. They should be used only for screening purposes to indicate tasks or tests that might be affected by limited vision.

Visual Range of Motion

Assessing visual ROM is important for analyzing whether the patient is able to scan the environment effectively. Limitations in lateral, upward, or downward gaze will affect the therapist's placement of test and ADL materials and will affect the patient's ability to use visual information in the environment. Visual ROM is tested by asking the patient to follow a moving target with the eyes without moving the head. The therapist slowly traces the letter *H* in the air approximately 16 inches from the patient's face using a finger, a pencil, or a dowel rod. The therapist observes to ensure that the patient is able to move the eyes to the extreme right, left, top, and bottom of the eye socket (Figure 3-4). If hemianopia makes it difficult to follow the target, the patient may be asked to move the eyes as far as possible to the right, left, up, and down. Some patients may be unable to follow the instructions because of impulsivity or language deficits. For these patients the therapist can observe eye movement during functional activities.

Limitations in ocular ROM can complicate performance of ADL or tests. For instance, when eating a meal, a patient with limited downward gaze may show

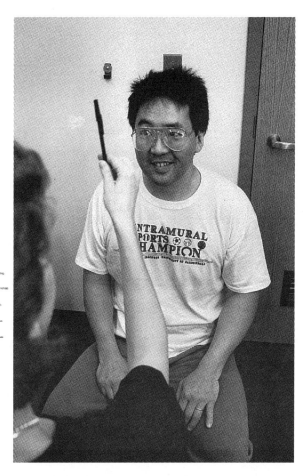

Figure 3-4 This patient is able to follow a moving target throughout the full ROM, without head motion, with the left eye. The right eye shows incomplete visual ROM.

decreased attention because of multiple task demands. The patient not only must concentrate on the motor and perceptual aspects of performing the task with one hand while attending to perceptual cues such as the location of the food, but also must compensate for visual defects. Frustration may result from the numerous demands imposed by a previously simple task. The patient may be unable to see cues that normally serve to guide performance, such as the location of the food, the table edge, or utensils. Proper positioning of items may improve function significantly and lessen the impact of ocular ROM deficits. The therapist then can more clearly isolate the cognitive and perceptual limitations that may also be affecting performance.

Saccades

Saccades, or the ability to alternate gaze rapidly and accurately between two points, is important in efficiently scanning the environment. Difficulty in using saccadic eye movement will affect reading, mobility, and performance in visually stimulating environments. Relevant visual details may be neglected and subsequent processing errors made. Saccades are tested by asking the patient to alternate his or her gaze between two points while the therapist observes the quality of response. The therapist positions two objects (for instance, a red pen and a black pen) and asks the patient to look first at one and then the other object (Abreu 1987) (Figures 3-5, 3-6, and 3-7). Commands should be short, since the patient's speed and accuracy of response are important. For example, the OT can say "red," then "black." The interval of time between commands should vary, so that the patient does not anticipate the command. The positions of the two objects should be varied, so that movement in all visual quadrants can be observed. In the report, the therapist should describe the speed and accuracy of the patient's response in each quadrant.

This test is difficult to use with patients who are impulsive and who lack motor persistence. It is almost impossible for them to maintain their gaze on one object until the therapist gives the command to look at the other stimulus. It is also difficult to explain this test to patients with language deficits; therefore, it should be used selectively with patients who are cognitively and linguistically able to cooperate. As suggested previously, observation during function can be used when the patient is unable to participate in formal testing. The speed and accuracy of eye movements can be observed when a patient is searching for a person or object in a room or when alternating gaze between two objects during a functional task.

Pursuit

Pursuit of a target is important in eye-hand coordination tasks involving a moving object. For instance, catching a ball, stopping a pencil from rolling off a

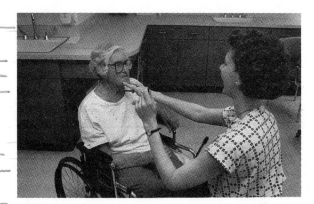

Figure 3-6 Cues are provided to remind the patient to look straight ahead.

table, or watching a child requires smooth, accurate visual pursuit. Pursuit can be evaluated during the ocular ROM evaluation by observing the quality of eye movements when the patient is following a moving target. The control and smoothness with which the eyes move in each quadrant should be documented. When the patient is unable to cooperate with formal testing, the eye movements can be observed during activities that require visual monitoring of a moving object.

Tactile Sensory Testing

Prior to performing body awareness tests that require tactile or somatosensory integration, basic responses to tactile stimuli must be determined. Some of these tests are performed by the OT as part of the upper extremity evaluation. Consultation with a physical therapist or review of the chart may provide useful information about the patient's lower extremity and trunk sensation. In addition, a brief evaluation of response to a light touch on the face is helpful. Tactile discrimination tests listed

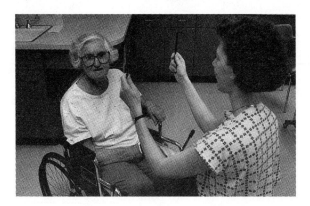

Figure 3-5 Saccades are tested by asking the patient to look at the red or black pen on command.

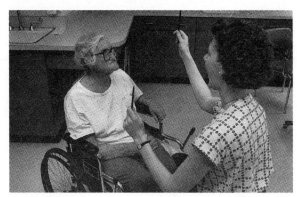

Figure 3-7 Motor impersistence prevents the patient from maintaining the requested head position.

in the perceptual guide (Chapter 11) should not be given if primary sensory deficits are present.

The upper extremity sensory evaluation performed by OTs at the Rehabilitation Institute of Chicago (RIC) includes tests for sharp/dull discrimination, proprioception, response to hot/cold in functional activities, and stereognosis or two-point discrimination. These tests are given to detect difficulties that may interfere with safety, motor control, motor retraining, or speed of performance. Aphasic patients are asked to point to picture cards or objects during the sharp/dull discrimination and stereognosis testing. When a patient is unable to copy a limb position during proprioceptive testing because of hemiplegia or motor-planning problems, he or she is asked to indicate whether the joint is moving up or down by giving a verbal response, using a gesture, or by pointing to directional arrows. If tactile sensory tests show normal or nearly normal performance, yet movement remains uncoordinated or objects are frequently dropped, further testing using tactile perceptual tests may be indicated.

As in all other evaluations of a CVA patient, the therapist must be alert to the influence of cognitive, perceptual, psychosocial, and motor deficits on sensory test performance. Some patients may be unable to attend to or appreciate the abstract nature of the tests used to assess sensation. They may not comprehend the instructions, may guess at responses, may show motor impersistence that prevents them from keeping their eyes closed, or may find the procedure irrelevant and may not participate fully. In these cases the therapist can modify the approach and ask the patient to describe the sensation in the hand or indicate whether he or she can feel the therapist's touch. Other observations during function will also prove valuable. For instance, does the patient need to watch the hand when performing a fine motor task? Does the patient maintain proper force when grasping an object? Can the patient manipulate objects in the hand? When touched, does he or she acknowledge the stimulation? Does the patient appear to respond only to pain? Is the patient aware of the position of his or her arm during activities, or does it become twisted or forgotten? Although some of these symptoms may be difficult to distinguish from tactile inattention, careful observation may provide clues about tactile sensory deficits versus tactile perceptual deficits.

Auditory and Receptive Language Deficits

Just as awareness of primary visual sensory problems is important prior to cognitive and perceptual evaluation, so is awareness of auditory or receptive language deficits. Decreased hearing will cause difficulty in following verbal instructions, especially in a noisy environment. The increased effort required by a patient with auditory acuity problems may result in more rapid fatigue and difficulty in sustaining attention. Misperception of words due to decreased acuity or receptive aphasia may result in incorrect performance of an evaluation activity.

Although OTs do not usually evaluate auditory acuity, information may be found in the patient's medical record and through discussion with the patient or family. When possible, discussion with the audiologist or speech and language pathologist provides more detailed data about auditory and receptive language skills. Since hearing deficits are common and can affect function, routine evaluation of elderly patients by an audiologist soon after admission to a rehabilitation facility is suggested. If access to these resources is limited, the OT can ask the patient to respond to simple one-step commands, such as "shake your head no," or "give me the pencil." The therapist must be careful to avoid gestural cues that would allow the patient to respond without clearly hearing the instructions. Long commands should be avoided due to the need for more advanced attentional and motor planning skills. If the patient is unable to respond to simple verbal commands, the therapist must determine whether the difficulty is due to impaired auditory acuity, poor attention, motor planning deficits, receptive language disturbance, or noncompliance.

Specific knowledge about the patient's ability to hear and understand spoken language can help us to modify the testing environment, change our tone of voice, use amplification aids, use nonverbal cues, provide written directions, simplify instructions, or use demonstration as appropriate to enhance performance. An electronic amplification device that resembles a small radio with earphones can be used in the clinic to help some patients with conductive hearing loss to hear instructions. This device is available from Radio Shack and other vendors for a nominal charge. The speech pathologist and audiologist often can provide tips that will facilitate each patient's performance; therefore, consultation with them is recommended whenever possible.

EXPRESSIVE LANGUAGE DEFICITS

Information from the speech and language pathologist regarding expressive language deficits can be just as helpful as input about receptive language skills. He or she may be able to shorten the time spent on evaluation and lessen the patient's frustration by suggesting an optimal method of communication. When this consultation is not possible before beginning the cognitive and perceptual evaluation, the therapist must experiment with different communication methods. The patient may be able to shake the head yes and no, point to simple words or pictures, or use other gestures to communicate. It is important to remember, however, that motor-planning deficits may interfere with accurate use of gestures. To help facilitate the participation of patients with aphasia, many of the evaluations that are found in the RIC occupational therapy cognitive and perceptual protocol were chosen to minimize the need for sophisticated language skills whenever possible.

MOTOR FUNCTION

This manual is not intended to describe assessment of motor skills; however, the relationship of motor deficits to cognitive and perceptual assessment should be considered. The presence of hemiplegia may influence the types of tests that the patient can perform. For instance, the Allen Cognitive Level Test is best performed by using two hands. Although the leather-lacing activity can be modified by using a clamp to stabilize the work, patients may respond negatively to the added difficulty that one-handed performance imposes. For this reason, most of the tests recommended in the RIC cognitive and perceptual protocol can be performed unilaterally.

A second factor to consider in relation to motor performance is the demand that decreased upper extremity strength and decreased functional mobility impose on the cognitive and perceptual systems. When the patient is faced with learning new ways to perform old habits, demands are placed on cognitive skills. Increased attention and problem solving are required. He or she must learn how the changed body interacts with the environment and must be aware of factors that were not previously relevant. For instance, area rugs that were not problematic prior to the CVA now cause potential safety concerns. Wheelchairs and their operation now must be mastered.

A new patient may be labeled as impulsive because he or she does not lock the wheelchair brakes. While this may be an accurate assessment, we must also consider how motor learning occurs. A new patient who has been confined largely to bed or given maximal assistance for transfers may not have had the opportunity to test the extent of his or her physical abilities safely and fully. The patient may not know that safety is compromised when the brakes are not locked. In addition, the patient may be unfamiliar with the movements required to operate this new equipment.

The first time an able-bodied person attempts to ski, he or she must learn about the body's capability and the operation of unfamiliar equipment in this new activity. Although the person is likely to fall, one would not say that judgment was impaired unless he or she started on the expert slope. People gradually learn how to be safe in a given activity and how to modify tasks to suit their physical abilities. Each person generally weighs the risks against the benefits of attempting a task in order to make an effective judgment. Just like the novice skier, the stroke patient needs time to learn about the new equipment he or she has been given and about how the body operates within the limitations that the CVA has imposed.

Patients who have not had the opportunity to test their limits or are anxious to resume independence may attempt activities that we consider dangerous. The therapist must help patients learn about themselves in a gradual and safe manner rather than labeling them as impulsive and restricting opportunities to explore the new constraints of their bodies. This process takes time and can be facilitated through careful selection of activities that challenge each patient and by discussing or demonstrating ways to improve performance.

Motor deficits can also influence perceptual processes. When the presence of hemiplegia dictates that new methods to perform tasks must be learned, motor-planning deficits may become apparent. Patients who are motorically capable of using the accustomed method to perform self-care skills often do not demonstrate apraxia. More advanced motor-planning skills are called into play when new patterns of motion must be learned to perform previously habitual tasks. For instance, any patient who demonstrates significant hemiplegia with loss of upper extremity, lower extremity, and trunk control will have difficulty with bed mobility. When motor-planning deficits are also present, the patient may use movement patterns that are counterproductive and may appear to be resistive. The frustration experienced by both the patient and the caregivers may result in interaction that is less than therapeutic. In treatment it is often helpful to improve motor control. When movement can be restored, function will improve and the effects of motor planning deficits will decrease because the patient can use familiar methods to perform daily tasks.

Motor deficits also impair learning and problem solving by limiting the patient's ability to actively manipulate and explore the environment. Trial-and-error problem solving is often accompanied by manipulation of objects. Thus, the motorically impaired patient who is cognitively unable to perform the high-level mental calculations necessary for covert thinking and is unable to manipulate items effectively is left with restricted strategies for problem solving.

The influence of poor postural control and balance on cognitive and perceptual evaluation must also be considered. Poor posture may reduce the patient's ability to attend to relevant factors in the environment. If the patient's eyes are frequently directed at the lap because of poor head control, or if he or she is constantly falling to the left, the ability to interact meaningfully will be lessened. In addition, when the patient performs a self-care task such as dressing, which requires a great deal of mobility and postural control, the ability to process cognitive and perceptual information may be decreased because a large amount of attentional capacity may be directed to the task of maintaining balance. Because each person can handle a limited amount of system stress, fear of falling may interfere with the ability to solve dressing problems. It is quite possible that problem-solving skills will be enhanced when motoric demands are decreased or when posture is improved through positioning devices.

The OT is in a unique position to evaluate the ways in which various performance factors interact in a functional activity. The therapist can determine how motoric demands, coupled with cognitive and perceptual requirements, affect decision making. Valuable information can then be provided about how to modify the various sensory processing, cognitive, perceptual, and motor demands of a task in order to make performance less stressful as well as more effective for the patient.

In summary, before testing particular cognitive and perceptual skills, the therapist should be aware of the patient's primary sensory status. When evaluating performance, the impact of psychosocial, motor, and sensory changes must be considered along with the effects of cognitive and perceptual deficits. Since these factors interact in performance, the therapist must be aware of the demands he or she is placing on the patient and use skilled activity analysis to determine which components are most interfering with a positive outcome. After the deficits that most affect function are carefully defined, a comprehensive treatment plan can be developed.

Chapter 4

Cognitive and Perceptual Evaluation Techniques

COGNITIVE AND PERCEPTUAL EVALUATION OVERVIEW

A thorough cognitive and perceptual evaluation allows the therapist to identify strengths and deficits in the cognitive areas of arousal, attention, memory, orientation, and problem solving and in the perceptual areas of visual perception, body awareness, and motor planning. Although there are many schemes for categorizing cognitive and perceptual skills, the areas described in this chapter were thought to be most critical to independent functioning. The second edition of *Uniform Terminology for Occupational Therapy* (AOTA 1989) was consulted, and approved terminology was used whenever possible. Many of the cognitive and perceptual categories have been further divided to describe more clearly particular kinds of problems. For example, the category of attention is further divided into subcategories of sustained attention, selective attention, and alternating attention. The broad categories are intended to help the therapist organize and conceptualize information, whereas the examination of specific problem areas assists in treatment planning. A thorough understanding of cognitive and perceptual deficits can help the therapist determine realistic goals in both self-care and component skill areas. The remainder of this chapter explains each skill tested, the relationship of that skill to function, and why particular tests were chosen.

As stated earlier in this book, cognitive and perceptual evaluation should occur within the context of activity whenever possible. The selected activity should correspond with the patient's previous interests and roles

as well as with his or her current abilities. For example, severely impaired patients with arousal deficits can be evaluated through observation of responses to various types of sensory stimulation during a simple oral/facial hygiene task. More functional patients can be challenged to use attention, memory, visual perceptual, body awareness, motor-planning, and problem-solving skills in a variety of tasks that range from putting on a shirt to a complex community shopping trip. The setting that is selected for the evaluation and the difficulty of the tasks that are introduced can be adjusted to correspond to the capabilities of the patient. Thus, functional observation can provide many opportunities to detect cognitive and perceptual strengths and deficits that will affect future independence. Specific examples of behaviors that can be observed during meaningful activities are provided in the evaluation guide (Chapters 10 and 11).

Following observations of function, tests may be used as needed to clarify observations or provide quantitative data for baseline measurements. These tests are explained briefly in this chapter. Further instructions and information pertinent to their use are provided in the evaluation guide (Chapters 10 and 11).

EVALUATIONS FOR COGNITION

Arousal

Description

Arousal can be defined as a state of readiness to receive information from the environment. An increased level of arousal can enhance sensitivity to stimulation.

This function is regulated by the brain area defined by Luria (1973) as "functional unit: one." In this area, the subcortex and brain stem are primarily responsible for mediating arousal, but interaction with the cortex is also demonstrated. The reticular formation in particular helps to maintain cortical tone and the waking state. Vizzetti (1989) describes three types of arousal: (1) Internal arousal is the activation of processes to maintain respiration and digestion as well as to stimulate unconditioned reflexes such as sexual behavior and hunger. (2) External arousal is the activation of processes to orient oneself to stimuli in the environment. This type of arousal is necessary for awareness of changes in the environment and to compare events with previous experiences. This comparison with the past requires a close association with mechanisms of memory. (3) Intentions arousal is the activation of processes required to maintain the energy and motivation necessary to carry out activity. Siev et al. (1986) describe alertness as a prerequisite for attention. Arousal clearly is important for function, since work, self-care, and leisure cannot occur without proper awareness of the environment.

Functional Implications

Many cerebrovascular accident (CVA) patients treated in a rehabilitation setting are alert enough to respond to external stimuli and maintain intentions necessary to participate in activities of daily living (ADL) tasks or clinic treatment. Occasionally, however, more severely involved patients display impaired arousal and alertness. Correct levels of arousal provide a heightened level of awareness when a person is in a potentially hazardous situation or allow a relaxed awareness of one's surroundings when unwinding at home. An appropriate level of arousal is critical to any higher cognitive or perceptual activity and can be considered the first level in the attention continuum. Because other activities and evaluations cannot be presented until alertness is established, it is important to obtain as much information as possible about the types of stimuli that enhance performance.

Evaluation

The Rehabilitation Institute of Chicago (RIC) cognitive and perceptual evaluation does not use formal tests for evaluation of arousal. Instead, structured observations of the patient's responses to various forms of sensory stimulation provide a helpful baseline for treatment. When the patient's level of arousal is low, the therapist should attempt to define whether verbal, visual, olfactory, tactile, or vestibular stimulation seems to optimize his or her performance or whether novel stimulation is more effective than familiar activities in producing a response. This is accomplished by evaluating the patient during a variety of simple activities at various times of the day and by using various types of sensory stimulation.

Since a patient with impaired arousal will demonstrate severe cognitive deficits, it is important to choose tasks that are engaging, are not demeaning, and provide challenges appropriate to his or her capabilities. Components of self-care tasks such as bringing a washcloth to the face, bringing food to the mouth, or using lotion can be effective for eliciting behavior. When a task is too difficult, the patient may "shut down" and be unable to participate. On the other hand, a task that is too easy may be considered demeaning and may result in a refusal to participate. Careful selection of activities based on the patient's presentation and responses can facilitate the evaluation process.

After observing arousal, it is important to document the following:

- the amount of stimulation required to elicit responsive behavior
- the types of activities that best enhance arousal
- the type of stimulation that is most effective
- the length of time during which improved alertness is maintained
- the time of day that the patient is most alert

Attention

Description

Attention progresses on a continuum that, at the most basic level, begins with sustained attention, proceeds to selective attention, and culminates with alternating attention. Each of these categories is considered important for treatment planning and can be described as follows:

1. Sustained attention is the ability to maintain a consistent response during a continuous, repetitive activity. Sustained attention is observed through tasks that require focused responses in a quiet environment for at least one minute (Lezak 1983).
2. Selective attention is the ability to focus on a task while screening out distractions.
3. Alternating attention is the mental ability to move flexibly between tasks having different cognitive requirements. For example, to listen to and then write a message or to cut vegetables while monitoring food cooking requires alternating attention.

Divided attention is a controversial category that is sometimes described as a separate type of attention. It relates to the ability to respond simultaneously to multiple tasks. Some therapists believe that this skill actually represents very rapidly alternating attention. It is generally believed that this type of attention can occur only when one or both of the activities have become automatic and when different sensory systems are being used. For example, it is possible to carry on a conversation while driving, but it is not generally possible to carry on a meaningful conversation while trying to learn new information. Since this category is controversial, it was not included in the RIC occupational therapy evaluation protocol. For the purposes of this protocol, divided attention is evaluated with alternating attention.

Functional Implications

All aspects of attention have relevance to self-care. Sustained attention allows us to direct our efforts toward a simple repetitive task until it is completed. For a patient with cognitive or perceptual problems that make even a simple task difficult, all of his or her attention may be required to focus on a simple repetitive task such as eating. For a less involved patient, sustained attention may be challenged during a higher-level repetitive task such as balancing a checkbook, reading, or counting stitches in a needlework project. By its definition, sustained attention takes place in a quiet environment and does not require screening out distractions; it simply requires maintained focus on one activity.

Selective attention, the ability to screen distractions, allows a person to attend to repetitive activities performed in a distracting environment, such as a busy therapy department or a community setting. For example, attending to exercises, eating, or performing a leisure activity while distractions are present requires selective attention. Work tasks such as sorting mail, typing, or working on an assembly line while ignoring the distractions of people talking and telephones ringing are other activities that require this skill.

Alternating attention is necessary when a person is engaged in two activities or in a task with multiple simultaneous steps. For instance, when preparing a meal, a person might be chopping vegetables while periodically attending to food cooking on the stove. A mother must constantly shift her attention from a task she is performing to monitor the activity of her child. Tasks such as attending to hazards in the environment while looking for a particular store in the community, knitting while watching television, or talking on the telephone while writing a message require rapid alternating attention. Parts of these tasks are accomplished through au-

tomatic motor programs, yet at various critical points, attention is required to ensure that the activity is completed successfully. Evaluation of attention is important because this cognitive skill is frequently impaired after a stroke and because one must be able to attend to relevant aspects of a task before higher-level information processing can be expected.

Evaluation

It is clear that attention is necessary for all self-care tasks. Understanding the specific types of attention deficits that a patient experiences can help the occupational therapist (OT) choose activities and a setting that will best enhance performance. It is important to observe both auditory and visual attention, since the patient may perform better by using one modality rather than the other. To challenge various patients effectively, the RIC cognitive assessment protocol suggests observations and tests that can be used with severely involved patients as well as tests that can be used with minimally affected patients.

Sustained Attention. A patient who has difficulty in sustaining attention should be evaluated in a quiet, nondistracting environment. Observations of repetitive functional tasks such as feeding, bathing, shaving (Figure 4-1), or putting away dishes can be used. Higher-level patients can be challenged to look up numbers in the telephone book, find a computer disk (Figure 4-2), balance a checkbook (Figure 4-3), or file work-related material. Any repetitive task that can be performed in a quiet environment and is appropriate to the patient's roles or interests can be used to evaluate sustained attention. It is important to choose activities that provide intellectual challenge commensurate with the patient's capacity. If not enough challenge is provided, the therapist may incorrectly assume that attention is sufficient to perform required tasks. If too little challenge is pro-

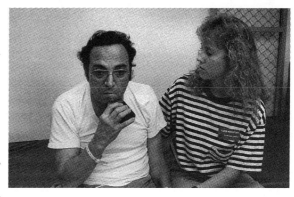

Figure 4-1 The ability to sustain attention to a simple functional task can be observed during basic ADL.

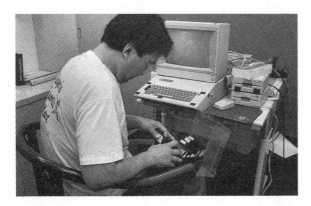

Figure 4-2 Finding a computer disk requires sustained attention and provides cognitive challenge suitable for a higher-level patient.

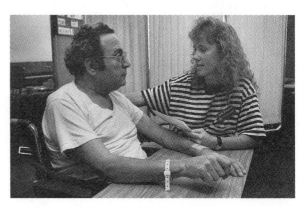

Figure 4-4 During the Random Letter Test for sustained auditory attention, the patient responds by tapping when the target letter is heard.

vided, the patient may lose attention because of boredom. Proper activity selection is therefore crucial.

When needed, tests that require auditory or visual vigilance are available. Sustained auditory attention can be evaluated by requiring the patient to listen to a list of letters and to indicate when the target letter is heard (Figure 4-4). Strub and Black's Random Letter Test (1985) is used, since scoring criteria are available. This task consists of 60 letters read at the rate of one per second. The letters are arranged so that target letters are repeated in several instances. This helps detect the patient's ability to sustain responses when required, as well as to stop responding appropriately. The patient must have sufficient receptive language skills to distinguish letters and to comprehend the directions. A patient with severe aphasia would be unable to participate in this test.

Visual vigilance can be tested in a similar way by

presenting a series of 60 cards with various shapes printed on each (Abreu 1987). The patient is asked to respond to the target shape (Figure 4-5). This task requires some basic visual perceptual skills in order to recognize the correct shape; therefore, the ability to distinguish the shapes should be tested prior to giving the test.

The Letter Cancellation Test described in the unilateral visual neglect section of this chapter also requires sustained attention. This test requires that the patient scan a page and mark all of the target letters. The task can be made more complex by decreasing the distance between the letters or by using two target letters. The test selected for the RIC protocol is a Letter Cancellation task described by Diller et al. (1974). Lezak (1983) indicates that difficulties on this test are associated with unilateral inattention in left-side hemiplegics and with temporal processing deficits in right-side hemiplegics.

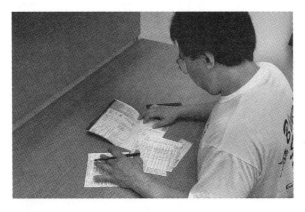

Figure 4-3 Balancing a checkbook requires sustained attention during a difficult cognitive task.

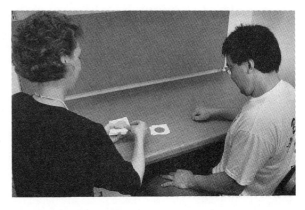

Figure 4-5 The Visual Vigilance Test assesses sustained visual attention.

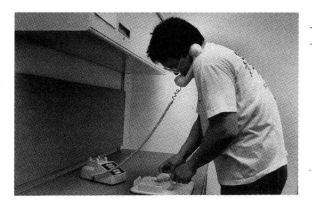

Figure 4-6 Alternating attention is required to attend to a cooking task while conversing.

Scattered errors throughout the page or an increase in errors toward the end of the test can indicate difficulties in sustaining attention.

Selective Attention. Selective attention is tested by requiring the patient to attend to a repetitive activity in a distracting environment. Functional activity suggestions include bringing the patient to the clinic to observe shaving, evaluating feeding in the dining area, or asking the patient to locate a particular food item in the grocery store.

Although the RIC cognitive evaluation relies primarily on functional observations for evaluating selective attention, the Random Letter Test, the Visual Vigilance Test, or the Letter Cancellation Test can be administered first in a quiet place and then in a distracting environment in order to identify the patient's ability to screen distractions. The Stroop Test might be useful in some settings; however, it was thought to be too difficult for most of our patients. It is a very hard standardized test of selective attention that consists of color words (i.e., *red, blue, green*) printed in ink of a color that does not correspond to the word (Jensen and Rohwer 1966; Logan 1980). For instance, the word *red* might be printed in green ink. The patient is asked to name the color of ink rather than to read the word. This requires inhibition of one's natural tendency to read the words.

Alternating Attention. Alternating attention should be tested when a patient demonstrates high-level skills and the potential to return to home making, community, work, or school activities. Any activity that requires attending to several factors can be used to observe alternating attention. For example, the patient may be asked to cook a multi-step meal that requires preparing several dishes simultaneously; or, at a higher level, the patient may be asked to attend to a radio show while sorting items or to carry on a conversation while cooking (Figure 4-6). The ability to alternate attention between relevant events in the clinic and the task at hand can also be observed.

Alternating attention may also be evaluated through tests. The Trail Making Test is supported by Lezak (1983), Reitan (1958), Sareen and Strauss (1991), and Abreu (1987). This test requires a patient to connect numbers sequentially (Part A) (Figure 4-7) or letters and numbers (Part B) (Figure 4-8) arranged randomly on a page. Heaton and Pendleton (1981) feel that poor performance on this test may correlate with difficulty following new procedures or adapting to changing expectations. Some of the literature cited by Lezak (1983) links performance on Part A to vocational potential. Part B requires mental tracking and switching between a numerical series and an alphabetical series. Differences in performance between Part A and Part B can indicate difficulties following a mental sequence or shifting between two types of cognitive activity. Because Part B requires recognition of numbers and letters, visual scanning, and shifting attention, careful observation of the patient's responses on both Part A and Part B is important to determine whether the language component, the ability to search for and organize spatial information, or the capacity to shift attention causes the most difficulty. Like other tests requiring response speed, this evaluation is influenced by age (Lezak 1983). Norms that account for age are available.

The Symbol Digit Modalities Test, a standardized instrument, is also reported as a measure of complex attention requiring concentration, visual search, and visual shifting (Lezak 1983). This test requires the patient to use a code to assign numbers to symbols (Figure 4-9). Visual perceptual skills, attention, and language abilities related to reading are tested, since both the instructions and the task are quite complex. Because numbers are substituted for symbols, both the right and left hemispheres are activated. The right hemisphere is primarily responsible for the interpretation of symbols while the left hemisphere is responsible for language. The required integration of the two hemispheres makes this test very sensitive (Smith 1982). It is suitable for use only with relatively functional patients who have the potential to return to work, home care, or community activities.

The OT has an important role in evaluating attention, since functional activities require a wide range of attentional skills. The OT is able to observe the patient's capacity to attend during simple or complex tasks and in quiet or distracting environments. By choosing the right combination of complexity and dis-

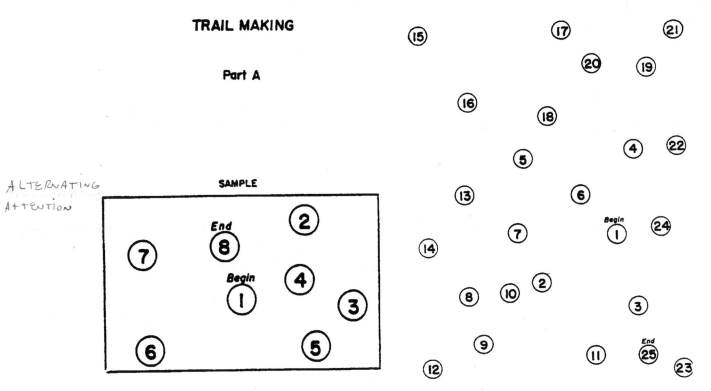

Figure 4-7 The Trail Making Test. Part A, a task using visual spatial and attentional skills, requires the patient to connect the numbers sequentially. *Source:* Reprinted from *Army Individual Test Battery, Manual of Directions and Scoring*, US Army Adjutant General's Office, 1944.

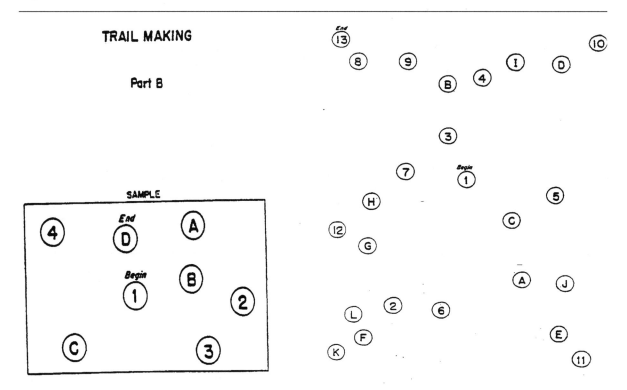

Figure 4-8 The Trail Making Test. Part B requires the patient to connect the letters and numbers sequentially. Alternating attention is required to keep both sequences in order. *Source:* Reprinted from *Army Individual Test Battery, Manual of Directions and Scoring*, US Army Adjutant General's Office, 1944.

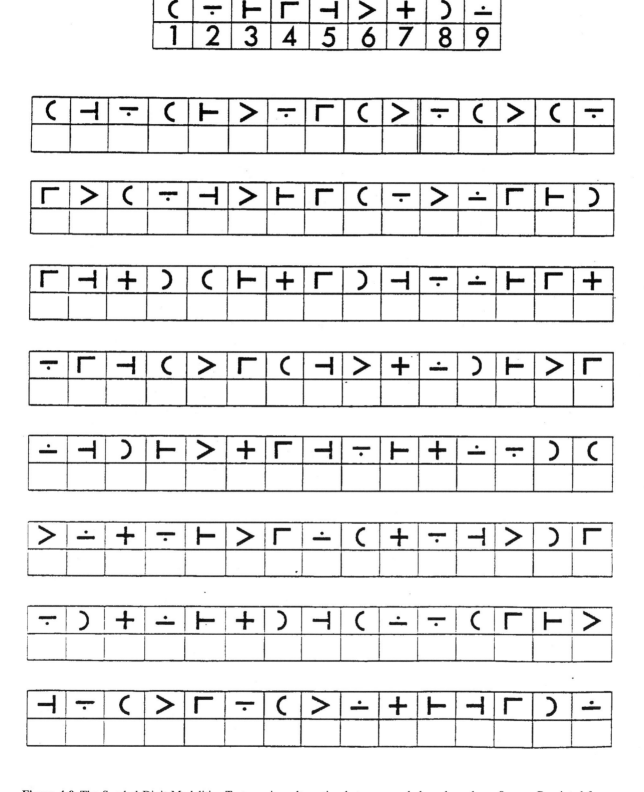

Figure 4-9 The Symbol Digit Modalities Test requires alternating between symbols and numbers. *Source:* Reprinted from *Symbol Digit Modalities Test* by Aaron Smith with permission of Western Psychological Services, © 1982.

traction, the therapist can challenge a person while allowing successful task performance.

Memory

Description

Memory is classified in various ways by various authors. For the purposes of the RIC protocol, it can be defined as the ability to take in, store, and retrieve information (Morse 1986). Memory can be assessed through various parameters, including the length of time the information is stored, the sensory modality that is used to obtain the information, or the type of information that is being stored. Each of these classification systems can be helpful and thus will be described.

Time Classification. Time guidelines and the stages of memory are described differently by various authors. The RIC protocol uses the following stages and time guidelines:

1. Sensory memory, encoding, or acquisition phase: 1 to 30 seconds (Luria 1980). This initial phase of memory is described by some as the period of imprinting during which large amounts of sensory information enter the brain. Decreased arousal or damaged sensory receptor sites in the brain affect this stage of memory.

2. Short-term memory: 30 seconds to 1 minute. Although Zoltan et al. (1986) define time guidelines as 20 to 40 seconds, and Ranka and Chapparo (1987) identify time guidelines as 20 to 60 seconds, for consistency within the departmental standards, a guideline of 30 to 60 seconds was used. During the short-term memory phase, the average person can remember approximately seven chunks of information, plus or minus two chunks (Kimble 1985). For example, a person can generally remember a seven-digit number; however, remembering only a five-digit number or a number as long as nine digits is also considered normal.

3. Long-term memory: over 1 minute. When information is considered important enough, it is rehearsed and sent to long-term storage. Information can remain here for a long period of time; however, it gradually fades if it is not used.

4. Distant, or remote, memory refers to stored events from one's past life (Boll et al. 1981). After brain injury, some patients are incapable of new learning; however, they retain information from the past that can be used in a therapeutic context.

Sensory Modality Classification. Possibly more useful to the OT than the time classification for memory is classification by types of stimuli. Visual, auditory, tactile/kinesthetic, and other sensory information is recorded in memory. By varying the modalities used for teaching, the OT is able to observe whether recall is best facilitated by presentation of information verbally, visually, or through tactile/kinesthetic senses. Visual memory allows us to remember things we have seen, auditory memory allows us to remember what we have heard, and tactile/kinesthetic memory enables us to remember sequences of movement. Declarative memory, the ability to remember facts, relies heavily on auditory or visual memory. Procedural memory, or the ability to retain habitual patterns of behavior, requires tactile/kinesthetic processing. Episodic memory, which allows us to remember emotionally charged events, can rely on input from a variety of senses. The emotional overtones connected with this type of memory cause it to be retained longer and more vividly.

Functional Implications

The OT must determine how memory deficits affect daily life (Brooks and Lincoln 1984) and which types of memory are most affected. Difficulty in retaining new information, learning new procedures, remembering dates or names, remembering directions, and recalling the locations of items are functional problems related to memory deficits. Each of these difficulties may be caused by problems in a specific type of memory. To understand functional implications, it is helpful for the OT to determine what stage of memory and which modality is most affected. This helps predict the types of learning strategies that may be most helpful.

Functionally, immediate memory, the stage of sensory imprinting, is a necessary step prior to moving information to short-term storage. Unless the information is registered for a brief time, it cannot move into storage for later retrieval.

Short-term memory allows us to sort useful information from irrelevant information. Because it would be impossible to store every experience, that first 60 seconds is used to compare information to past experiences and determine whether it is helpful to retain or discard the information.

Short-term memory also allows a person to remember information for brief periods. For instance, it may be useful to remember a name briefly during a social event, but if there is no expectation of seeing that person again, the information may not be transferred to long-term memory. The ability to perform a routine household chore requires short-term memory to recall which steps have been completed. When the therapist is aware that a patient is unable to retain information for brief periods, the patient would not be expected to store that information for future use. Cues and structure will be required for performance.

Long-term memory is necessary for storage of information that will be used in the future. This type of memory is critical for remembering new techniques, learning new information, or retaining instructions. In addition, to learn from experiences, one must compare a recent event to information from the past. After comparing similarities and differences between events and outcomes, a person can decide which strategies were beneficial and which were detrimental. The next time a similar situation arises, these insights can be applied. For some patients who lack the capacity to learn new information, reminiscing and reliance on previously learned information may be helpful in treatment.

Evaluation

Functional observations can be used to assess the patient's ability to remember information immediately, within an hour, and from day to day, or to recall past biographical and personal historical information. For example, the therapist can note whether the patient is able to remember a name or can remember treatment activities from day to day.

It is important first to be sure that the patient is attentive to the information presented. The therapist should have an awareness of the patient's attentional skills and present the information in an environment conducive to learning. Repetition should be provided to ensure that information is learned. In addition, the OT should be convinced that the patient found the information relevant enough to commit to memory. After a given period of time (one hour, one day), the patient can be re-evaluated to determine how much information was retained (Erickson and Scott 1977). Being aware that the patient has undergone a traumatic, life-challenging event and is adjusting to an unfamiliar environment, the therapist considers whether the patient's memory is reduced as a result of stress, cognitive changes, or a combination of these factors.

During observations of memory, the OT should be conscious of the way information is presented: verbally, visually, or tactile/kinesthetically. Although OTs tend to use a multisensory approach, for evaluation purposes it is helpful to test each sensory system separately in order to define the modalities that are most and least helpful for remembering. For example, verbal instructions can be used one time to teach a concept; another time demonstration can be tried. Another situation might lend itself to written or pictorial instructions. By noting which modalities resulted in the best learning,

the therapist can structure future treatment sessions accordingly.

Tests can be used when functional observations are unclear about the types of learning problems evidenced. A test for immediate auditory memory is the Digit Repetition Test (Strub and Black 1985), in which numbers up to nine digits long are read to the patient. Randt et al. (1980) also support use of number repetition for evaluation of memory. The patient then repeats the numbers to the therapist. This test is also considered a test of attention. Short-term visual memory can be tested by asking the patient to look at pictures of functional objects (Figure 4-10). The stimulus card is then removed, and the patient is asked to list verbally the pictures recalled or to point to them on a response card (Figure 4-11). When pointing is used, the task is easier because recognition rather than free recall is required. Long-term memory can be assessed by asking the patient to remember for increasing periods of time information such as a shopping list or instructions specific to treatment.

Orientation

Description

Orientation is a skill that requires integration of attention, memory, and perception. The RIC cognitive protocol examines orientation to self, significant others, place, and time. Orientation is easily assessed in an informal or formal manner and provides a baseline understanding of cognitive function. Because a disoriented patient usually shows other forms of cerebral dysfunction (Lezak 1983), it is important to note deficits in orientation so that other evaluations can be tailored to determine the underlying causes of disorientation. If the underlying problems that contribute to disorientation are identified, the therapist can suggest interventions. For example, if a patient is disoriented to place because of inability to attend to visual cues in the environment, strategies to enhance attention to relevant details may be effective; a patient who is disoriented because of memory problems may benefit from learning memory-retrieval strategies.

Orientation to time includes awareness of the date and season, as well as the ability to estimate the passage of time. Studies have shown that hospitalized patients without neurological deficits are generally accurate within two days of the correct date (Benton 1983d), but CVA patients frequently show a very distorted awareness of the date.

Topographical orientation contributes to orientation to place and is defined as the ability to follow a familiar route or to follow a new route when the opportunity to

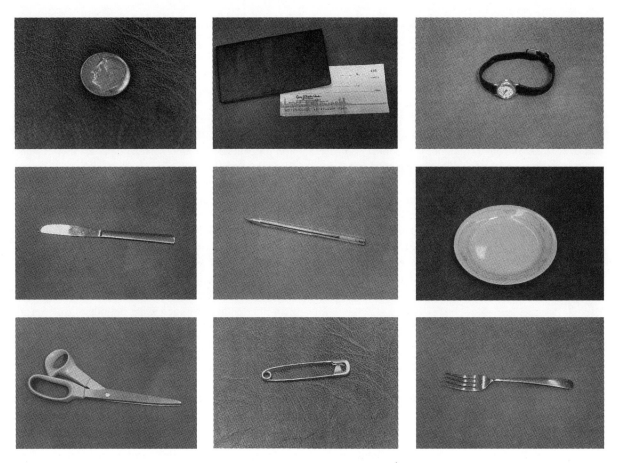

Figure 4-10 Short-term visual memory is tested by asking the patient to remember the objects on this card.

become familiar with it has been given. In addition, the ability to describe the relationship of one place to another in one's house or hometown would demonstrate topographical orientation. Topographical orientation has been recognized as a visuospatial function (Benton 1985; Bouska et al. 1985). For the purposes of logical classification and because it also involves memory, evaluation suggestions have been included in the orientation section. When a patient demonstrates difficulty in finding his or her way, problems with visual spatial awareness should be considered and distinguished from memory problems.

Functional Implications

Orientation to person is the most basic form of orientation. It is unusual to encounter a patient who is not oriented to self in a rehabilitation setting unless significant arousal deficits are present. A person who is disoriented to people around him or her may not interact appropriately with family, with hospital personnel, or with caregivers. Because disorientation to others may cause extreme confusion and lack of cooperation,

awareness of this problem will assist the team and the patient's family in their interactions with the patient.

Poor awareness of time, date, and season can contribute to general confusion and poor judgment when a patient is participating in community-level activities. In a structured hospital setting a patient's inability to estimate the passage of time is often overlooked. The patient may request meals at inappropriate times, become anxious when anticipating a visitor who is not due to arrive until later, or be unprepared for an appointment because the concept of time is not internalized. This problem can contribute to difficulties at home or in any setting that is less structured than the hospital.

A person who is not oriented to place may show similar problems in interacting within the environment and may have unfounded expectations about how the day should proceed. For example, one patient who was disoriented to place believed he was in his office. He frequently commanded staff to perform various duties and became upset when he was not allowed to inspect certain rooms in his business. It was helpful to understand his disorientation when dealing with his frustra-

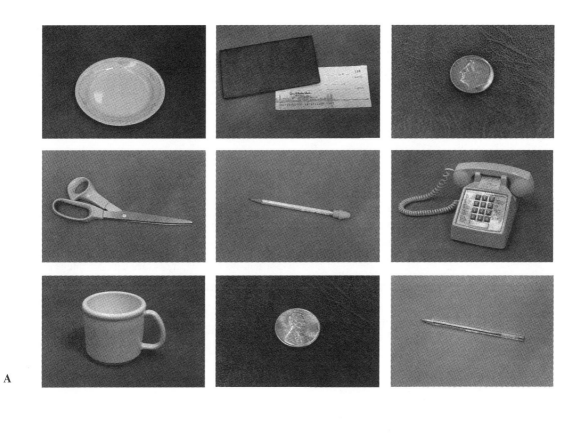

A

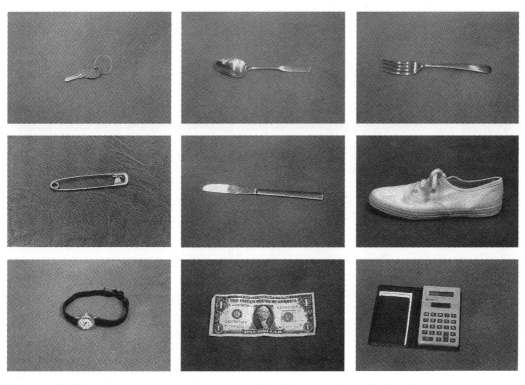

B

Figure 4-11, A and B The patient can point to response cards if unable to recall verbally the objects presented.

tions and the defensive feelings he often elicited in staff.

Evaluation

Orientation is evaluated by asking questions that relate to person, place, and time, or by observing the patient's interaction with others. Formal interview questions are suggested in the evaluation guide (Chapter 10); however, when possible, the OT is encouraged to use a more conversational approach to gain the needed information. The use of a formal orientation interview can be interrogational in tone and can cause the patient to become defensive, especially when orientation is poor. The patient can also be asked to estimate the passage of one minute in order to evaluate more specifically a patient's internal awareness of the passage of time. Topographical orientation is considered a visual spatial skill with a memory component. It is tested by asking the patient to locate areas within the

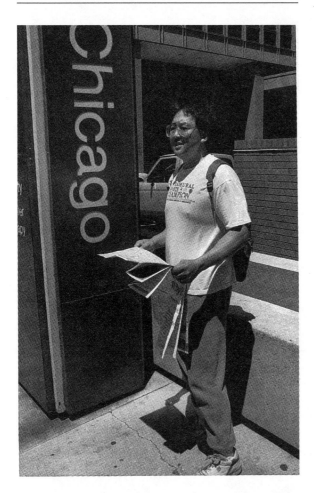

Figure 4-12 High-level patients can be tested for topographical orientation by using a map in the community.

room, on the nursing unit, or within the clinic. High-level patients may be asked to draw a floor plan, use a map in the community (Figure 4-12), plan a bus trip, or navigate in an unfamiliar building. The RIC protocol contains suggestions for orientation questions as well as various options for observing time awareness and topographical orientation.

Problem Solving

Description

As occupational therapists we are most concerned with how cognitive skills are used to perform self-care tasks. When predicting the level of independence a patient will attain, the area of problem solving is very important. Various authors describe problem solving in various ways. Lezak (1983) describes many of the higher-level processes inherent in problem solving as components of executive function. She believes that executive functioning serves to organize and express cognitive skills in activity. Although each of these systems of classification is useful in the intended situation, for the purposes of this occupational therapy cognitive evaluation, problem solving is considered the highest-level cognitive skill.

Problem solving requires the integration of many cognitive skills, such as attention, memory, organization, planning, and judgment (Zoltan et al. 1986). Evaluation of problem solving therefore entails analysis of component skills such as memory and attention as well as analysis of the processes by which a decision is reached. The evaluation protocol thus suggests observation of the following process skills:

- identifying the problem
- generating solutions
- planning an action
- implementing the plan
- monitoring the effectiveness of the plan
- reaching an effective outcome

Because integration of various cognitive and perceptual skills is required, effective problem solving implies that the component skills are adequate to meet the challenge of the problem, and that these skills are integrated to allow solutions that are appropriate to the unique characteristics of the situation. It is therefore important to allow the patient to encounter problems that correspond in difficulty to those that will be experienced on discharge. Although the evaluation of low-functioning patients focuses on component skills, the evaluation of high-level patients focuses on integrated problem solving and on detecting the underlying problems that interfere with effectiveness.

Allen (1985) describes a six-level cognitive hierarchy in which the top two levels relate to problem-solving behaviors. Exploratory actions (level 5) are problem-solving methods characterized by overt trial-and-error procedures. The highest level, planned actions, requires preplanning and consideration of the consequences of an action. These classifications are helpful for describing two ways in which problem solving occurs. The patient with a trial-and-error style may need to experience failure before being able to identify a problem, whereas the patient with a covert style of problem solving is able to anticipate possible problems. Similarly, the patient with a trial-and-error approach may not generate solutions or identify a plan until engaged in the task. Then, through trial and error, various methods can be attempted until a successful outcome is reached. The covert problem solver, functioning at a higher level, can identify various alternatives, formulate a plan, and monitor progress toward the goal. This type of problem solving is more efficient; however, it is unrealistic for many patients with cognitive limitations.

Functional Implications

Problem-solving skills are necessary for any level of independence. Unless problem-solving skills are present, the patient will be unable to apply learned skills to new situations. For example, problem solving is used to decide how to open a package with one hand or how to attract the attention of a caregiver. Problem-solving skills of a higher level are needed to plan for appropriate child care or to consider vocational possibilities following a CVA. When a patient effectively solves problems, his or her behavior is safe, efficient, and flexible. At the highest level, the patient is able to apply concepts to new situations and generate unique solutions to problems. A patient functioning in this way is able to collaborate with the therapist in treatment and has potential for living independently.

Evaluation

Patients who show poor arousal, severe attentional deficits, significant memory and orientation limitations, or serious perceptual difficulties should not be tested for problem-solving skills. Their basic cognitive and perceptual deficits interfere with identifying relevant features of the problem or considering realistic alternatives, thus making them unable to perform the steps necessary for problem solving. The therapist can comment on safety and problem identification but should focus the evaluation on the component cognitive and perceptual skills that are precursors for effective problem solving.

The preferred method of evaluation for problem solving is observation, since OTs have the unique ability to view performance of ADL tasks that will be relevant upon discharge. It is important that the therapist relinquish the teaching role during this part of the evaluation in order to give the patient some freedom to solve problems. The therapist should select tasks that will challenge the patient's problem-solving skills without jeopardizing safety or creating undue frustration. By allowing the patient to experience uncertainty and asking him or her to estimate the probable outcomes of actions, the OT can evaluate the patient's ability to generate solutions and to examine covertly their effectiveness (Vizzetti 1987).

When the occupational therapist must provide recommendations for the patient's potential to live alone, the ability to solve problems becomes very important. Functional activities that approximate those which must be performed outside the hospital must be emphasized. In addition, component skills that may significantly impair problem solving and decision making should be carefully examined (Alexander 1988).

Planning can be assessed by asking the patient to describe how a solution might be achieved. Once the plan is initiated, the patient is observed to determine how well the previously generated solutions and plans are used and how well the plan is modified to meet changing environmental factors or unforeseen problems. Because safe and effective problem solving relies on so many cognitive and perceptual skills, careful observation of performance is necessary to define underlying cause(s) of difficulty.

During the initial evaluation period, time constraints and the patient's desire to focus on basic self-care performance may make observation of problem solving in challenging situations difficult. For example, the high-level patient who has demonstrated good problem-solving skills during basic ADL tasks may not perform as well during community-level work or home care tasks. Although problem solving may have been adequate for simple self-care, the complex problems presented in more abstract or challenging tasks often are not evaluated during the initial phase of rehabilitation. Because information about complex problem solving is helpful when setting realistic goals and predicting future independence, various assessment methods are suggested.

Several tests can be used to observe higher-level problem-solving strategies during the initial evaluation phase. The patient can be asked to solve verbally a series of hypothetical problems. These situations are meant to depict real problems that might be encountered. Responses can give insight into the patient's ability to define problems and generate alternative solutions. Verbal problem solving does not give an indication of how this plan would actually be implemented or whether the plan would be adjusted spontaneously if it was not effective. Thus caution must be used in interpreting the patient's response. A plausible response would indicate adequate problem identification and generation of solutions but would not provide information about implementation. Failure to give a good response would indicate difficulty with basic skills such as identifying problems or generating solutions.

The patient's organizational skills can be observed through their approach to the Three-Dimensional Block Design Test (Benton 1983e) or copying the Rey (1964) Complex Figure Test. Both tests are described in the visual construction portion of this chapter. According to Lezak (1983), various observations about a patient's problem-solving strategies can be made. High-level patients who retain conceptual skills will be able to visualize a form as a whole and work rapidly to reproduce it. Other patients may make a few incorrect choices, but they will refer to the model as a whole in order to reproduce it accurately. Those with more average skills will use a trial-and-error approach. In the block design test, for example, they will compare each block with the model before proceeding. They may never view the design as a whole, but they will use an orderly piece-by-piece approach to solving the problem. Organization of the task, awareness of errors, and impulsive behavior can be observed.

A simple, nonstandardized activity has also been used successfully to observe the patient's ability to generate solutions, test the solutions overtly or covertly, and reach a creative solution. The patient is asked to place a wooden block on a small, upright bulletin board by using materials such as a safety pin, rubber band, tack, small box, or small cup (Figure 4-13). There are several ways of solving the problem. For instance, the

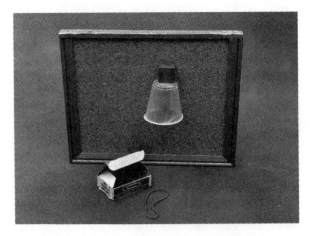

Figure 4-14 Placing the block on a cup that is tacked to the board is one solution to the bulletin board problem.

box or cup can be tacked to the board and then the block can be placed on it (Figure 4-14). The patient is able to ask for physical assistance if needed, but the activity can be accomplished with one hand. These tests are not meant to substitute for observation of problem-solving skills in functional activities, but to provide some structured methods of observation early in the evaluation process.

EVALUATIONS FOR VISUAL PERCEPTION

This category includes many tests of visual perceptual function. Visual perception is one of the most widely studied and important perceptual systems. Adults rely more heavily on this sense than on any other. Faulty visual information is powerful; any OT who has issued prism glasses knows that altered visual perception initially can be very confusing, but adaptation soon occurs. The person changes the way in which he or she relates to the environment according to the changed visual information. It is clear that faulty visual information caused by perceptual deficits also can alter function.

The RIC perceptual evaluation protocol examines the following four categories of visual perception:

1. unilateral visual inattention
2. visual spatial awareness
3. visual analysis and synthesis
4. visual construction

The first two categories describe purely perceptual processes and the last two categories require the integration of cognitive and perceptual skills. The final category, visual construction, also involves motor responses and thus is the most complex of the visual perceptual skills. The categories are listed in a hierar-

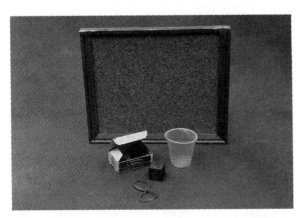

Figure 4-13 The bulletin board problem asks the patient to find a method to place a wooden block on the face of a vertical cork board.

chical manner, since a deficit at a lower level will have an impact on performance at a higher skill level.

Unilateral Visual Inattention

Description

Unilateral visual inattention has been discussed extensively in the literature, yet disagreement remains about the true nature of the deficit. Although some therapists feel that it is primarily an attentional problem, others feel that faulty visual control and registration are the primary causes of the deficit. Gianutsos et al. (1983) nicely combine several theories. They believe that there are three factors responsible for visual imperception. The first factor is left spatial hemi-imperception, which causes difficulty in returning to a fixed starting point in the left visual field, inefficient visual searching, and difficulty in monitoring the left visual field. The second factor is lateral eye movement inefficiency, which negatively affects the ability to monitor both the right and left visual fields quickly. Problems with ocular efficiency interfere with optimal visual scanning. The third factor is foveal hemi-imperception, which is related to difficulty in reading the beginning or end of a word. This deficit is believed to be due to a primary impairment of the foveal visual field.

Functional Implications

Many authors cite the correlations between tests of unilateral visual inattention and ADL function. For example, Denes et al. (1982) state that unilateral spatial neglect is a crucial factor contributing to decreased ADL and social functioning in left-side hemiplegics. Other authors, including Wilson et al. (1987) and Kotila et al. (1986), reinforce the negative impact of unilateral neglect on ADL function. Gianutsos et al. (1983) focused on more subtle forms of visual imperception and felt that these subtle problems have an impact on safety, especially on high-level tasks such as driving, when speed and accuracy are critical. Unilateral inattention is also associated with other visual perceptual deficits, possibly because it interferes with accurate visual imagery. Clinically, the therapist is aware of the wide range of problems in self-care function that are evident in patients with unilateral visual neglect. Both subtle and more overt difficulties with visual awareness can be seen in activities ranging from neglect of items during dressing or feeding, to difficulty maneuvering in the clinic, to problems reading instructions, to unawareness of critical factors in the environment during community-level tasks.

Evaluation

Various types of activities and tests can be used to detect unilateral visual inattention. Since unilateral visual inattention is such a widely discussed topic, there is significant support for the use of functional observations, drawing and copying tasks, crossing-out tasks, and tasks involving high-level processing and speed. The perceptual evaluation guide (Chapter 11) provides guidelines for observation of unilateral visual attention and provides directions for test activities. Preliminary information may be obtained through observation. When necessary to confirm clinical observations, tests may be given. These tests graphically display problems with unilateral attention and often help the patient and family "see" the deficit. The therapist can help the patient by explaining how tests correlate to functional problems and by pointing out these problems when they occur during activity. Each type of activity and a rationale for their use in the occupational therapy evaluation process are described.

Functional Observations. Although there is some controversy regarding the use of functional tasks for evaluating unilateral visual inattention due to questionable sensitivity, especially when deficits are mild, Wilson et al. (1987) strongly support the use of behavioral observations. They developed the Rivermead Behavioral Inattention Test, which includes items such as eating a meal (simulation), dialing a telephone, reading a menu, telling and setting time, sorting coins, copying an address, and following a map. They found that the most sensitive portions of the battery included setting the time, copying an address, reading a menu, and describing eight items on a life-sized photograph of a meal. This test has been shown to be reliable and valid, and it may be inferred that similar observations during actual self-care performance are also valid for detecting more overt forms of unilateral neglect. Arnadottir (1990), an Icelandic OT, also advocates using functional observations for evaluation of unilateral inattention, and she has described her methods thoroughly in her book, *The Brain and Behavior: Assessing Cortical Dysfunction through Activities of Daily Living.*

Despite the fact that some authors feel that functional observations are not sensitive to unilateral visual inattention, clinical experience indicates that they are a valuable method, especially when treatment goals relate to basic self-care. If the therapist is vigilant during the observations of both simple and more complex functional tasks, he or she can readily identify problems with unilateral visual attention (Figures 4-15 and 4-16). These deficits can be noted for the purposes of the evaluation, but—more important—they can be described to the patient or the family. Evaluation and

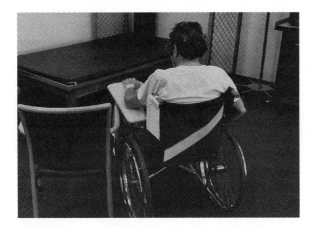

Figure 4-15 Left-side visual inattention is demonstrated as the patient bumps an obstacle with the wheelchair.

treatment can be combined, and the patient profits directly from the evaluation period.

Line Bisection. Schenkenberg's Line Bisection Test (Figure 4-17) was chosen because it is easy to administer, is easy for the patient to understand, and is supported in the literature. Schenkenberg and associates (1980) studied the use of their Line Bisection Test for evaluating unilateral visual inattention. Through comparison with other tests of unilateral neglect, they found this test effective. Schenkenberg et al. recommended using the tool in conjunction with other tests such as symmetrical drawings and tests for memory of designs. The subject is asked to draw a mark in the center of 20 lines of varying lengths placed in various positions on the page. Occupational therapists Van Deusen and Harlowe (1987) also recommend the Schenkenberg test as a method of differentiating unilateral neglect from

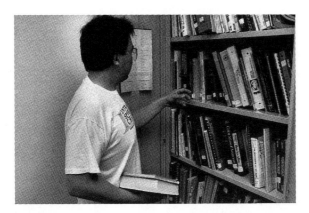

Figure 4-16 This patient demonstrated subtle right-side visual inattention when locating a book in the library, a complex task that demands concentration and visual scanning.

other types of visual perceptual dysfunction and suggest that it would be a good addition to an occupational therapy cognitive perceptual evaluation.

Although the Line Bisection Test is recommended, analysis of the results is somewhat cumbersome. In their study of four groups of 20 patients, Schenkenberg et al. (1980) found that the left-placed lines and the center lines were the most discriminative for left neglect. Most control patients and right-side hemiplegics did not deviate more than 5 percent from the true center of these lines. Van Deusen and Harlow (1987) studied 93 older adults and found that the mean score on the test was close to zero with a standard deviation of 5.55 for left-side lines and 4.35 for right-side lines. The mathematical method of scoring the test described by Schenkenberg et al. and Van Deusen and Harlowe requires measuring the lines from the left edge to the patient's mark and then calculating a percentage deviation using the following formula: % Deviation = (measured left half − true half)/(true half) × 100. Since this formula and the calculations involved created negative incentives for using the test, transparent overlays showing the true center and standard deviations for each line were created to simplify scoring. Van Deusen and Harlowe state that 1 standard deviation from the norm can be considered a mild impairment, 2 standard deviations indicate moderate impairment, and 3 standard deviations show severe impairment.

Drawing and Copying Tasks. Many authors cite the use of drawing and copying tasks as a means of identifying unilateral visual neglect. Lezak (1983) suggests that bilaterally symmetrical models are particularly helpful in observing unilateral neglect. She also describes the use of free-hand drawings of a clock for eliciting unilateral neglect. Riddoch and Humphreys (1983) state that drawings of a clock, a person, and a bicycle are sensitive to left-side visual neglect.

Campbell and Oxbury (1976), Zarit and Kahn (1974), Abreu (1987), and Schenkenberg et al. (1980) use drawing and copying tasks as part of a battery to identify unilateral neglect. Campbell and Oxbury (1976) found that, five months after the initial evaluation, many patients learned to compensate for neglect in drawing; however, strong preferences for right-side responses in visual recognition tasks remained. Some authors have associated these responses with neglect. It may be inferred that drawings are less sensitive than more complex tests in detecting unilateral neglect. Lezak (1983) also cautions that relatively simple drawings may not identify milder forms of neglect. Van Deusen and Harlowe (1987) found that clinical observations in activities such as drawing a person correlated

Figure 4-17 The Schenkenberg Line Bisection Test requires that the patient put a mark at the center of each line. *Source:* Reprinted with permission from *Neurology* (1980;30:513), Copyright © 1980, AdvanStar Communications.

highly with other perceptual scores but the Schenkenberg Line Bisection Test did not. They therefore felt that drawings were not pure indicators of unilateral visual inattention.

Drawing and copying tasks are included in the RIC occupational therapy perceptual battery primarily as a measure of visual constructive skills. Because the literature also supports their use in observing unilateral inattention, we have included suggestions for interpretation in our unilateral inattention protocol. The tasks offer a variety of levels of difficulty. Simple design copying is the most basic task, followed by drawing a familiar object from memory. Copying the Rey figure, a complex task requiring organization and attention to detail, provides even more challenge. Exceptionally high-level patients can be asked to draw the Rey Figure from memory immediately after copying the design. Whenever possible, drawing and copying tasks should be combined with line bisection or functional observations to describe more accurately unilateral visual neglect.

Crossing-Out Tasks. Albert's Test (1973), a modification of Denny-Brown's test, consists of 40 lines placed in a standard, nonlinear array on a sheet of paper (Figure 4-18). The patient is asked to mark each line. Damasio and associates (1980) used this test in their study of neglect. Fullerton et al. (1986) also report use of this test and believe that it is helpful because of its ease of interpretation and simplicity. To score the test, the unmarked lines are counted. Albert considered all missed lines as an error of neglect. Thirty control subjects showed a mean score of zero. Fullerton and his colleagues (1986) compared the number of missed lines on each half of the page. If more than 70 percent of the unmarked lines are on one half of the page, unilateral visual neglect exists. Thus one unmarked line on the left side of the page would indicate unilateral inattention, but an unmarked line on each side of the page would not. An advantage of this test is its ease of scoring and administration to even relatively low-functioning patients. Fullerton and his associates found that the test was closely correlated with functional recovery.

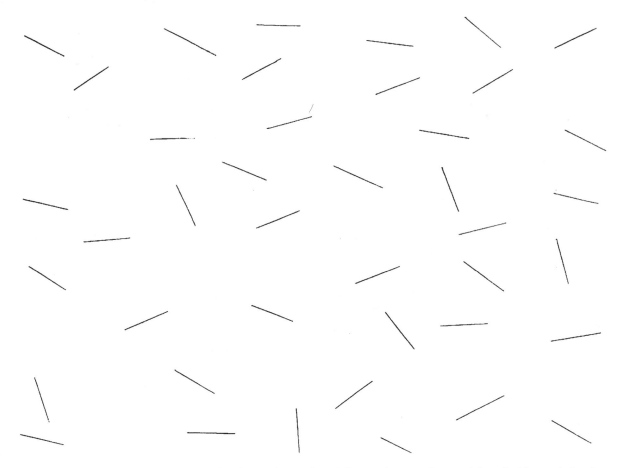

Figure 4-18 During Albert's Test, the patient is asked to mark each line on the page. *Source:* Adapted with permission from *Lancet* (1986;430), Copyright © 1986, Lancet Ltd.

In a study of 66 brain-injured patients and 30 control subjects, Albert (1973) found that visual field defects and neglect are not necessarily related and that when they do occur together they occur most often in patients with left-side hemiplegia. He found that visual inattention is highly correlated with visual construction difficulties and with tests of visual spatial organization in left-side hemiplegics. He also found that a high frequency of both right-side and left-side brain-damaged patients shows neglect. Right-side hemiplegics had a 30 percent incidence and left-side hemiplegics had a 37 percent incidence; left-side hemiplegics, however, showed more severe deficits. After studying the response patterns of patients with localized lesions, Albert concluded that various factors can be responsible for neglect, including decreased

- attention
- reception of visual stimuli
- integration of visual information
- oculomotor function
- immediate recall

Fullerton and his colleagues (1986) studied 205 stroke patients, using a battery of tests. They found that Albert's Test was a significant predictor of unilateral visual neglect and of function six months after stroke.

Abreu (1987), among other authors, suggests presenting the patient with a typed array of letters and asking him or her to mark all the *O*s. She feels that the small print found in a letter cancellation task is helpful in eliciting neglect because of the demands it places on the scanning system. Heilman and Watson (1978) support the idea that crossing-out tasks involving words or letters cause an increase in symptoms of left neglect. This may be due to the fact that the left hemisphere processes verbal material and promotes an orienting response to the right. Because of the demand on language skills, the Letter Cancellation Test may be inappropriate for some aphasic patients suspected of having unilateral neglect. The Letter Cancellation Test (Figure 4-19) (Diller et al. 1974) is included in the RIC battery because it is challenging and relevant to reading for higher-level patients.

```
B E I F H E H F E G I C H E I C B D A C H F B E D A C D A F C I H C F E B A F E A C F C H B D C F G H E

C A H E F A C D C F E H B F C A D E H A E I E G D E G H B C A G C I E H C I E F H I C D B C G F D E B A

E B C A F C B E H F A E F E G C H G D E H B A E G D A C H E B A E D G C D A F C B I F E A D C B E A C G


C D G A C H E F B C A F E A B F C H D E F C G A C B E D C F A H E H E F D I C H B I E B C A H C D E F B

A C B C G B I E H A C A F C I C A B E G F B E F A E A B G C G F A C D B E B C H F E A D H C A I E F E G

E D H B C A D G E A D F E B E I G A C G E D A C H G E D C A B A E F B C H D A C G B E H C D F E H A I E
```

TRIAL

```
F C B E H B A C G D E H I E G D C D A F C G I E C D A F C G I D F B C A H
```

Letter Cancellation Test: Cancel the "Cs" and "Es"

Figure 4-19 The Letter Cancellation Test challenges high-level patients to cross out the designated letters. *Source:* Reprinted from *Studies in Cognition and Rehabilitation in Hemiplegia*, Rehabilitation Monograph No 50, by L Diller et al with permission of New York University Medical Center Institute of Rehabilitation Medicine, © 1974.

High-Level Speed and Complexity Tasks. Gianutsos et al. (1983) feel that more subtle forms of visual imperception can be difficult to detect by using methods such as confrontation, drawing and copying, cancellation tasks, and line bisection. They believe that patients often are unaware of the absence of vision. Because these deficits frequently persist despite recovery in other areas, the patient who reaches a relatively independent level may be at risk when participating in an activity that requires rapid visual processing, such as driving. Gianutsos et al. suggest several high-level tasks that combine complexity and speed. Recommended tasks include a paper and pencil word search activity and a computer program requiring rapid reading of words in various positions on the screen. They have also developed computerized tasks that do not require reading numbers or letters. It is believed that at least one task involving speed and complexity is a useful addition to an evaluation of high-level patients who may return to independent community activities or driving. Currently the Reaction Time Measure of Visual Field (Gianutsos and Klitzner 1981) is recommended. The patient is asked to respond to numbers presented at various places on the screen by pushing a key or hand-held switch. The response time is calculated for various visual fields.

Visual Spatial Awareness

Description

Abreu (1987) defines spatial awareness as the ability to detect subtle or gross differences in position, direc-

tions, angles, and rotation. This includes the ability to orient one's body in space and to perceive the position of objects in relation to oneself (Siev et al. 1986; Colarusso and Hammill 1972). Accurately perceiving visual spatial relationships is inherent in tasks such as drawing to verbal command, copying a picture, or copying a block design (Lezak 1983; Filskor and Boll 1981). These tasks also include a motor execution and planning component.

Functional Implications

A person with visual spatial deficits may show difficulty locating objects in space, estimating an object's size, or judging his or her distance from an object (Bouska et al. 1985). Specifically, an individual with a visual spatial deficit might have difficulty with reading, counting, correctly orienting a functional object prior to use, or following a route from one place to another (Bouska et al. 1985). Bernspang et al. (1989) found that visual factors such as spatial relations are important predictors of long-term self-care function. It is difficult to test pure spatial judgment in functional tasks, because all activities require motor performance. The therapist must infer from the way in which the patient performs whether the underlying cause is difficulty with spatial judgment. For instance, a patient may rotate an item several times to determine the correct orientation or may be unaware of a mispositioned item. A test such as The Cross Test or Benton's Judgment of Line Orientation (1983b) that does not require a motor response can help delineate whether the problem relates more to the spatial or performance aspect of the task. This information helps the therapist decide on the best course of treatment. For visual spatial problems, simplification of visual information in the environment may be helpful, while hand over hand guidance and chaining techniques may be more appropriate for motor performance deficits.

Evaluation

Since pure spatial judgment is a visual skill, it is almost impossible to test in its pure form during function. All functional tasks require motor output as well as visual awareness of spatial orientation. Patients who misalign clothing, orient objects incorrectly, or have difficulty positioning one part of an object in relation to another during construction tasks may be suspected of demonstrating spatial orientation difficulties. A test that does not require motor output is useful in determining whether the constructional deficit is due to spatial orientation or motor-planning problems.

The Cross Test was used in a study by Kim et al. (1984) as a measure of visual spatial ability. The Cross Test can be completed by a simple motor or verbal response to the question "are the two crosses in the same location?" (Figure 4-20). It is a simple test that is administered more quickly than Benton's Judgment of Line Orientation Test; however, it does not have estab-

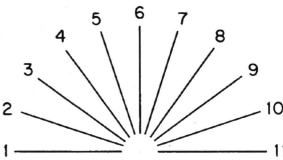

Figure 4-21 The Judgment of Line Orientation Test is a pure test of visual spatial skills. *Source:* Reprinted from *Contributors to Neuropsychological Assessment: A Clinical Manual* (pp 44–53) by A Benton with permission of Oxford University Press, © 1983.

lished norms. The Cross Test is suggested as a quick screening tool.

Benton's Judgment of Line Orientation Test can be considered a pure measure of visual spatial awareness because it does not require a sophisticated motor response (Benton 1983b; Benton et al. 1979). This 30-item test involves visually matching two stimulus lines oriented at various angles to a labeled array (Figure 4-21). The patient can point to or verbally identify his or her response. Norms and test retest reliability for Benton's test were established on 137 normal subjects divided into six age- and sex-matched groups. The test was also given to 100 patients. By comparing results with the location of the lesion, Benton found that al-

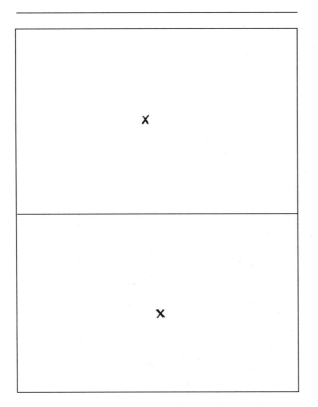

Figure 4-20 The Cross Test is a screening evaluation for visual spatial skills.

most all of the errors were made by patients with posterior lesions, while Benton's test can be used for more discriminative testing. Both tests aim to isolate visual spatial awareness as the sole component being evaluated.

EVALUATIONS FOR VISUAL ANALYSIS AND SYNTHESIS

Description

Visual analysis and synthesis was chosen as a broad evaluation category based on the work of Bouska et al. (1985). They include this category in their classification of visual perceptual skills. They believe that an understanding of similarities and differences and of relationships of parts to each other is required to analyze complex visual information. In addition, cognitive skills such as reasoning and deduction are required. For high-level patients, test materials therefore should challenge the patient's ability to make fine visual distinctions, analyze foreground from background, recognize items based on incomplete information, and synthesize elements into a whole.

Functional Implications

It is thought that these higher-level visual skills have significant impact on a person's ability to function in complex situations. Visual analysis is required to pick out an item from a cabinet or a drawer, to process vital information in the environment, to perceive subtle distinctions between two faces, or to recognize familiar landmarks. A therapist with a good understanding of a patient's visual perceptual deficits will be more likely to set realistic goals, can help the caretakers and patient understand how particular problems relate to function, and can plan treatment that addresses specific deficits.

Visual Analysis

Visual analysis is the ability to determine the relevant aspects of a visual presentation and then to analyze how the information is like or different from other information. This skill allows us to detect similarities and differences between items (visual discrimination) and to detect relevant information from a cluttered background (figure-ground analysis).

Visual Discrimination

Description. Visual discrimination refers to the ability to detect differences and similarities between objects, thereby determining whether they are alike or different. Benton (1983f) reviews studies that indicate that impairment in simple visual discrimination is not fre-

quent in patients with brain damage; however, complex visual discrimination is often impaired. In addition, he states that form discrimination is correlated with visual construction.

Evaluation. A nonstandardized screening task, consisting of simple and more complex shapes that the patient must match, has been devised (Figure 4-22). When subtle difficulties are noted or suspected, The Visual Form Discrimination Test, a more in-depth test designed by Benton (1983f), can also be performed (Figure 4-23). This test, which requires the patient to determine which of the response stimuli are the same as the target stimuli, was selected because it is relatively brief yet has standardized directions, well-established reliability, and has been shown to be valid.

Figure-Ground Analysis

Description. Figure-ground analysis requires carefully studying a picture or setting and separating the relevant foreground information from the irrelevant background information. Although very simple figure-ground tasks such as finding a white shirt on a white sheet may relate more to visual attention, complex figure-ground tasks can provide information about visual analysis. Benton (1985) describes studies showing that figure-ground deficits have been found in patients with focal brain damage as well as in patients with right parietal damage or left hemisphere damage with aphasia. No significant association was found between visual field deficits and performance on figure-ground tests.

Evaluation. Siev et al. (1986) suggest a functional test of figure-ground skill. The RIC perceptual protocol

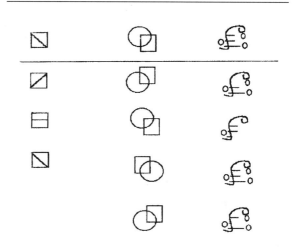

Figure 4-22 The Visual Discrimination Screening Form is used to assess the patient's ability to analyze the critical features of a form and match it correctly. *Source:* Adapted from *Rehabilitation of Perceptual-Cognitive Dysfunction* (pp 118–120) by B Abreu, with permission of B Abreu, © 1987.

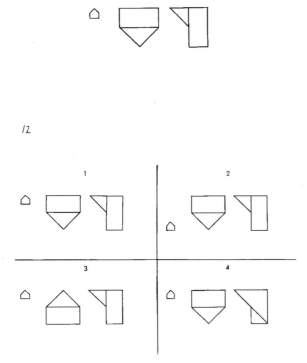

Figure 4-23 The Visual Form Discrimination Test is a standardized assessment. *Source:* Reprinted from *Contributions to Neuropsychological Assessment: A Clinical Manual* (p 58) by A Benton with permission of Oxford University Press, © 1983.

suggests some activities that may be observed to determine whether high-level visual processing is affected. The degree of difficulty must be analyzed when testing this area through function. Picking out a brush in a fairly empty drawer will not require the same degree of visual discrimination, analysis, or synthesis as will be required for scanning a well-stocked grocery store shelf

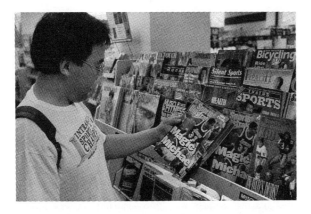

Figure 4-24 Visual analysis is required to evaluate the critical features of an item and locate it on a rack.

for a can of chicken noodle soup or searching a rack for a particular magazine (Figure 4-24). Many of the visual discrimination, analysis, and synthesis challenges encountered in basic ADL tasks during the initial evaluation will not be as challenging as some of the complex formal test items. Abreu (1987) states that a patient may be able to do well on a test that requires him or her to find 1 object out of 25 but may do poorly on locating a geometrical shape in an embedded figure. The amount of detail and concentration make the second task more analytical than the first. Patients who will have reason to perform complicated visual analysis or synthesis because of the nature of their work or leisure activities may benefit from testing with complex materials if deficits are suspected.

Several figure-ground pictures were compiled as a screening tool designed to be administered quickly (Figure 4-25). This test is not standardized. The Ayres Figure-Ground Test (1978) requires more time, but it does have limited norms for adults and can be used to test figure-ground skills further in patients who show possible deficits during screening or functional activities (Figure 4-26). The Ayres test is recommended by Lezak (1983), who feels that its test items, which range from simple imbedded figures to complex geometrical shapes, are appropriate and challenging for adults. She believes that its simple administration and the inclusion of both familiar objects and geometrical forms make it a valuable tool. Siev et al. (1986) also recommend the Ayres Figure-Ground Test and provide pilot data showing normative scores for adults. These norms are included in the perceptual evaluation guide (Chapter 11) to assist the therapist in interpretation of the patient's performance.

Visual Synthesis

Description

Benton (1985) describes patients who can identify a single visual stimulus but are unable "to integrate separate elements into a meaningful whole." These patients may be able to identify details in a picture, but they cannot derive meaning from those features. This problem is one of visual synthesis. Visual closure is considered a type of visual synthesis.

Functional Implications

A person who is unable to synthesize visual information will have difficulty in environments that present significant amounts of visual stimulation. In a room, for instance, they may be able to describe various elements but cannot use that information to describe the main activity taking place. If part of an object is obstructed,

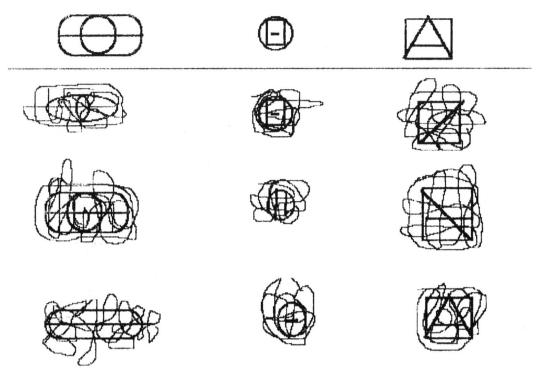

Figure 4-25 Visual analysis is required for this figure-ground screening test.

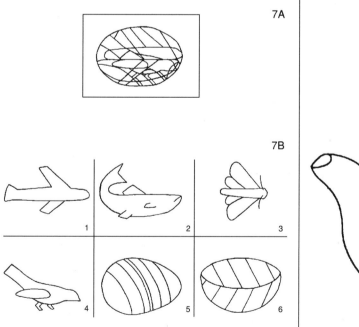

Figure 4-26 The Ayres Figure-Ground Test provides challenges to the high-level patient's ability to analyze complex visual information. *Source:* Reprinted from *Southern California Figure-Ground Visual Perception Test* by J Ayres with permission of Western Psychological Services, © 1978.

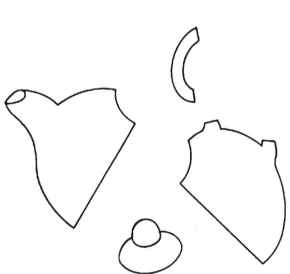

Figure 4-27 The Hooper Visual Organization Test requires synthesis of visual information in order to picture an object after viewing its parts. *Source:* Reprinted from *The Hooper Visual Organization Test* by HE Hooper with permission of Western Psychological Services, © 1983 (revised).

they may be unable to visualize the whole. For example, if a stop sign is partially occluded by vegetation, it may not be recognized.

Evaluation

The Hooper Visual Organization Test (1983) is designed to evaluate a patient's ability to mentally arrange parts of an object to form a whole (Figure 4-27). Bouska et al. (1985) describe the Hooper test as a standardized test of visual synthesis. It was chosen to help identify higher-level visual processing problems and to separate the visual perceptual from the constructional components of drawing, building, or functional tasks.

Although the Motor Free Visual Perceptual Test has been partially standardized and can be used to test some of the visual analysis and synthesis skills described above, it is currently used by speech and language pathologists at RIC. To prevent duplication, other tests were chosen for the occupational therapy perceptual battery.

Some of the standardized tests described above are occasionally used by the psychology department at RIC. Generally, psychological testing occurs later in the patient's stay and therefore is not helpful for initial planning. When an OT decides to use these standardized tests, plans must be discussed with the psychologist. Results are shared to prevent duplication of services while providing the necessary information to both disciplines.

Visual Construction

Description

Benton (1985, 175) states that "constructional praxis refers to any type of performance in which parts are put together or articulated to form a single entity or object."

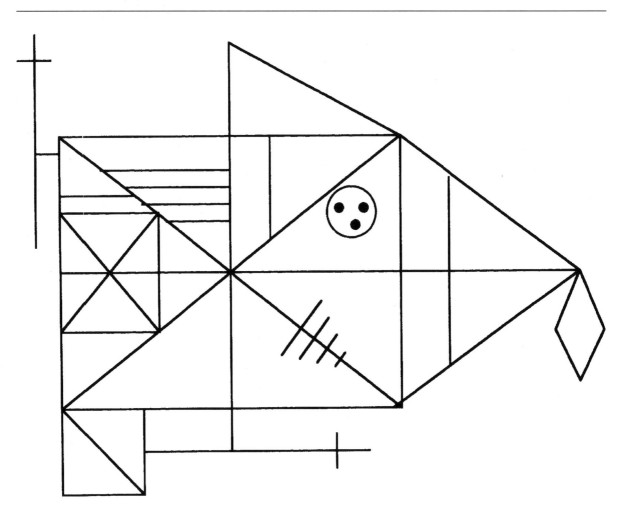

Figure 4-28 Copying the Rey Complex Figure is a difficult visual construction task. *Source:* Adapted from *Archives de Psychologie* (1944;30:206–356), Université de Genève.

It is the most complex of the visual perceptual skills, since it involves visual perception, visual analysis and synthesis, and motor output. Its complexity makes it a good indicator of function.

Functional Implications

Many functional tasks and clinic activities require putting parts together to form a whole. Dressing involves putting items of clothing in the correct position and sequence on the body. Setting the table requires that utensils, napkins, and dishes are arranged correctly. Loading a dishwasher, making a bed, tying a shoelace one-handed, organizing a cabinet, making a sandwich, and arranging flowers require visual construction skills. Craft activities frequently require complex visual construction skills. It is helpful to observe functional activities or visual construction tasks that are appropriate to the patient's interests and anticipated discharge setting.

Evaluation

Any of the functional tasks listed above can provide information about visual construction skills. Specific drawing, copying, and building tasks can also be used to observe visual construction quickly if adequate opportunities have not been present during ADL tasks. Asking a patient to draw a picture or copy a drawing is a fast, easy way to observe the patient's ability to perceive spatial relationships among the component parts and combine these parts accurately into a whole. Lezak (1983) indicates that copying tasks involve the immediate act of perception, whereas free drawing involves the more complex ability to create a visual image in one's mind and translate that image into a product. Although these tasks do involve motor responses, they are not as demanding as the motor requirements for ADL tasks. Thus, they may be more helpful in separating visual perceptual deficits from motor deficits.

Andrews et al. (1980) found that simple copying and drawing tasks were of value in screening stroke patients for perceptual deficits that were likely to impede recovery. Williams (1967) found that normal reproduction of a house, clock, and flower by stroke patients indicated a higher capacity to learn dressing skills. Baum and Hall (1981) found that copying and free drawing tasks were significant indicators of dressing ability in the head injured patient. This easily administered test is useful in gaining information about unilateral neglect, organization of a spatial task, perception of spatial relations, and visuoconstructive ability (Kaplan and Heir 1982; Oxbury et al. 1974; Benton 1985; Lezak 1983).

The RIC evaluation protocol suggests copying a house and flower for more involved patients, freehand

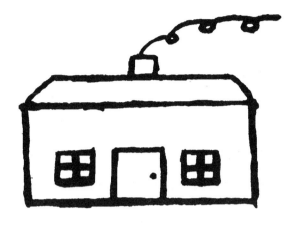

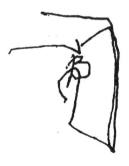

Figure 4-29 Severe unilateral visual neglect is demonstrated in this drawing.

drawing of a person and clock for more functional patients, and copying the Rey Complex Figure (Rey 1964) for the highest-level patients (Figure 4-28).

The therapist must interpret drawing performance to detect underlying deficits. Severe unilateral visual neglect may be noted by failure to include half of the object (Figure 4-29). Partial neglect may be seen when details on one half of the picture are missing or the

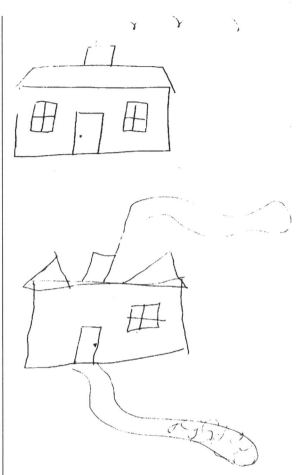

Figure 4-31 Incorrectly placed elements suggest visual spatial disturbances.

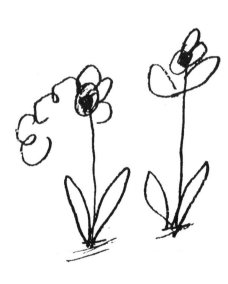

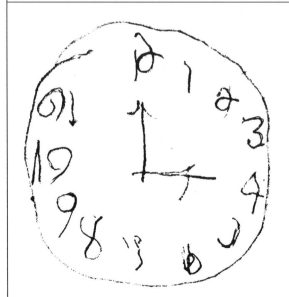

Figure 4-30 Missing details on the left half of this drawing indicate partial unilateral visual inattention.

Figure 4-32 Perseveration, suggestive of motor-planning deficits, is shown by the number "9" incorporated into subsequent numbers on the clock.

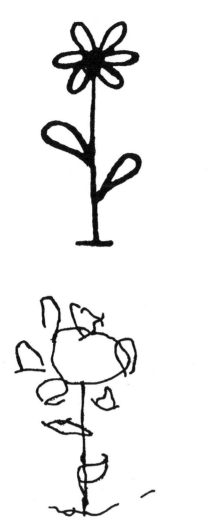

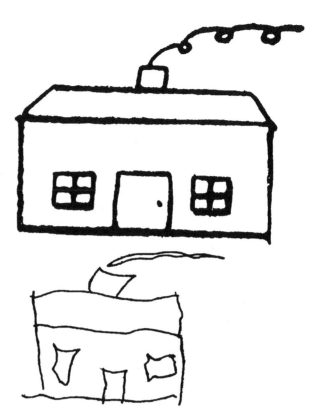

Figure 4-34 Lack of detail is characteristic of the right-side hemiplegic patient's drawing.

Figure 4-33 Rounded forms drawn by a right-side hemiplegic patient indicate possible motor-planning difficulties.

drawing is asymmetrical (Figure 4-30). Organization of spatial information may be lacking, as evidenced by a scattered approach to the task. This may indicate nonsystematic and poorly organized visual scanning processes (Moore and Warren 1990). The position of one part to another may be incorrect (i.e., rotated, unjoined, or misplaced), suggesting difficulty with spatial relations (Figure 4-31). Perseverative movements or rounded, poorly constructed shapes indicate possible motor-planning deficits (Figures 4-32 and 4-33). Lack of detail is also characteristic of the right-side hemiplegic patient's performance (Figure 4-34) (Filskov and Boll 1981).

Building and assembling tasks also involve visual construction and are often challenging for patients with brain damage. Lezak (1983) reports that these tasks involve spatial perception at both the conceptual level and the motor execution level. One must accurately perceive spatial relations among the component parts, plan the task, sustain attention to the activity, and correctly orient one's hand and the object to construct the design. Kaplan and Hier (1982) note a significant correlation between performance on a block design test and improvement in self-care scores.

The RIC occupational therapy perceptual protocol provides a nonstandardized three-, five-, and ten-block design that the patient is asked to copy (Figure 4-35). This test is intended as a screening tool and is not complex enough to detect subtle difficulties. Benton's Three-Dimensional Block Design Test is a more sophisticated and extensive evaluation consisting of a six-, an eight-, and a fifteen-block design that can be copied from either a photograph or a model (Figure 4-36). The test was standardized on four groups of 30 patients, and norms were derived from 100 adult control patients from a medical surgical service. Benton (1983e) found that age and education affected performance in the control population when the design was created from the photograph. Although construction of the design from a photograph was more difficult, scoring was not modified. Therefore, test performances from a model and from a photograph are scored in the same way. Preliminary studies of 40 patients show that the photographic presentation may be more sensitive in eliciting performance deficits in mildly impaired left-side hemiplegic patients. Either method of presentation can elicit difficulties in both right-side and left-side hemiplegic patients. Benton feels that right-side hemiplegics generally show performance problems related to language and motor-planning problems, whereas left-side hemiplegics have difficulty because of visual perceptual deficits.

Because visual construction tasks require a variety of skills, it may be difficult to determine the underlying cause of the problem. Careful observation of performance often points to a particular deficit. If reasons for the patient's difficulties seem unclear, more specific tests for motor-planning, spatial relations, visual attention, or visual analysis and synthesis deficits can be used to delineate the problem. Some therapists might argue that the lack of specificity of constructional tests is a detriment. However, the complex nature of the tasks is probably what makes them so predictive of performance in functional activities that require many of the same skills. The value of these constructive tests lies in their correlation with functional outcome (specifically dressing ability) (Brown and Hall 1981), their ease of administration, and their potential to provide information about several kinds of perceptual problems.

EVALUATIONS FOR BODY AWARENESS

Description

Body awareness is defined for the purposes of this protocol as the ability to integrate sensory information in order to appreciate tactile sensation, the relationship of body parts to the whole, and the orientation of the body in space. It is conceived as an integrated category

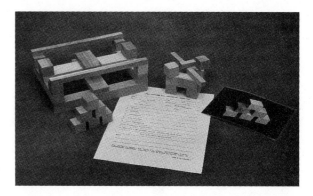

Figure 4-36 For high-level patients, the standardized Three-Dimensional Block Design Test provides challenge.

encompassing many types of sensory processing, just as visual perception involves many subskills.

Functional Implications

Therapists know that patients with poor body awareness demonstrate problems in performing mobility activities, maintaining posture during dynamic tasks such as dressing, using both sides of the body together, and planning new movements. Warren (1981) suggests a relationship between body scheme disturbances and functional skills. She states that disorders in body scheme contribute to the presence of dressing apraxia. There is less information about body awareness than about visual and cognitive processing in the neuropsychological and occupational therapy literature. From a clinician's viewpoint, however, body awareness is very important for understanding the patient's abilities and deficits in a holistic manner. OTs are interested in the interaction of mind and body in purposeful activity. Information about body awareness helps define problems that interfere with efficient performance of activity.

Evaluation

With the exception of tactile sensation and perception, most often body awareness can be evaluated through functional observations. As with other cognitive and perceptual areas, the tests listed are intended to be used only when functional observations are unclear or when treatment planning can be enhanced by gaining information about a very specialized function such as tactile discrimination. A wide range of tests is described to detect a variety of problems, but the OT must carefully select those tests that are relevant to treatment.

Since body awareness is conceptualized as an integration of various sensory and perceptual components, the screening tests and more formal tests address a variety of skills. Tactile sensation, estimation of midline,

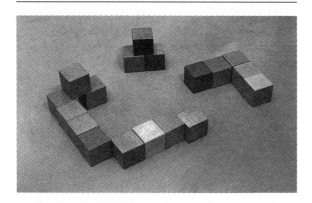

Figure 4-35 This three-dimensional visual construction task is used as a screening activity.

attention to unilateral and bilateral tactile stimulation, integration of both body sides, body visualization, and right-left discrimination tests can help identify basic problems with body awareness. More discriminative functions such as finger identification, tactile form perception, and graphesthesia can also be tested. Prior to testing discrete tactile integration functions, adequate sensation must be ascertained through formal sensory testing.

Unilateral Tactile Inattention

Description

Tactile inattention often occurs with parietal lobe dysfunction and is frequently associated with visual and auditory inattention (Lezak 1983). It is characterized by inattention to one side of the body, with the level of inattention disproportionate to the degree of sensory loss. Thus a person with mild sensory deficits may fail to attend to an arm, twisting or bumping it without concern. A patient with no sensory deficits may extinguish sensations on the affected side when competing information is presented on the sound side. It is therefore important to observe responses to double simultaneous stimulation, because a patient may learn to attend when tactile stimuli are presented to one body side but may continue to show difficulty when stimuli are presented to both body sides simultaneously. A test for bilateral integration is therefore included in this portion of the evaluation.

Functional Implications

Unilateral tactile inattention is included in this category because, clinically, failure to attend to both body sides affects many self-care tasks, including dressing, hygiene, and safety in higher-level tasks. In addition, failure to use both body sides in function despite motoric and sensory capacity to do so will affect the speed and efficiency of motor performance in all bilateral tasks. Bilateral integration deficits may be especially detrimental in activities such as sports, leisure, or work tasks.

Evaluation

Unilateral tactile inattention can be observed when patients fail to attend to the affected side for safety or hygiene. More subtle forms of inattention may be evident when patients with motor return and adequate sensation fail to use the affected limb. They may lose their grasp when attempting to carry an object and walk, or when concentrating on another aspect of the task.

Testing a patient for tactile inattention can help the therapist detect extinction of a stimulus when a competing stimulus is presented to the nonaffected side of the body. The Bilateral Simultaneous Stimulation Test is a short assessment that can be used for screening. The Face-Hand Test is a more discriminative test to be used when subtle forms of inattention are suspected of interfering with function. Both tests are supported by the literature and have norms available for scoring (Goldman 1966; Schwartz et al. 1977; Lezak 1983) (Figure 4-37). When a patient shows good motor function and the potential to use the affected limb in self-care, bilateral integration can be evaluated by observing the use of the limbs together in a bilateral task (Figure 4-38) or by using a modified version of a test described by Roach and Kephart (1966). The patient is asked to make a large circle in the air, first with one arm, then the other, and then with both arms simultaneously. When a significant discrepancy is seen during bilateral versus unilateral movement, bilateral integration deficits can be suspected (Figures 4-39 and 4-40).

Tactile Discrimination

Description

Tactile discrimination refers to the ability to process discrete tactile information in order to judge the shape, texture, size, form, location, and direction of movement

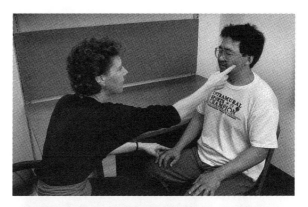

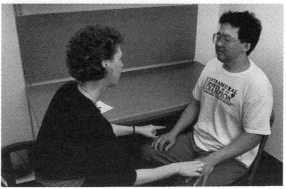

Figure 4-37 The Face-Hand Test is used to detect unilateral tactile inattention.

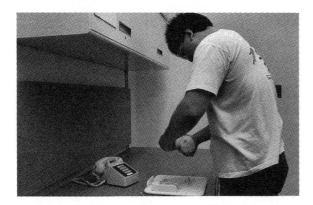

Figure 4-38 Bilateral integration can be observed through functional tasks that require the use of both sides of the body together.

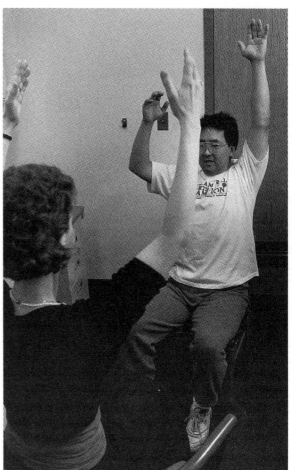

Figure 4-40 When the patient is asked to make bilateral circles, the right arm lags because of problems in sustaining the attention required to produce full motion of the right arm.

of the stimulus. It is used in manual form discrimination and graphesthesia. Benton (1983c) reports that deficits in tactile form perception are generally believed to reflect disease in the parietal lobe.

Functional Implications

Tests requiring a high degree of tactile discrimination are included in the RIC perceptual protocol because it is thought that knowledge of higher-level tactile processing can help a therapist understand the reasons for a patient's difficulty with tasks requiring fine tactile discrimination; the therapist then can evaluate whether the deficits might respond to remediation or whether compensation techniques must be taught. For example, these tests were very helpful in determining whether a blind person who recently had a stroke would be able to continue to use tactile discrimination to read Braille and explore her surroundings. Test re-

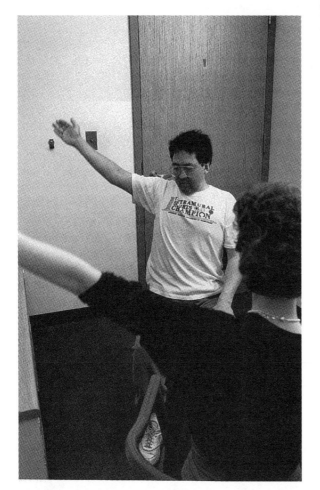

Figure 4-39 During unilateral movement, the patient shows good motor control and nearly full range of motion with the affected right arm.

sults might clarify coordination deficits that do not appear to be due to motor-control problems. If poor tactile processing is identified, visual and auditory information might be more helpful when skills are taught. If tactile discrimination is identified as a perceptual strength, manual exploration might be used to compensate for other perceptual losses.

Evaluation

Benton's Tactile Form Perception Test (1983c) measures one aspect of tactile processing. In this test the patient actively explores a raised design and forms a mental image of the shape (Figures 4-41 and 4-42). He or she responds by pointing to the perceived shape on a multiple-choice card. Difficulty on this test is associated with other tasks that measure "spatial thinking." A graphesthesia test is also included because it is thought to measure an ability different from that measured by the tactile form perception test. Graphesthesia tests the ability to recognize moving tactile spatial information given by an outside source, whereas the tactile form perception test requires that the patient actively explore a stationary item. This distinction may be important in determining whether a patient's difficulty lies more in the ability to respond to tactile information imposed by the environment or in the ability to explore his or her surroundings tactilely. The first problem may be related to tactile inattention, while the second may be caused by difficulty in spatially organizing the information to form a whole. Use of other tests to measure attention and spatial skills may help to confirm or deny such a hypothesis. If a patient has difficulty with both tests, either problem may be the root. The therapist could

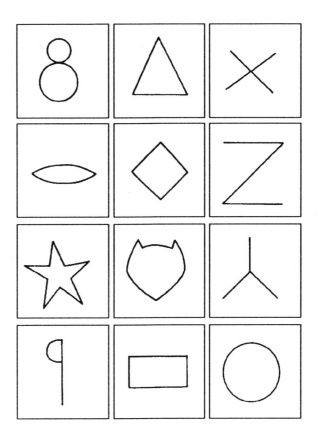

Figure 4-42 After feeling the sandpaper shapes, the patient points to the figure that was detected. *Source:* Reprinted from *Contributions to Neuropsychological Assessment: A Clinical Manual* by A Benton with permission of Oxford University Press, © 1983.

plan treatment that incorporates active tactile exploration, provides tactile input, emphasizes tactile attention, or promotes spatial awareness, depending on test performance and the suspected cause of the difficulty.

Right-Left Discrimination

Description

Impairment in right-left discrimination may be attributed to either a language deficit or a cognitive deficit (Abreu 1987). Right and left orientation involves verbal, sensory, conceptual, and visual spatial components (Abreu 1987; Benton 1985). The individual must understand the verbal labels of *right* and *left* in order to apply these labels. In addition, the person must possess an intuitive awareness of the differences between the two body sides. This involves sensory discrimination. Conceptually, the individual must use the right and left labels on his or her own body as well as on another person or within the environment. Visual spatial ability is

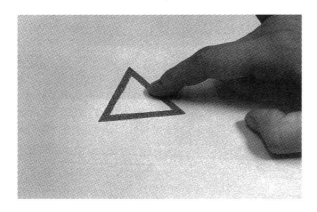

Figure 4-41 Tactile discrimination can be tested using the Tactile Form Perception Test. *Source:* Test from Contributions to Neuropsychological Assessment: A Clinical Manual by A Benton, Oxford University Press, © 1983.

brought into play when determining right and left on a confronting person or on objects in the environment. When labeling right and left on a person facing him or her, the patient must be able mentally to reverse the person to apply the appropriate term.

Functional Implications

Right-left discrimination is used during direction following and in higher-level tasks such as driving. Bouska et al. (1985) suggest that treatment should address disorders in body scheme and right-left discrimination prior to progressing to treatment for visual spatial deficits. They believe that patients need to internalize a spatial understanding of self before being able to make judgments regarding the spatial orientation of objects around them.

Evaluation

Formal tests generally are not necessary, since a patient's response to right-left directions can be observed during activities. If the therapist has failed to note this ability and feels that following these verbal directions will be important to daily activities, nonstandardized right-left questions can be used to assess the patient's understanding of these words.

Midline Orientation

Description

Midline orientation refers to a person's ability to perceive an upright, symmetrical posture. A patient who lacks midline orientation often sits tilted to one side and seems unaware of the faulty position. Motor loss may compound this problem further, but it is the patient's perception of an upright position that is being evaluated, not the motoric ability to assume it.

Functional Implications

Poor midline awareness affects all ADL tasks. Patients who cannot perceive an upright position will fall during unsupported sitting. They will be unable to align their bodies properly for functional activities, and the stable base necessary for controlled movement will be disrupted.

Evaluation

The therapist determines the patient's estimation of midline by clinical observation and not by a standardized test. Most often, the therapist will be able to judge the patient's awareness of midline through observation during functional mobility. Occasionally, a more systematic approach may be needed to separate motor deficits from perceptual deficits interfering with up-

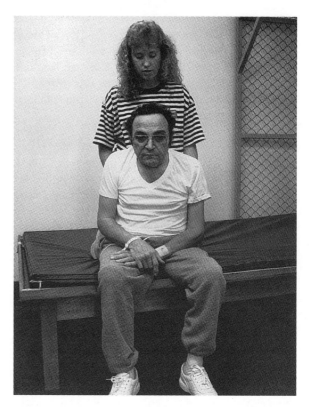

Figure 4-43 Midline orientation is evaluated by asking the patient to indicate when he has reached a "straight" or upright position.

right posture. One documented test of estimation of midline exists, the Body Center Test (Diller et al. 1974), but the test requires more time than the results warrant. Our battery therefore describes a series of nonstandardized, specific steps to use in determining a midline orientation problem (Figure 4-43).

EVALUATIONS FOR MOTOR PLANNING

Description

Motor planning is described in many ways by many authors. Various hypotheses exist about the mechanisms underlying motor-planning deficits. Some explanations of motor planning are so broad that almost any area of the brain and any type of brain dysfunction could affect motor planning. While in some senses this is true, since all aspects of sensory perception, integration, and cognition work together in a complex way to produce an effective motor response, this definition does not describe the particular deficits seen in hemiplegia—most often in right-side hemiplegics.

In adult hemiplegics with particular types of brain dysfunction, there appears to be a specific constellation of problems that can be tested. These motor-planning problems result in behavior that is qualitatively different from the behavior of hemiplegics with poor spatial relations awareness, and it is also different from the behavior of patients with general dementia. The specific motor-planning deficits of right-side hemiplegic patients are distinct from other perceptual and cognitive problems. This protocol uses test procedures designed to identify this specific deficit and its underlying causes.

Classification of Motor-Planning Deficits

The classification system proposed by Roy (1983) provides a framework consistent with the OT's interest in multisensory processing, yet it is specific enough to describe the particular problems noted in stroke patients. Roy describes two broad systems responsible for motor planning: the conceptual system and the production system.

Conceptual System. The conceptual system is used to determine the perceptual characteristics of an object and how it can be used, to understand how an action might be performed, and to visualize or rehearse the steps of a task. Language may play a part in conceptualization by giving labels to actions, objects, and their use. The conceptual aspects of a task come into play when a new action is learned and all steps must be compared with previous activities, visualized, and/or mentally rehearsed. For example, to paddle in the bow of a canoe, a person might rehearse, "Place the paddle forward, keep the paddle perpendicular, push with the top hand, rotate the torso, remove the paddle near the hip, and turn the blade slightly while returning to the starting position." The novice must visualize, verbalize, and rehearse each step. Once learned, this sequence is very natural and requires little thought unless water or wind conditions change.

Conceptualization is also required when a new tool is used to perform a familiar action (e.g., when using a nail file to turn a small screw). In this kind of task the person must analyze the demands of the activity and the characteristics of various tools. This analysis can lead the person to choose an object that has the characteristics needed to perform the job. Roy feels that patients with a deficit in conceptualization may be those with receptive language disorders.

Production System. The second system described by Roy is the production system. Within this system there is a low-level system that is able to carry out well-learned movement sequences and patterns of movement at an automatic level. Little conscious thought is required. Background tone and postural adaptations are made to promote effective movement patterns. This type of movement is probably controlled at a subcortical level. The body responds to the environment and to objects to produce the correct action with little thought. Neural feedback loops provide information about the effectiveness of an action, and adjustments take place subconsciously. Within an action sequence there are critical points when attention to the task is necessary in order to ensure the correct outcome.

For instance, if a person prepares a cup of coffee with cream and sugar in the same place and in the same manner every day, the activity becomes routine. If he or she then decides to eliminate cream for health reasons, a conscious effort must be made to alter the normal sequence of action. If the person is distracted at the critical point, cream might be added despite the best intentions. At these critical points, cortical systems come into play to modify routine movement pattern and produce purposeful, goal-directed action.

Temporal-sequential disorders are believed to be a production problem common in apraxia. Right-side hemiplegic patients are found to make bigger errors when asked to perform actions in a particular sequential order. In addition, they tend to perseverate during activity. Patients who showed perseveration during motor activities were asked to arrange pictures in order of occurrence, a task that does not require skilled motoric sequencing. Perseveration was dramatically reduced. This finding suggests that perseveration is a production problem, not a conceptual problem (Roy and Square 1985).

Roy and Square (1985) also state that problems in spatially orienting an object or a limb for use are not due to a conceptual problem but are due to a production problem. They cite research that shows that a patient usually is able to recognize an incorrect action performed by another but may have difficulty performing that action. This may be due to poor perception of his or her body in space, which causes difficulty in moving the limbs in the correct direction.

Decreased fine motor control is sometimes noted in conjunction with motor-planning deficits. This is believed to result from pure motor difficulties and is not considered a problem in sequencing or conceptualizing movement patterns (Roy and Square 1985).

Functional Implications

Motor-planning deficits affect all function. The most severe conceptual disturbances prevent the patient from using utensils or tools properly, interfere with the use of adapted equipment, and limit the patient's ability to learn new methods to compensate for hemiplegia. Whenever possible, familiar motor patterns should be used. Patients who have the potential to regain lost mo-

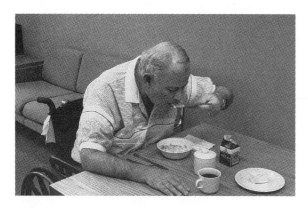

Figure 4-44 Awkward limb position, suggestive of motor-planning deficits, is noted as this patient brings cereal to his mouth.

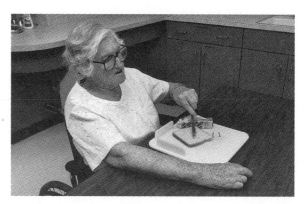

Figure 4-45 This patient with motor-planning problems is improperly orienting the knife and is using a stabbing motion when attempting to butter her bread.

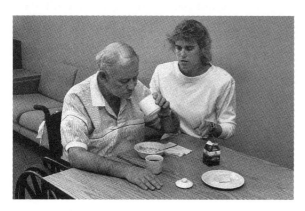

Figure 4-46 Sequencing difficulties are seen as the patient, attempting to sweeten his coffee, picks up the sugar bowl.

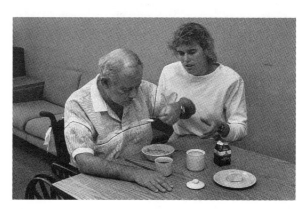

Figure 4-47 The patient then tries to eat the sugar, perseverating on actions used previously for eating.

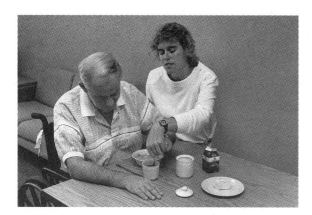

Figure 4-48 Manual guidance is required to redirect the patient's action.

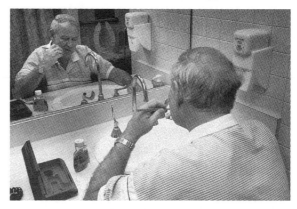

Figure 4-49 Awkward limb position is due to motor-planning deficits, which confound the patient's attempt to learn new motor patterns with his nondominant extremity.

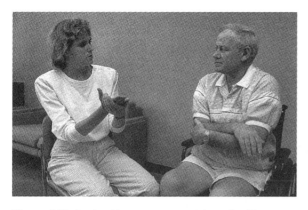

Figure 4-50 During his attempt to copy the unfamiliar motor patterns required for range-of-motion exercise, motor-planning problems are demonstrated repeatedly.

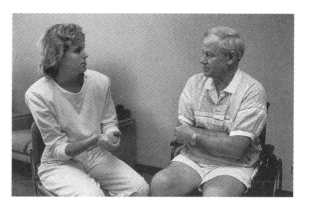

Figure 4-51 Perseveration is noted as the patient persists in assuming the previous position.

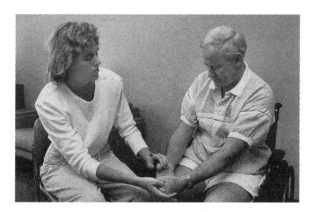

Figure 4-52 Hand-over-hand assistance is required to correct the movement.

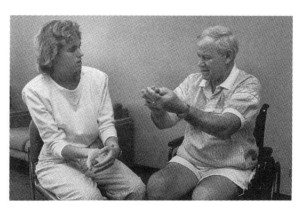

Figure 4-53 The patient substitutes gross body movements for the requested fine finger movements.

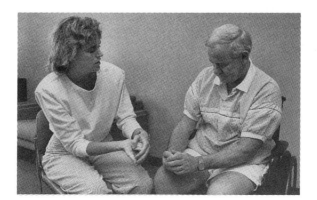

Figure 4-54 Finally, a measure of success is achieved.

tor function should be treated aggressively, since improved motor function will allow them to perform tasks by using familiar movement patterns and thus diminish the impact of motor-planning deficits.

Patients who show production problems may have a tendency to perseverate or sequence a task improperly. Since their deficits are less severe, they profit more from repetition, practice, and the opportunity to use an action in a variety of settings. For example, if a patient is learning to open a drawer, the opportunity should be given to open drawers in the clinic, in the hospital room, and at home; by practicing in many environments, generalization is more likely to occur.

Evaluation

The RIC occupational therapy cognitive perceptual evaluation provides assessments for each of the cognitive, sensory, and perceptual skills that influence motor planning. Evaluation of these skill areas allows the therapist to identify component skill deficits that affect skilled movement. In addition, suggestions are provided for evaluating conceptual and production functions holistically. The OT is in a unique position to evaluate motor-planning skills in the context of everyday activities. Functionally, the therapist can observe the patient's ability to imitate familiar gestures, such as waving "hi" or blowing on hot food. The ability to recognize the function of and use of common objects during ADL tasks frequently is impaired in patients with motor-planning deficits. Functional observations of activities requiring use of tools or utensils are therefore stressed. Finally, production problems are evaluated by noting

- improper orientation of an object (Figures 4-44 and 4-45)
- perseveration or sequencing difficulties during functional tasks (Figures 4-46, 4-47, and 4-48)
- difficulty when attempting to learn new activities such as use of the nondominant hand (Figure 4-49) or wheelchair propulsion

More structured assessments can also be made by asking the patient to copy unfamiliar movements (Figures 4-50 to 4-54). The influence of language on motor planning can be assessed first by testing the patient without providing verbal cues, then by giving cues to assist performance. The specific nature of the deficits should be documented. For example, descriptions of the presence of perseveration, the influence of verbal cues on performance, and the differences between execution of gross and fine movements will provide information useful in treatment.

Part II

Goal Writing and Treatment Planning

Chapter 5

General Considerations for Goal Writing and Treatment Planning

Goal writing and treatment planning begin when sufficient evaluation data have been gathered to form an accurate picture of the patient. Plans are based on the patient's goals, diagnosis, current medical status, previous roles, and present level of function in self-care and component skill areas. In addition, the therapist's experiences with similar patients and knowledge of expected outcomes are reflected in the objectives. Continual formal and informal re-evaluations occur during the entire treatment process, resulting in program changes. Modification of goals based on the patient's responses is essential to relevant, high-quality treatment. The skilled occupational therapist (OT) uses observation and evaluation skills to make predictions about function; however, he or she remains sensitive to changes or lack of changes that signal a need to modify the original plans.

The treatment-planning process is ongoing and involves the following steps:

1. evaluating skill deficits
2. analyzing the impact of component skill deficits on function
3. setting realistic functional and component skill goals
4. planning treatment to address mutual goals
5. implementing treatment plans
6. evaluating the effectiveness of treatment

Each step in this process is valuable. The process occurs formally when documentation is updated. It should also occur informally each time the patient is treated. Attention to the goals will help guide treatment and will ensure that the therapist recognizes when changes in the goals or plans are necessary.

EVALUATING SKILL DEFICITS

The evaluation process as described in Chapter 2 is the first step in establishing goals and planning treatment. Information about the patient's previous roles, current status, and desired outcome is gathered through observation of self-care performance, formal evaluation, discussion with the patient and significant others, chart review, and consultation with other disciplines. Observation of self-care performance provides the necessary baseline for establishing functional goals. In addition, it provides information not available from other types of evaluation (Bowman 1990) and allows the therapist to analyze how cognitive, perceptual, psychosocial, and motor-performance deficits act singly and in combination to affect function.

On the basis of observations of function, the therapist can focus the formal aspects of the evaluation on factors that significantly affect self-care performance. Formal evaluations of cognitive, perceptual, and motor status are performed as needed to clarify observations made during self-care tasks, to quantify baseline performance so that future gains can be measured, and/or to provide challenges that were not available in the chosen functional activities. When carefully selected, formal evaluations can be time-efficient and can contribute to the information pool that the therapist will use to direct treatment.

Discussion about goals, interests, and outcome expectations with the patient and family are very important to the treatment-planning process. The occupational therapy literature frequently cites the importance of family and/or patient involvement in care (Levin and Gitlin 1990; Allen et al. 1989). Whenever possible, the patient should be directly involved in goal setting. A patient may be unable to participate actively in goal setting when the cerebrovascular accident (CVA) has resulted in significant cognitive and perceptual impairments. If possible, family members should then be consulted to determine previous interests and functional skills that they perceive to be important.

Chart review can provide background information and helpful medical details, and consultation with other members of the team can offer in-depth information related to their specialties. For instance, the social worker may be able to indicate a possible discharge destination or describe the social support system available to the patient.

ANALYZING THE IMPACT OF COMPONENT SKILL DEFICITS ON FUNCTION

Through evaluation, observation, and discussion the therapist identifies a complex variety of deficits that influence performance. In many cases, the CVA patient's problem areas will be numerous. The therapist first must decide which functional areas are realistic to address and then decide which component skill deficits most affect those self-care activities. To decide which functional areas will be addressed, the therapist looks at the patient's current self-care status and goals, the goals of the family, and the types and severity of component skill deficits. Therapists often attempt to focus on too many functional activities, leading to frustration for both the OT and the patient. Instead, several key areas of performance should be prioritized.

A minimally responsive patient might work toward self-feeding and simple oral/facial hygiene, with caregiver teaching about how to perform basic self-care and physical maintenance activities. An alert but confused patient might work toward increased independence in basic self-care skills such as dressing, grooming, bathing, and toileting. Caretaker instruction would focus on clarifying when and how to assist the patient in these activities as well as how to structure higher-level tasks such as community trips. An alert patient who demonstrates little confusion might focus on complete independence in all basic self-care activities and

begin to address meal preparation, community living skills, home maintenance, leisure activities, or work skills when applicable.

Frequently the therapist will prioritize basic self-care goals during in-patient hospitalization. These basic skills can be refined and more advanced self-care abilities developed through outpatient treatment. Although general guidelines can be given for functional areas that are appropriate for patients at various levels of function, each person's unique combination of psychosocial, physical, medical, cognitive, and perceptual factors make defining a treatment focus an exercise in clinical problem solving.

Once functional areas of focus have been determined, the therapist's mission is to identify the factors that most impede function and that can respond to therapeutic intervention. Refined clinical problem-solving skills assist in this process by allowing the therapist to integrate patient observations with knowledge of stroke pathology, the manifestations of various perceptual and cognitive deficits, and an understanding of the patient's interests and sociocultural background. Complex decisions about behavior must be made. When a patient is participating minimally in therapy, for example, the OT must make an informed hypothesis about the cause. Is the patient depressed because of the catastrophic change in his or her life situation? Is a frontal lobe lesion contributing to a lack of initiative and goal-directed behavior? Is arousal or attention impaired? Do severe visual perceptual deficits interfere with the ability to comprehend and master the environment, leading to an unwillingness to attempt such a difficult process? If visual perceptual problems are interfering, which ones are most limiting? Do motor-planning problems make all performance efforts ineffective and frustrating? If so, are the problems in conceptualization or execution? Does the patient's culture reinforce dependency for disabled and elderly people? Does medication or the medical condition contribute to lethargy? On the basis of numerous observations; information from tests; chart data; and discussions with the team, patient, and family, the therapist can discard unlikely hypotheses and focus on the most likely causes of a given behavior.

It is evident that the more relevant information the therapist has, and the more systematically and thoroughly the causes of behavior are examined, the more likely it is that the probable reason or reasons for the dysfunction will be defined. Many of the behaviors observed in therapy can have multiple causes. It is important for the therapist to be aware of a wide range of possible contributing factors so that decisions about which factors to emphasize are well founded.

Having sorted through complex information and having reached a decision about a probable underlying cause, it must be determined whether that problem is amenable to occupational therapy intervention. For instance, if the primary deficit causing poor participation is lethargy due to medication and medical status, the physician can be informed of the patient's difficulties in treatment. The OT will not be able to remedy the problem, but he or she will be better able to understand the patient's lethargy. If it is believed that the primary deficit or deficits can be improved through occupational therapy treatment, goals can be established.

For example, when a patient has difficulty attending to any task for longer than several minutes, it is probable that severe attentional deficits are present. Although this patient will also have difficulty with most other cognitive and perceptual abilities, the therapist will prioritize attention, since improvements in this skill should enhance performance in other areas. For a more advanced patient who has difficulty with community-level tasks because of unilateral visual inattention, visual spatial perception deficits, difficulty with selective attention, and poor problem-solving skills, the therapist may decide that visual attention and selective attention are the primary deficits that are limiting function. When the primary deficits have been identified and the functional areas of focus have been defined, goals can be set.

SETTING REALISTIC FUNCTIONAL AND COMPONENT SKILL GOALS

Setting realistic goals is one of the biggest challenges faced by the therapist. He or she must integrate many pieces of information about the patient's physical, cognitive and perceptual deficit areas, psychosocial skills, cultural background, social supports, and previous level of function. The therapist then must analyze the patient profile based on experiences with similar patients as well as knowledge of the clinical condition. Fleming (1991) describes three levels of problem solving used by occupational therapists: procedural reasoning, interactive reasoning, and conditional reasoning. Procedural reasoning is used to define a problem, make a prognosis, and determine treatment. Interactive reasoning is used to better understand the patient as an individual. Conditional reasoning is used to understand the patient in the context of his or her experience of disability and in the social or cultural system to which he or she belongs. It is also used to imagine a possible future for the patient. Procedural reasoning and conditional reasoning are especially helpful in the goal setting process. Umphred (1983) highlights the impor-

tance of understanding a patient's pre-existing patterns of behavior when setting goals. For example, an architecture student who enjoyed sports but did not like to read probably has well developed right parietal-occipital lobes with good visual spatial ability. This type of patient would learn best by seeing and doing. If a stroke damages the patient's most developed part of the brain, learning new strategies becomes more difficult. Knowledge of previous activity preferences and cognitive strengths can help in setting realistic goals and in planning effective treatment. The therapist who can successfully integrate many factors related to the patient's present and future function will be able to establish the most realistic goals.

Functional goal setting should always be the starting point for treatment planning. The occupational therapy department at the Rehabilitation Institute of Chicago (RIC) uses the RIC-Functional Assessment Scale (RIC-FAS) to set functional goals. The RIC-FAS is designed to be compatible with the Functional Independence Measures developed by the American Congress of Rehabilitation Medicine. The RIC-FAS is a seven-point scale that considers both physical and cognitive limitations when establishing a level of assistance. The levels of assistance range from dependent (level 1), to independent (level 7). This scale is described in detail in Chapter 12. These ratings may be used to set long-term or short-term goals.

Long-term goals (LTGs) are predictive of the patient's functional status at discharge. Short-term goals (STGs) are established for two-week periods. At times the RIC-FAS goals are not specific enough to describe the expected outcome. The goals can then be tailored to meet the patient's needs. For example, a patient may be rated at a moderate assist level in upper extremity dressing, requiring moderate amounts of physical assistance as well as cuing. Because of the severity of the stroke, this person is not expected to progress to the minimal assistance level. A qualitative goal thus might be established: The patient will put on a shirt with frequent cues but without physical assistance. This goal would reflect that the amount of physical assistance has decreased, although supervision is still required. A goal might also be established for a portion of a task when completion of the entire activity is not possible for the patient. For instance, overall, a patient may require maximal assistance (level 2) to complete all of the subskills associated with grooming. The average amount of assistance required for all subskills combined is used to determine the overall rating for grooming. The patient may require maximal assistance (level 2) for oral hygiene and shaving, with moderate hand-over-hand assistance (level 3) necessary for face washing and hair combing. One LTG might be: The patient will wash the face with cues for sequencing and assistance for wringing the cloth. A person who is nearly independent in performing a task such as one-dish hot meal preparation, requiring assistance only for unpredictable events such as dropping a utensil or running out of an ingredient, would be rated independent with set up or distant supervision (level 6). The goal might be: The patient will show problem solving sufficient for independently handling unpredictable occurrences during meal preparation (level 7). Long-term goals should always clearly describe a functional end point that is relevant to the patient's anticipated discharge situation and can be measured easily by any OT evaluating the patient.

Short-term goals address components of performance related to each LTG. They may break a functional skill into smaller steps. To reach the LTG of independence with setup in feeding, a patient with motor-planning problems interfering with object use might have STGs that progress as follows. The patient will

1. require minimal assistance and frequent cues for correct utensil use.
2. require intermittent cues for correct utensil use.
3. require occasional cues for correct utensil use.

An impulsive patient currently needing minimal assistance and intermittent supervision (level 4) may have a goal of requiring distant supervision (level 3) for toileting. A component of that goal might be to demonstrate awareness of physical limitations that inhibit safety. The STGs can be stated as follows. The patient will

1. identify one or two physical deficits that affect safety in the bathroom.
2. use modified techniques to ensure safe management of clothing in the bathroom.
3. identify situations in which assistance should be requested, e.g., clothing is twisted.

In many cases, similar STGs will be appropriate for several LTGs. Problem-solving skills, for example, will be required for all basic self-care activities when a novel situation arises and for home management, meal preparation, and community-level tasks. A patient may have LTGs in each of these functional areas. Alternately, it may be helpful to write a long-term component goal for problem solving. This LTG might read: The patient will demonstrate problem-solving skills adequate to perform self-care, home management, meal preparation, and community-level skills independently

(level 7). The STGs might include the following. The patient will

1. identify at least two strategies for meeting problems encountered in basic self-care.
2. identify at least two strategies for solving problems encountered in complex daily living tasks.
3. select and implement problem-solving strategies with verbal encouragement from the therapist.
4. select and implement problem-solving strategies independently.
5. identify positive and negative outcomes resulting from a chosen plan and suggest changes that might be made in the future.
6. monitor the effectiveness of the plan during the activity and modify the approach as needed to ensure success.

Although setting long-term component skill goals may not be necessary for the experienced clinician who can easily consider a range of functional and component skills and ensure a logical progression toward independence, it may be helpful to a newer therapist to write LTGs for key component areas to ensure that they are addressed in a systematic manner.

In summary, the therapist first should address LTGs in functional areas, then LTGs for component skills when necessary to organize complex factors into a rational plan. Finally, STGs for functional and component skills should be written. The needs of the patient will be the primary factor in establishing goals, but external forces also must be considered.

Payment sources provide guidelines for goals. It is required by Medicare that

- goals reflect significant functional improvement (especially improvement that will decrease the amount of care needed by the patient)
- the desires of the patient and family are being considered
- skilled intervention is required to meet the goals
- reasonable expectations of achievement are present

The OT's role delineation within each facility also influences the types of goals that are established. For instance, at RIC, the physical therapy department orders bathing equipment and practices transfers. Its goals reflect the patient's anticipated ability to use this equipment and his or her expected level of independence in all transfers; occupational therapy's goals address all of the factors required for bathing, including the physical aspects of adjusting the water, washing and drying the body, entering and exiting the tub, and demonstrating safety in reaching or bending in a wet environment. When the OT's LTGs clearly describe the functional behaviors that must be displayed to accomplish the goal and the STGs relate directly to these LTGs, they will serve as a realistic and helpful guide for treatment. Specific suggestions for goal writing are found in Chapter 12.

PLANNING TREATMENT TO ADDRESS MUTUAL GOALS

Patients, families, and caretakers will show varying abilities and interests in participating in goal setting. The therapist should be sensitive to their level of comfort, knowledge of the disability, and willingness to become involved. For those patients, families, and caretakers who show a sophisticated level of understanding and a desire to be involved in care, the therapist should provide many opportunities for input. When caretakers clearly are unable emotionally or intellectually to assist with the process, the therapist should not be judgmental in evaluating them. It may prove useful to discuss an appropriate level of involvement with the social worker, psychologist, and/or the rest of the team.

Family members can often be valuable allies in the goal setting process. When a family is able to state clear goals for therapy and appears to base these objectives on a reasonable knowledge of the disability, the patient's previous and current interests and abilities, and a knowledge of their own resources, efforts should be made to accommodate these goals and to discuss other areas of concern as appropriate. For instance, a family of a low-functioning patient may prioritize self-feeding and bowel and bladder regulation. While the therapist may evaluate the feasibility of improving performance in other activities of daily living and should discuss findings and other possible goal areas, treatment should focus on the priorities described by the family.

When occupational therapy goals and patient or family goals are congruent, establishing an effective plan is facilitated. When a conflict occurs, the therapist must be more diplomatic and creative in planning. If the OT discovers differences between his or her goals and those of the patient or family, he or she should attempt to identify possible reasons for the conflict: Does the patient and family have adequate information about the CVA and recovery process? Are they able to recognize cognitive, behavioral, perceptual, motor, and functional deficits and adjust goals based on the realities of these limitations? Are they able to appreciate small changes in component or functional skills as acceptable

measures of progress? Are they willing to make adaptations to accommodate current limitations, or are they focused solely on regaining the previous level of function? Are their values different from the therapist's? If so, are these values influenced by socioeconomic differences, sexual role definitions, or cultural variations? When the reasons for the conflict are defined, the therapist can use education, demonstration, and discussion to address some of the barriers.

After self-evaluation to ensure objectivity and appreciation of differences in roles, cultural expectations, and values, the therapist may attempt to persuade the patient and family of his or her beliefs. Arguments can be presented about the value of the goal and its potential benefit. Education can be provided to improve awareness of the effects of CVA and the recovery process. Discussion with other stroke survivors, the physician, the social worker, the psychiatrist, or other team members can be suggested to promote understanding. The OT can work with the patient to help him or her overcome fears or problem areas that prevent engaging in a particular activity. Finally, the OT can negotiate to have the patient participate in a particular goal area in exchange for an equal amount of time spent on another interest.

Similarly, if conflicts exist between the goals of the patient and those of the family, efforts at negotiation and involvement of other team members, specifically the social worker and the psychologist, may be helpful. When the patient is competent to make decisions, his or her desires should be weighted more heavily than those of the family, but assisting them to discuss their differences and try to arrive at mutual goals will facilitate adjustment when the patient returns home. For instance, if the family desires that the patient be independent in self-care and the patient believes that the family owes him or her assistance because of the disability, conditions are right for conflict. Often, differences in goals become more evident after the patient has returned home and is entering outpatient treatment. Mutual goal setting with the patient and the family can be especially beneficial at that time.

Conflict between goal areas sometimes arises when the OT attempts to balance functional goals with component skill areas. A patient frequently is willing to focus on motor performance but resists self-care activities, preferring to "wait until my arm and leg work better" before practicing. Although reasons for this reluctance may vary from patient to patient, it is accepted that delayed participation in self-care leads to increased dependence. The OT should be assertive in promoting involvement in basic self-care when the assessment indicates that this involvement is reasonable. Therapists must remember, however, that patients may have standards different than theirs in the areas of cleanliness, the need for independence, or acceptable levels of modification. The therapist should recognize the possibility that his or her own cultural biases are preventing full appreciation of other customs (Barney 1991). The OT should be sensitive to the patient's interests while actively working to promote optimum function in the areas of dressing, grooming, eating, toileting, and bathing. Interactive reasoning skills described by Flemming (1991) can be useful in understanding the patient and modifying the approach to maximize participation.

When considering a goal for a skill that is highly influenced by interests, values, and previous roles, the therapist should be open to the patient's and family's wishes. Clearly it would be unwise to establish a meal preparation goal for a patient if the family intends to perform this task and the patient no longer desires to cook. The therapist may believe that this is a good goal for the patient and that it would give purpose and structure to the day; however, until the patient also values this activity, it should be approached cautiously. Significant unresolved discord between the therapist's and the patient's or family's goals may indicate a need for a change in therapists or discontinuation of occupational therapy. Ultimately, however, the patient and the family have the right to decide whether a particular goal should be addressed.

PLANNING TREATMENT

Treatment plans should flow naturally from the established LTGs and STGs. They should address the main limiting factors that interfere with function while simultaneously providing opportunities to practice the component skills in functional activities. As Dunn and McGourty (1989) state, "Activities that are therapeutic but that do not relate to both a Performance Area and one or more Performance Components are not considered to be occupational therapy" (p. 817). Just as clinical problem-solving abilities are required for goal setting, they are needed to plan treatment. To integrate the interests and abilities of the patient effectively with techniques that have a foundation in science and are accepted forms of occupational therapy practice requires sensitivity to the patient and a strong knowledge base.

Treatment plans are based on assumptions about the most effective way to address the causes underlying the patient's deficits. To maximize effectiveness, the therapist should consider

- how the patient responds
- the cost of time and materials

- the support a particular technique or frame of reference has received inside and outside the profession
- his or her qualification to deliver the type of treatment adequately
- whether the treatment needlessly duplicates services provided by other disciplines
- how carry-over will be supported outside the therapy session

The treatment activities must be continually modified to promote active participation, challenge, and success.

Although an initial version of the treatment plan will be documented in the patient's note, the plan should be refined continually and adjusted according to the patient's response. A written plan provides a framework by which to begin treatment and prompts the OT to consider the theoretical basis for treatment. Understanding various frames of reference is important to providing a rational base from which to make treatment decisions. These theoretical frames of reference are discussed in Chapter 6. A written plan also serves as a foundation for treatment when another therapist will be working with the patient. It must always remain flexible, however, and amenable to change based on the patient's response. Frequent reflection on the established goals helps to ensure that each therapy session addresses primary skill areas.

Consider a patient who is working toward independence in self-feeding. The evaluation indicates that the following problems interfere with feeding: decreased left-side awareness, poor selective attention, and impaired left upper extremity function. The patient currently requires moderate assistance (level 3), and the goal is independence with setup (level 5). The treatment plan could include practice with feeding (functional approach); modification of the environment to minimize distractions, and positioning of food for optimal visual awareness during mealtime (compensation); introduction of graded distractions in clinical tasks to promote selective attention (cognitive remediation); positioning of items toward the left during clinical activities (cognitive remediation); incorporation of rolling, bending, and reaching in various planes for objects on the left side during clinical activities (sensory integration); cuing for use of the left upper extremity as a passive assist during meals (compensation and functional approach); and promotion of normal movement by inhibiting tone, increasing proximal stability, and facilitating controlled movement (Bobath approach). These techniques must be prioritized and combined with activities designed to address other goal areas so that each treatment session is unique, but focused.

The therapist selects the areas that are most inhibiting function, analyzes various therapeutic activities, and chooses those that effectively address several components simultaneously at a level that is challenging but not impossible for the patient. It is clear that treatment is effective when the patient is fully engaged in the task, when goal-directed benefits can be seen after each intervention, and when improvements in function occur. More specific information about cognitive and perceptual treatment planning and implementation is given in subsequent chapters.

EVALUATING THE EFFECTIVENESS OF TREATMENT

As described above, the therapist continually must monitor the effectiveness of techniques used and adjust treatment accordingly. In addition to ongoing monitoring, periodic re-evaluation is also important. This re-evaluation generally is accomplished by observing the functional areas that have been prioritized in goals. When these goals are written clearly in functional, measurable terms, the patient's progress can be documented easily.

Generally, well-written component goals will serve as the measure of progress in the areas of cognition and perception. Occasionally, however, formal re-evaluation may be appropriate to measure progress in these component skills. Re-evaluation using formal tests may be performed when specific information about changes in cognition or perception can

- help the family or patient acknowledge progress
- help the patient understand areas that continue to require improvement
- provide information useful to the therapist, an employer, or the family when predicting the ability to resume former roles

Many of the tests described in this protocol are limited to a single version. The therapist must realize that, by using the same test as a re-evaluation, improved performance may reflect the practice effect rather than actual improvement in the underlying skill. Benton (1983a,b,c,e,f) provides two versions of most tests, which have been statistically proven to be comparable. The therapist can use one version for the initial evaluation and the other version for the re-evaluation, thereby decreasing the influence of the practice effect.

For the discharge evaluation, it is recommended that the therapist observe changes in functional performance and in the cognitive and perceptual component skills that have influenced progress. The evaluations that are described for cognition and perception generally are used to detect problems in certain component skills and are not meant primarily to measure progress. An exception would be made if research was being conducted to correlate changes in measured cognitive and perceptual skills with functional changes. The OT should measure the outcome of treatment by the functional gains that have been made and by attainment of the goals that were established. Descriptions of how improvement in various activity components led to progress in self-care skills should be clearly stated. A well-written discharge evaluation that addresses functional improvements provides documentation that helps to ensure third-party reimbursement and serves as a reference point if the patient returns for outpatient or inpatient therapy in the future.

A thorough evaluation, well-written and realistic goals, and sensitive and effective treatment ensure that occupational therapy intervention produces positive results. For some patients, the therapist's efforts may be directed primarily at caregiver instruction; for others, the patient and the therapist become partners working to solve problems that interfere with full independence.

Frames of Reference and General Principles for Cognitive and Perceptual Treatment

CONSIDERATION OF VARIOUS FRAMES OF REFERENCE

In a large occupational therapy department it is not practical or helpful to demand that all therapists use the same model of treatment. Until research provides better information about the most effective forms of treatment, the art and science of occupational therapy rely heavily on the skills of the therapist and his or her relationship with the patient. The occupational therapist (OT) must believe strongly in his or her treatment methods and the ability to produce change in the patient. Confidence in the treatment methods used helps the patient establish trust in the therapist and can positively affect the outcome of treatment. Based on the patient's needs and the therapist's skills, many treatment models can be used effectively. The therapist must carefully select a model that addresses the goals of the patient and that utilizes his or her skills. The OT can then approach the patient confidently, since he or she has a clear rationale for treatment, is certain of the ability to deliver treatment effectively, and is ready to modify the approach if the optimal outcome is not achieved.

The OT should be aware of the treatment model used when intervening in the areas of cognition and perception. A model that reflects the skills and limitations of the patient should be selected. In addition, the model should be efficient in terms of time and outcomes. To choose an effective model, it is important to be aware of some of the frames of reference and the premises that underlie each approach. The cognitive and perceptual treatment literature identifies frames of reference used specifically by occupational therapy as well as models that have been borrowed from other disciplines.

Occupational therapy literature describes various frames of reference that can be useful in treating cognitive and perceptual dysfunction. Mosey (1986), in her book *Psychosocial Components of Occupational Therapy*, describes three frames of reference. The analytical framework, which deals with intrapsychic content, is appropriate for use with psychiatric patients. The developmental frame of reference states that behavior is influenced by mastery of a previous level, that progress occurs in distinct stages, and that the environment and activity can be used to stimulate development. Neurorehabilitation theories, such as those proposed by Bobath and Rood, belong to the developmental frame of reference. The acquisitional frame of reference states that behavior is influenced by interaction with the environment, that one's skills influence feelings about oneself, that improvement in skills occurs in a quantitative manner with no specific developmental stages for an area of function, and that adaptive behavior is enhanced when the environment is appropriately designed for learning that skill. The model of human occupation and many cognitive remediation approaches belong to the acquisitional frame of reference.

Various treatment models that belong to the developmental and acquisitional frames of reference are described.

Developmental Frame of Reference

There are two neurotherapy approaches within the developmental framework: sensorimotor and sensory integration (Price 1980). The sensorimotor theorists include Brunnstrom, Rood, Kabat, and Bobath. Their treatment approaches are applicable to a broad range of disabilities and ages and emphasize the effect of sensory input on motor output. Higher cortical processes are not emphasized. Sensory integration was developed specifically for the evaluation and treatment of learning-disabled children. Currently there are no evaluation methods suitable for measuring sensory integrative dysfunction in neurologically impaired adults.

Sensorimotor Approach

In treating the cognitively or perceptually impaired stroke patient, sensorimotor techniques can be used. They are beneficial for restoring more normal motor function. This allows more active exploration and interaction with the environment, thus promoting improved cognitive and perceptual skills. The importance of controlled sensory input to promote optimal motor output is emphasized. Selected sensory input logically assists in fostering better body awareness, including awareness of midline, awareness of the affected body side, and tactile discrimination. It is believed that improved awareness of one's body in space is a prerequisite to understanding the relationships of objects to oneself or of objects to each other. Improved body awareness, therefore, theoretically could assist in developing visual spatial skills. Although it is not stressed in this approach, vestibular stimulation occurs through movement when the patient assumes various developmental positions. Vestibular stimulation is thought to enhance many cognitive and perceptual processes because of the numerous connections of this system with other areas of the brain (Moore and Warren 1990).

Sensory Integrative Approach

Price (1980) notes the importance of sensory input in normalizing body concept and movement in stroke patients. She believes that sensory integrative theory may also prove valuable in remedying the confusion seen in the elderly after surgery, immobilization, and confinement. She believes that therapists using the sensory integrative approach with adults should have refined observational skills to describe problem areas accurately, develop specific techniques that are effective with adults, and have formal training in sensory integrative theory. Ottenbacher (1982) cautions that there are no well-designed studies that evaluate the effectiveness of sensory integrative treatment with geriatric or CVA patients.

Acquisitional Frame of Reference

Many examples of acquisitional models are found in the literature. They include skill training approaches, perceptual motor training and perceptual motor therapy, the functional approach, and the human occupation approach. While having different names and different features, all of the acquisitional models emphasize training particular skills. Some of the models are more cortical, while others address underlying neurological systems. This distinction is important when the OT is choosing an approach for a particular patient. If neurological reports and results of tests lead the therapist to believe that the patient's problems are more cortical in nature, emphasis might be on using educational strategies and a cognitive remediation approach in combination with functional activities. If damage to underlying neural mechanisms is suspected, approaches designed to provide controlled sensory stimulation and mild vestibular stimulation might be more appropriate.

Skill Training Approaches

The transfer-of-training approach described by Zoltan et al. (1986) asserts that practice of a component skill such as visual-spatial awareness will result in carry-over to functional tasks. Therapists who employ table-top activities, spatial tasks such as copying peg designs, or visual-perceptual computer programs are using this approach. At the Rehabilitation Institute of Chicago (RIC), this type of treatment is used very cautiously because it is often meaningless to the patient. Occasionally, paper-and-pencil tasks, scanning activities, computer activities, or puzzles are used when they relate to previous interests and when the patient is able to understand the rationale for their use.

Abreu and Toglia (1987) describe a model of cognitive rehabilitation that emphasizes teaching the patient to handle increasing amounts of data by developing strategies to organize and structure the information. Treatment is graded to increase gradually the demands on information processing. They identify three phases of treatment that correspond to the three functional brain units described by Luria (1973). Treatment phase one addresses deficits in functional unit one, which regulates wakefulness and responsiveness to stimuli. Treatment at this level stresses automatic tasks that require little processing and reinforce attention to the environment. Phase two focuses on deficits in analyzing, coding, and storing information. Activities are chosen that require moderate processing in order to discriminate, organize, and manipulate environmental information. Phase three focuses on treatment for deficits resulting from damage to the third functional unit described by Luria. At this level, treatment addresses concentration, organization of thoughts, and analysis of problems during complex activities.

Abreu and Toglia advocate analyzing the patient's level of function. On the basis of presentation, the therapist may

- teach the patient strategies to enhance performance
- use the physical, social, and cultural environment to increase or decrease cognitive demands according to the patient's abilities
- provide proper positioning or movement to enhance performance

Their philosophy is easily applied to treatment of a patient who has had a cerebrovascular accident (CVA), and provides a rationale for using various types of activities according to the site of lesion and the patient's clinical presentation.

When carefully considered and selected based on the patient's interests and needs, transfer of training activities may prove useful. Toglia (1991) offers many suggestions for enhancing carry-over and grading cognitive activities. She advocates carefully analyzing a task, grading components, practicing these components in many environments, enhancing patient awareness of problems, providing processing strategies, and relating new information to more familiar concepts. Patients who are very concrete and show severely impaired cognitive skills may be able to participate only in near transfer tasks, in which only one or two characteristics of the task are changed. Patients at this level benefit from repetition of the same task, in the same way, in the same environment.

Intermediate transfer occurs when the patient is able to successfully recognize the similarities between tasks when up to six surface task characteristics, such as color, shape, size, or position in space, are changed. Patients at this level may benefit from introducing slight changes in the task. The therapist can then help the patient understand how the new task is like the former activity.

Far transfer occurs when the task is different from the original activity; however, underlying principles remain the same. The therapist can help a patient at this level by exposing him or her to a variety of activities

that require a particular strategy. The patient can be assisted to understand the similarities and can be cued to use the relevant strategy.

Very far transfer occurs when generalization occurs to everyday tasks. Often this level of transfer is not evident in a therapy setting, but affects the patient's ability to function independently. While carefully selecting and grading treatment activities to emphasize certain strategies, patients are encouraged to anticipate and detect errors. The goal is gradual reduction of the therapist's cues and reliance on self-cuing. Toglia (1991) acknowledges that this approach would probably not be appropriate for patients with significant cognitive or language impairments.

The transfer-of-training approach is used in the cognitive remediation/retraining procedures reported by Diller and Gordon (1981). Remediation and retraining are procedures that address the skills necessary for problem solving and performance of familiar or advanced activities. Diller and Gordon describe techniques such as behavior modification, verbal and nonverbal cuing, use of mnemonic devices, and visual scanning training.

Soderback and Normell (1986) describe a transfer-of-training approach that they call "intellectual function training." Their program consists of eight card games plus 900 pages of training materials arranged in the following six sections: visual perception, spatial ability, verbal ability, numerical ability, memory, and logic. The activities are intended to be appropriate to occupational therapy intervention and relevant to everyday life. The therapist's role in training is to offer encouragement and provide strategies to enhance performance. Repetition of similar activities is recommended until the strategies are incorporated spontaneously.

Soderback (1988a) found that this training was more beneficial than the "rehabilitation approach," a more activity-based program, in improving cognitive and perceptual skills as measured by paper-and-pencil tests; but transfer of these skills to functional tasks was not optimal. She found that patients trained in functional tasks, however, were able to transfer their learning to theoretical test situations. She advises combining intellectual functional training with functional skill remediation and recommends further study of the carry-over of abstract learning activities to function.

The *Cognitive Rehabilitation Workbook*, by Doughtery and Radomski (1987), is a collection of training materials available to OTs. It contains training units to address practical skills such as computations; checkbook management; time management; meal planning; giving directions; and using telephones, calendars, and newspapers. The intent of these activities is to help the patient learn specific skills as well as more general work behaviors.

Perceptual Motor Training and Perceptual Motor Therapy

Price (1980) describes perceptual motor training as a direct form of remediation. Training exercises based on educational principles are provided to overcome perceptual deficits. Price feels that this classroom approach to treatment is best provided by educators, not therapists. She also describes perceptual motor therapy, which uses sensory input to enhance perception and motor output. Tactile, vibratory, and proprioceptive input is provided, while vestibular stimulation occurs through motor activity. This form of treatment is often applied in conjunction with sensorimotor therapy and may be useful in the treatment of adults.

Carr and Shepherd (1987, 1989) are physical therapists who use a learning approach to retraining motor skills. They believe in analyzing movement to detect deficits that interfere with function, repetitive practice of the impaired motions, helping the patient analyze movement, and providing verbal input or feedback to facilitate learning. Each motion that is practiced is then used within a functional activity to enhance carry-over. Although they emphasize motor function, their techniques can be used during motor re-education activities to enhance analytical skills, body awareness, memory, and motor-planning abilities in the more alert CVA patient.

Functional Approach

The functional approach described by Zoltan et al. (1986) also belongs to the acquisitional frame of reference, since it emphasizes quantitative improvement of specific functional skills. This model stresses repetition, compensation, and practice in a particular skill area. Although it does not address the underlying cause of dysfunction, it is practical and offers immediate benefit to the patient, whose emotional status and level of independence improve as functional gains are made. In a study of 67 CVA patients, 19 of whom were assigned to the "intellectual housework training" group, Soderback (1988b) found that this method was successful for improving verbal, numerical, praxis, memory, and logical functions. The treatment consisted of maintaining attention, locating objects, reading recipes, following verbal directions, using utensils, estimating amounts of ingredients, remembering ingredients, and simultaneously attending to two courses while participating in meal preparation activities. The benefits of using functional activities is further described later in this chapter.

Human Occupation Approach

The Model of Human Occupation is another model that belongs to the acquisitional frame of reference. This model, described in Chapter 3, is based on the belief that the human functions as an open system. There are several assumptions about this system:

- that it changes according to interaction with the environment
- that what one does influences what one becomes
- that, as an open system, a person interacts with the environment through a cycle consisting of four phases

These phases are

1. intake: bringing in information or energy from the environment
2. throughput: taking information and energy and making it part of oneself
3. output: acting on the environment to produce change
4. feedback: receiving information about one's actions

As an open system, humans have a desire to explore and master their environment. This is accomplished through the volitional subsystem, which motivates us to act; the habituation subsystem, which helps us organize our behavior into routines; and the performance subsystem, which contains the basic musculoskeletal and neurological skills needed to act (Kielhofner and Burke 1985).

This model has not been widely applied to adults with neurological deficits, and its evaluation tools rely heavily on verbal interview techniques, which may not be appropriate for many stroke patients. The concepts of the volitional, habituation, and performance subsystems can be useful in ensuring that all relevant aspects of care are addressed. Many CVA patients are severely involved at the performance level, and a great deal of the inpatient rehabilitation stay is devoted to remedying these deficits. A skilled and effective therapist must move beyond the skill-building level to optimize performance at the habituation and volitional levels as well.

Influencing habits is important to improvement in basic and complex self-care tasks. Techniques for self-management must become routine; otherwise, the patient will experience ongoing frustration about the amount of effort that is required to perform previously automatic tasks. When the OT can encourage the patient to continue his or her efforts through the frustrating period of relearning old habits, there is a greater likelihood of ongoing carry-over of skills. Often, mastery of a skill is not accomplished during the inpatient stay, and the assistance of the family, home health therapists, and/or outpatient therapists may be needed to provide encouragement and training to ensure that techniques become habitual.

The volitional subsystem is also important in treating an adult who has had a stroke. Again, the patient may easily lose motivation as difficulty is encountered with previously routine activities. The desire to explore and master the environment may be limited by the perceptual and cognitive deficits now experienced. The self-concept that has been formed during a lifetime may be changed significantly as alterations in previously meaningful roles and relationships are faced. The effective therapist must work to enhance the patient's sense of accomplishment and assist in assuming meaningful roles while recognizing the limitations that affect performance.

Examples of Patient Treatment Using Various Models

Each of these models of treatment may be effective if used in a thoughtful way to address a specific patient need. For instance, a patient who has physical deficits but is alert, is oriented, and is registering most sensory information correctly may respond well to the motor-relearning approach of Carr and Shepherd (1987, 1989). The patient is asked to concentrate on movement patterns, attend to ineffective characteristics, remember correct behaviors, and eventually use problem-solving skills to analyze his or her own movement. Although the emphasis is on motor performance, many cognitive skills are also being trained.

For a patient who has been a visual learner and enjoys academic activities, paper-and-pencil tasks might be appropriate if the activity is carefully chosen to address functional areas that will be used in daily life. For example, computations and checkbook management will be meaningful to a patient who has taken pride in directing home finances, but they would be inappropriate for a person who has no interest in this area and is able to delegate the task to someone else.

More abstract transfer-of-training activities such as pegboards and puzzles generally are not useful when presented to the patient at a table top. If used, the patient's responses must be carefully monitored, their purpose explained thoroughly to both the patient and the family, and the activity should be combined with movement to promote better integration of the information.

Paper-and-pencil tasks or perceptual training activities can be used to teach strategies such as systematic scanning, carefully checking one's work, or the use of mnemonic devices. These strategies should also be called upon in activities that integrate the senses in a more complex way. For instance, when academic activities are used to teach a skill, the patient should then be challenged to use the technique in a relevant self-care task.

Patients who demonstrate difficulty with basic sensory registration and integration should be provided with activities that use a sensory integrative framework or a perceptual motor therapy approach. The therapist should select tasks that provide controlled multisensory stimulation. Movement and tactile exploration will be incorporated to maximize learning and assist in integration of information.

The functional approach should be a prominent part of each patient's treatment plan. It can be combined with other techniques to facilitate carry-over and generalization to activities of daily living (ADL). In some cases, functional activities can be used alone when a patient will have a very short stay, when he or she is opposed to clinic activities, or when he or she is unable to understand their purpose. The functional approach allows the therapist to provide graded sensory stimulation, purposeful movement, and opportunities for cognitive skill development in a concrete, relevant manner.

The Model of Human Occupation or other occupational behavior frames of reference describe the essential elements of occupational therapy practice. They can be used as an overall philosophy into which more specific skill training fits. While focusing on sensory registration, integration, or higher-level thought processes, the therapist must ensure that treatment is relevant to the patient's goals, that the previous life style is considered, that the patient's belief in self is enhanced, and that he or she is helped to form habits or skills that can facilitate performance.

GENERAL APPROACHES TO TREATMENT

Understanding Neurological Function

The nervous system is very complex. To treat disorders effectively, the therapist must have an understanding of brain functions, neural plasticity, and the interaction of various neural systems. Although a thorough description of the neurology underlying various pathologies is beyond the scope of this book, principles to consider when planning treatment are discussed.

Location of Lesion and Common Symptoms

Knowledge of the location of the patient's stroke and the usual problems that accompany lesions in a particular location can help the therapist select relevant evaluations and predict functional difficulty.

Thrombosis and embolism are frequent causes of stroke. By restricting blood supply to a particular part of the brain through narrowing of the vessel or blockage, damage in a specific location occurs. Hemorrhages in the brain also cause strokes; however, the damage is more diffuse because of the formation of clots and the pressure exerted on adjacent brain tissue. Lacunar infarcts, which are small cerebral lesions, result in motor or sensory disturbances without overt cognitive or perceptual changes (Miller 1983). Patients with this type of stroke are able to participate fully in goal setting and problem solving.

Occlusion of major arteries in the brain results in predictable symptoms. Occlusion of the middle cerebral artery results in contralateral hemiplegia, hemisensory loss, and hemianopia. In addition, dominant hemisphere lesions are accompanied by expressive and/or receptive aphasia and apraxia, while nondominant hemisphere lesions result in visual spatial deficits, impaired body awareness, and visual construction deficits (Easton 1981). Since 85% of strokes are due to thrombotic or embolic occlusion of the middle cerebral artery (Roth 1988), these symptoms frequently are evident.

General symptoms of anterior cerebral artery occlusion include frontal lobe signs such as reduced behavioral control, decreased arousal and attention, contralateral hemiplegia, and mild hemisensory loss. The posterior cerebral artery lesions result in contralateral hemiplegia, hemianesthesia, and homonymous hemianopia. Aphasia results from a dominant hemisphere lesion and visual spatial deficits from a nondominant hemisphere lesion (Chusid 1973). Lesions of the internal carotid artery result in a combination of problems associated with anterior, middle, and posterior cerebral artery occlusion. Occlusion of the vertebrobasilar artery results in cranial nerve palsy and unilateral or bilateral motor, sensory, or cerebellar signs, depending on where the occlusion occurs (Easton 1991).

Beyond understanding the symptoms of particular lesions, several general principles of neurology are important to appropriate treatment planning. An understanding of the "hard wiring" and "soft wiring" of the central nervous system, general knowledge of brain plasticity, and an understanding of brain organization are helpful in determining which treatment approaches may best be used. These concepts of brain function are very involved and are best understood by those who study them intensely. In this chapter the information is discussed from a clinician's perspective. The reader should be aware that the material has been simplified to facilitate practical application.

Hard-Wired and Soft-Wired Systems

Farber and Moore (1990) discuss hard-wired and soft-wired components of the nervous system. The hard-wired system is determined through genetics and is the neurological framework that allows us to develop skills. This system programs reflexive behaviors that enable us to survive and begin to explore our world. Hard-wired systems are older phylogenetically and ontogenetically and mature earlier than do soft-wired systems. They are relatively resistant to damage in the adult, yet, once damaged, they are difficult to influence through rehabilitation techniques. According to Moore and Warren (1990), examples of behaviors mediated through hard-wired systems include the need for love and nurturance, the propensity to fight when necessary to defend oneself or one's family, the drive to reproduce, the drive to be upright and move, the need to learn, and the need to explore the environment. Balance responses and gross movement patterns are hard-wired, as are systems that allow humans to anticipate stimuli and prepare the body to respond efficiently to the environment. This subconscious use of preprogrammed patterns of movement allows us to concentrate on learning and exploring rather than on the motor aspects of a task. Humans also possess extensive hard wiring that promotes learning through sensory channels. This system is efficient, allowing learning to occur more quickly than through the motor system.

The soft-wired system is newer, is more flexible, and is modified by learning. This system develops through experience. It is more vulnerable to insult and deteriorates with age; however, it is also responsive to therapeutic intervention. Soft wiring allows us to learn fine coordination, speech, and various cognitive processes. Both the hard-wired and soft-wired systems are necessary for integrated human behavior (Moore and Warren 1990).

The concepts of hard and soft wiring suggest several implications for therapy. Treatment is more successful when it addresses learned behaviors rather than deficits in primary survival systems. Patients who have lost very basic programmed reflexes and behaviors have less potential for improvement than those who have lost learned patterns. Consequently, skills such as balance and basic sensory awareness may have less potential for improvement than learned skills such as planning a meal. Experience with CVA patients confirms this idea. Patients who show extensive sensory loss usually do not regain it, and those who show marked disturbances in arousal and exploratory behavior generally have less potential for independence. In contrast, patients with moderate motor loss frequently can regain fine control when they are able to use learning strategies to assist in reprogramming movement. Those with perceptual motor problems can be taught compensation techniques to improve performance. When very basic systems are disturbed, treatment goals are set at a lower level; when higher cortical processes are affected but lower skills are preserved, goals can be set at a higher level.

Neural Plasticity

Another important concept that can help guide treatment is neural plasticity. It is known that learning prompts changes in the nervous system throughout life and that an enriched and stimulating environment can help to maintain or improve mental capabilities in adults as well as children. When injured, the adult nervous system can improve (Bach-y-Rita 1980). One theory is that when a lesion occurs in one area, other multifunctional areas of that hemisphere may be able to take over some of its jobs. Certain areas of the brain are more general in their functions, especially the association areas of the cortex. Here, another pathway may become active to substitute for a lost function. Women and left-handed people have more generalized brain pathways; therefore, they are more likely to be able to substitute for injured areas following brain damage. There also is evidence that neurons cross over to specific areas in the opposite hemisphere when a defined area on one side of the brain is damaged (Moore and Warren 1990). Another factor contributing to brain plasticity is the ability of axons and dendrites to grow and develop new connections within the brain. Factors that can influence these responses include individual motivation, age, sex, handedness, area of the lesion, intelligence, and participation in structured treatment (Moore and Warren 1990). The fact that regeneration of damaged areas can occur lends support to the value of well-planned therapeutic intervention designed to help the brain reorganize information in a new, meaningful way. In determining treatment goals, the factors listed above must be kept in mind, since, if all other factors were equal, a motivated young woman would have more potential than a nonmotivated older man.

Functional Brain Units

Also important to planning treatment is an understanding of the general functional units of the brain. Luria's work (1973) helps to clarify brain organization. He describes three functional units (Figure 6-1). Unit one consists of the reticular formation, midbrain, thalamus, hypothalamus, uncus, and the fibers that connect it to the medial zones of the cortex. It is responsible for waking, attending to relevant stimuli, and selective at-

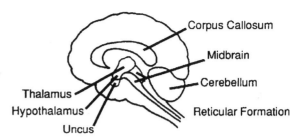

First Functional Unit

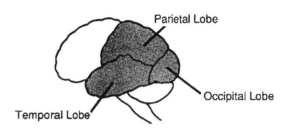

Second Functional Unit

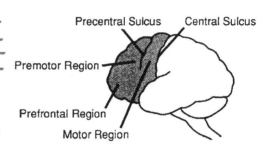

Third Functional Unit

Figure 6-1 Three functional brain units as described by Luria. *Source:* Redrawn with permission from *Scientific American* (1970;222(3):67), Copyright © 1970, Scientific American. Unit one consists of the reticular formation, midbrain, thalamus, hypothalamus, uncus, and the fibers that connect it to the medial zones of the cortex. Unit two contains the parietal, temporal, and occipital lobes. Unit three consists of the frontal lobe.

tention. Unit two contains the parietal, temporal, and occipital lobes. It is responsible for receiving, analyzing, and storing information. Unit three is formed by the frontal lobe and is concerned with programming, regulating, and verifying information.

These functional units do not correspond rigidly to the arterial blood flow within the brain. For example, the anterior cerebral artery supplies much of the frontal lobe (unit three); however, it also supplies a portion of the basal ganglia and the internal capsule (unit one) (Chusid 1973). The middle cerebral artery, often damaged in thrombotic or embolic strokes, supplies the thalamus, basal ganglia (unit one), the parietal lobe and the temporal lobe (unit two), and a portion of the frontal lobe (unit three). Symptoms vary depending on where the obstruction of the middle cerebral artery occurs. The therapist must be aware of the location of the lesion in order to predict the types of symptoms that might be expected. Lesions that affect the deepest, oldest areas of the brain are likely to produce unit one symptoms; lesions in the parietal, temporal, and occipital lobes produce unit two symptoms; and lesions in the frontal lobe produce unit three symptoms. Often a lesion will affect function in several levels; thus a combination of deficits will be noted.

First Functional Brain Unit. The first functional unit is nonspecific in nature; that is, it affects all sensory and motor systems equally. It is responsible for maintaining appropriate levels of cortical tone, allowing us to interact effectively in various situations. Three factors, internal metabolic processes, inflow of information, and influences from the medial aspect of the cortex, can increase its responsiveness.

Internal metabolic processes connected with respiration, digestion, food seeking, or sexual activity can influence arousal and attention. When hunger occurs, a person may show increased arousal in order to meet that need; conversely, the need may be inhibited to allow focus on a higher-level task relevant to the person. Following a meal, arousal may decrease to allow more effective digestion.

Information coming from the environment can also stimulate the first brain unit. A tonic, or background, state of arousal is mediated through lower levels of the reticular formation and is responsive to general sensory stimulation. Novel information elicits the orienting response, which provides increased levels of alertness. Increased attention allows a person to attend to, investigate, and compare events to previous experiences so that, if necessary, he or she can respond to changes in the environment. This form of activation occurs primarily in the thalamus and limbic system and is related to memory for the comparison of a current to a past event. When information is no longer new or novel, this system does not respond. If the person has decided to act on the information, the cortex will activate the first functional brain unit.

Signals sent from the medial aspect of the cortex represent the third type of stimulation that influences the arousal centers in the brain. The cortex sends information about goals, plans, and social intentions to the reticular formation, which in turn activates the correct amount of arousal. In this way, a person can be relaxed when intending to rock a child to sleep or alert when driving in a snowstorm.

Damage to this area of the brain can result in a general decrease in tone, slowness, disorientation, and a tendency toward an akinetic state. In addition, selective thinking is lost, leading to confabulation. Memory is impaired in all modalities equally because of the inability to screen irrelevant information. The brain is bombarded with irrelevant information that inhibits established memory traces.

It is evident that an understanding of this brain unit and its deficits can help in treating patients with low levels of arousal and attention. For instance, eliminating distractions may allow some information to be stored and retrieved from memory. Understanding that physiological processes such as hunger may improve arousal during feeding can help the therapist justify the value of basic self-care activities to himself or herself, the family, and other team members. The OT can interpret whether primitive behavior or inappropriate sexual conduct is a failure of this brain area to inhibit reflexive actions. This knowledge will help the OT understand the patient and teach techniques to modify the behavior. The therapist will be aware that a patient may respond momentarily to novel stimuli in the environment, but unless that stimulation has relevance, attention will not be maintained. Therefore, the importance of meaningful activity for low-functioning patients is heightened, since arousal will not be sustained unless the patient is involved enough to form basic plans or intentions. At times the patient's plans and intentions may be directed at avoiding the therapist's activities. In these cases, increased arousal will be seen, but it may be counterproductive as the patient becomes agitated. The therapist should seek to find activities that arouse the patient and allow him or her to remain involved through purposeful activity.

Second Functional Brain Unit. The second functional unit is concerned with receiving, storing, and interpreting sensory information. Luria (1973) describes three levels within this functional unit. The lowest level (primary level) is concerned with receiving and sending impulses, the secondary level is concerned with integrating and programming information, and the tertiary level is concerned with complex mental activity. The primary level of functional unit two is concerned with gathering specific sensory information and analyzing it. This occurs in the projection areas corresponding to each sensory modality. The parietal lobe gathers tactile kinesthetic information, the temporal lobe gathers auditory information, and the occipital lobe gathers visual information. The secondary level consists of the projection association area, where synthesis and coding of sensory information occur. The tertiary level is responsible for integrating information in a uniquely human way. This level of the brain is able to integrate several types of sensory input because it contains multimodal neurons that are able to respond to more than one kind of stimulus. It is capable of responding to general features of a situation and of spatially organizing discrete impulses to synthesize a whole. The coding and organizing of sensory information also allow us to remember experiences. This process allows us to give meaning to concrete sensory experiences by using abstract thought. A child uses sensory experiences to develop cognitive skills, but an adult categorizes sensory experiences into logical, cognitive schemes that provide meaning to experience. Thus, the higher levels of processing become dominant over the lower levels of sensory processing in the adult.

Lesions in this area of the brain result in impaired sensory processing related to the specific area of damage. For instance, lesions in the primary zone result in inability to receive sensory information, lesions in level two result in incorrect coding of information, and lesions in level three interfere with integration of sensory information. Walker (1989) states that within the visual system, lesions in level one result in visual field deficits; lesions in level two cause visual agnosias, reduced figure-ground perception, and decreased spatial awareness; and lesions in the right hemisphere at level three lead to unilateral spatial neglect and poor visual construction skills. Because the tertiary level of processing is dominant in adults and controls lower levels, it can compensate to some extent for lesions in the secondary zones of the adult brain (Luria 1973).

Third Functional Brain Unit. The third brain unit, devoted to programming, regulating, and verifying information, also consists of three divisions. The primary area is the motor cortex, which is an efferent system controlling movement. The secondary region is the premotor cortex, which helps to organize patterns of movement. The tertiary region is found in the prefrontal area and regulates behavior. Connections from this area are made throughout the cortex and lower levels of the brain, including the reticular formation, where it is able to facilitate and inhibit responses. Its far-reaching neural connections and its relationship with speech make it a powerful regulator of behavior. When a person engages in mental dialogue, he or she is using the frontal lobe.

Damage to this area results in a decreased ability to inhibit orienting responses to irrelevant information; thus the patient appears impulsive and stimulus-bound,

responding to any distraction that occurs. When in a nondistracting environment, however, the person with damage to this area may be able to retain information and delay a response.

A therapist who is aware of damage to this area of the brain would begin treatment in a quiet environment, gradually increasing the stimuli and teaching strategies to inhibit impulsive behavior. He or she might use sensory stimulation to activate areas in the intact second brain unit with the hope of influencing organization in the third. Cues and environmental structure may greatly improve function, therefore making caretaker teaching very important.

Some pertinent information about brain function and general treatments techniques have been presented. To enhance understanding, treatments for various cognitive and perceptual deficits are also described separately; however, the therapist must be aware of how they work together. In planning treatment, the OT should consider each deficit area and its relationship to others so that activities can address several component skills simultaneously.

Because CVA patients can present a complex array of problems, a therapist often will be confronted with challenging situations. He or she should be willing to seek assistance, use resources, or refer a patient to another therapist when his or her abilities do not match the needs of the patient. Therapists working with CVA patients must be willing to upgrade their skills continually and to remain aware of research in neurology that has an impact on treatment.

Using Functional Activities

One of the greatest strengths of occupational therapy treatment lies in the use of functional activities. Through functional activity, the OT provides treatment that is relevant to the patient and the family, valued by reimbursers, and effective in promoting independence. Furthermore, meaningful functional activities promote repetition, maintain interest, and require selective inhibition—factors that contribute to remediation of deficits following a stroke (Bach-y-Rita 1981). When the therapist is able to analyze the components of an activity and relate various treatment principles to an ADL session, he or she can enhance effectiveness and creatively use the skills of the profession. Too often, therapists become disenchanted with ADL tasks, preferring to focus on more glamorous neuromuscular, cognitive, or perceptual treatment techniques that are currently in vogue. Unfortunately, therapists frequently learn these techniques in a very skill-specific manner and do not learn to apply them to functional activities. The therapist is then faced with the difficult challenge of developing his or her own methods of incorporating the principles into ADL skills. Often the transition to function is not made and dynamic treatment is used in the clinic to address component skills, while ADL training becomes repetitive and routine. ADL training may become very technique-oriented without attention to the interaction of components. By combining specific cognitive or perceptual treatment techniques with self-care activities, the activities can be both more effective for the patient and more stimulating to the therapist.

Occasionally a patient is reluctant to resume functional activities. These tasks may be threatening, since they highlight the extent of the patient's dysfunction. Tasks that formerly were considered simple are now difficult and may be very damaging to self-image. The patient frequently refuses to participate in self-care and requests that a nurse dress him or her since "that is what they are paid to do." Often the therapist can attain the patient's confidence gradually and elicit participation by initially helping with a large part of the task, asking him or her to perform only those portions that can be completed successfully. As confidence builds, more active participation can be requested until an optimal level is achieved. If the patient's resistance to self-care is strong, the therapist may need to begin with a more component-oriented treatment program, perhaps focusing on motor skills that will aid independence. Later, as rapport is built, the OT can negotiate with the patient to perform part of the self-care in return for time spent on a component interest.

A very-low-functioning patient may be unable to accomplish any self-care activity effectively. Despite limited self-care goals, ADL may be used as a method of stimulation for these patients. The opportunities to use functional movement patterns during dressing, the sensory stimulation that occurs with oral/facial hygiene or eating, and the opportunities to follow simple commands are numerous. The skilled therapist can use ADL tasks as a meaningful treatment modality to stimulate basic sensory, vestibular, motor, and cognitive systems. Structured ADL treatment provides familiar, focused, controlled stimulation in a nondistracting environment and may be much more effective in integrating sensory input than stimulation programs provided in a clinic setting.

When ADL tasks are used as a treatment modality, the patient's achievement of task skills is secondary. Much of the ADL activity may be done for the patient; however, the therapist's careful use of sensory stimulation, motor facilitation, and cognitive and perceptual cues makes the task therapeutic. Unlike the nurse, who must dress, wash, and feed the patient within tight time constraints, the OT can encourage maximal participation, take time to use therapeutic touch, and structure the activity to improve involvement.

Grading ADL Activities

To use self-care activities as an effective treatment modality, the therapist first must choose relevant activities based on the patient's past life and current goals. He or she must then analyze the components of the chosen task. The cognitive, perceptual, motoric, and environmental demands of the task should be determined and matched with the skills of the patient. For example, the cognitive requirements of upper extremity dressing (UED) from a wheelchair in the patient's hospital room is analyzed below. In a treatment situation, the OT would also analyze information about the perceptual, motor, and environmental demands of a task in the same way. All of the information would then be synthesized into a single plan.

Analysis of the Cognitive Requirements of UED

Cognitive Demands	Patient Skills
1. Short-term memory (STM) and long-term memory (LTM) to learn adaptive techniques and location of objects in a new environment	1. Mildly impaired STM and LTM, with better visual than tactile/kinesthetic or auditory memory
2. Selective attention in a mildly distracting environment	2. Adequate selective attention
3. Identification of problem situations and alternative solutions to manage flaccid upper extremity and balance deficits	3. Unable to anticipate problems and persists in using an approach even when it is ineffective
4. Judgment to select the best solution	4. Unable to identify alternatives; therefore unable to use judgment
5. Organization and planning to approach task in an efficient manner	5. Shows poor anticipation of events and consequences, and does not organize or plan tasks

Based on analysis of the patient's strengths, deficits, and the demands of the task, the therapist plans treatment. The patient in the example above is allowed to experience problems associated with managing balance deficits and the flaccid upper extremity, and an opportunity is provided to discuss these difficulties immediately. The patient is encouraged to offer suggestions for improving performance. Visual demonstrations or diagrams are provided to compensate for memory deficits. The patient is prompted to identify a possible problem before it occurs, and to choose one solution to the problem. Finally, assistance is given as needed to help the patient carry out the plan. When the patient persists in using an ineffective approach to a problem, the therapist can stop the behavior and help him or her to analyze the situation. Structure and organization can be provided through cuing and by presenting each new step of the task in a sequential way. As awareness of deficits and the ability to select and implement solutions improves, the patient can be encouraged to organize the task more independently.

Effectively grading a task requires that the therapist be (1) sensitive to the multiple emotional, cognitive, motoric, and perceptual demands that an activity places on the nervous system; (2) aware of the structure provided; and (3) flexible so that changes can occur on the basis of the patient's response. All of the factors identified in the activity analysis must be balanced to provide a task that is challenging without producing undesirable stress responses. An activity that is optimally challenging will attract the patient's full attention. He or she will appear focused and interested. A task that is too demanding may result in more primitive patterns of motor behavior (Warren 1990), withdrawal, anxiety, or refusal to participate. Similarly, a task that is too easy may lead to lack of attention, boredom, or rejection of the activity. Careful analysis of the task and awareness of the patient's strengths, weaknesses, and interests allow the therapist to upgrade or downgrade the activity as needed.

The therapist should also be aware of the structure that is provided in therapy. At times, the OT may be unaware of the amount of assistance that is given. The way in which activities are set up or the cues that are unconsciously provided may improve the patient's performance significantly. For example, the therapist may observe the patient performing a meal preparation activity in the kitchen. Prior to the task all items are placed on shelves or in the refrigerator. The therapist asks the patient to come to the kitchen and prepare a tuna salad. No other cues are given until the patient asks for a chopping board. The therapist points out the general location of this item, and the patient continues to complete the task successfully.

Although the example above describes a relatively unstructured task, there are certain factors of which the therapist must be aware. The method of arranging the items in the cupboards and in the refrigerator may have been more organized and easier to manage than what the patient would encounter at home. On the other hand, a very systematic homemaker may well have a more convenient system in place. The therapist helped the patient locate the cutting board. This assistance is commonly given, since it is customary in both therapeutic and social situations to help someone find items in an unfamiliar setting. However, the OT also could have used this opportunity to observe the patient's ability to solve a problem independently. The therapist provided a cue to begin the task. While the patient may have expected such direction because the therapist has a responsibility for planning treatment, the OT must be sure to provide opportunities for the patient to initiate activities independently. If initiation of activities does not occur in the hospital setting, it may not occur at home. Finally, the hospital routine itself imposes structure. Schedules are provided and reminders are given that help the patient maintain a productive routine. An opportunity to experience unstructured time is valuable for a high-level patient who will be resuming complex daily living skills. When working with patients who are anticipating a return to unstructured, independent living, the therapist must gradually withdraw assistance to observe them in a natural setting. Home, community, and work site evaluations are especially helpful.

Using Clinic Activities

Clinic activities provide a useful adjunct to basic or complex ADL skill training. Through these activities the OT provides remediation or teaches compensation strategies for particular component skills that affect performance. Based on analysis of the tasks that the patient hopes to perform, and on knowledge of the patient's strengths and weaknesses, the OT can devise treatment to focus specifically on factors that significantly limit function. One of the first component areas that the OT might address is postural control. Because humans have an innate drive to remain upright against gravity, patients must be assisted to regain postural alignment before they will be able to focus on cognitive tasks (Warren 1990). Emphasis on postural control and mobility forms a foundation for treatment of patients who need controlled sensory input, vestibular stimulation, and the experience of their bodies moving in space before they will be able to relate to abstract cognitive or perceptual concepts. While the low- or moderate-level patient has a special need for controlled motion, all patients having motor loss can benefit. Whole-body movements are especially helpful in regaining awareness of the body in space, increasing arousal and attention, facilitating motor-planning skills, and integrating the two sides of the body.

Many patients who have had a CVA experience significant physical limitations. Movement becomes a conscious, rather than an automatic, activity. The conscious thought needed to perform previously preprogrammed activities occupies part of the brain's capacity to attend to and process information. The patient's attention, memory, perceptual motor integration, and problem-solving skills are used to relearn movement patterns. Motor re-education can therefore be a meaningful activity through which cognition and perception can be addressed. As the patient becomes more skilled, combining motor activities with other challenging cognitive perceptual tasks, such as playing a game or performing a self-care activity, can effectively increase the mental processing demands of the activity and provide additional challenge.

Whenever possible, the patient should be out of the wheelchair. He or she may sit on a regular chair, a mat, a bench, a rocker board, or a ball, depending on balance and the amount of challenge the therapist wants to provide. He or she may be asked to perform activities while rolling, standing, kneeling, half-kneeling, or in more dynamic positions requiring transitional movement. The greater the physical challenge, the more effort will be required to concentrate on a cognitive or perceptual activity. Challenge may be effective in promoting protective mechanisms in a patient who is not alert. Too much challenge will interfere with performance. The therapist must balance these factors carefully to provide optimal challenge.

Consider a patient who is learning one-handed skills in the kitchen. While performance at a standing level may be the ultimate goal, a patient who is very fearful in this position will be unable to learn new techniques. Initially, the learning may best take place while the patient is sitting in a chair at the kitchen table. Later, as the task is better integrated, and as control and confidence in standing improve, the same activity should be performed in an upright position. The increased demands of standing will increase the complexity and mental requirements of the task.

Prior to using more extreme developmental positions, the therapist must assess the impact of these techniques in relation to the frailty of the patient and in relation to medical problems, such as a cardiac condition or arthritis. Treatment should not focus on correction of longstanding postural problems, should not stress weak joint structures, and should use postures that are relevant to the patient's life style. For instance, a 75-year-old patient who has dispensed with activities performed on hands and knees, such as gardening and scrubbing the floor, does not need to work in the all-fours position. A younger stroke patient who intends to resume an active life style, however, can benefit from activities in a wide range of positions.

When the therapist is planning clinic activities, he or she should be attentive to the environment. Since a clinic can frequently be overly stimulating, unnecessary distractions should be decreased. Visual distractions may be limited with a curtain, with a screen, or by positioning the patient in a corner or toward a wall. Auditory distractions can be reduced by working in a quiet room. When the patient is able to focus on a task in a quiet environment, the therapist might choose to work on selective attention in a distracting setting. The clinic can be an excellent place in which to provide this challenge.

Activities generally should be selected to provide multisensory stimulation. It is common knowledge that it is much easier to remember an event that involves active participation than one that has been read about. The multiple stimulation that occurs through participation in an activity reinforces learning (Warren 1990). For example, if the therapist is teaching a one-handed technique, he or she does not merely describe the method but helps the patient use it in a variety of settings until the verbal instructions, demonstrations, and motor processes have been integrated effectively. Similarly, when working to improve a patient's ability to scan the left visual field, the OT could choose an activity that provides visual stimulation, whole-body movement, tactile stimulation, and auditory cues. He or she might ask the patient to take objects off a kitchen shelf or therapy counter, name each item, place them in a basket at knee height, wipe the shelf or counter, and replace the objects.

To use multisensory stimulation effectively, the therapist should use evaluation data to determine the channels that are currently helping the patient process information. For example, a patient with relatively intact visual and tactile processing but difficulty with language would perform best through demonstration. In addition, the therapist should try to ascertain the patient's previous learning style and use methods that correspond to his or her previous tactics when possible. A patient's work may give insight to learning preferences. For instance, a lawyer probably relied on language skills for learning, a carpenter may be more of a visual/kinesthetic learner, and a businessman might use auditory and visual skills.

A patient who effectively integrates sensory information and is working on a specific high-level cognitive skill, such as abstract problem solving, can benefit from treatment that facilitates independent thinking. At this level the patient must begin to generalize from previous experiences, and can base some new learning on previously established perceptual motor foundations. Although a child learns primarily through sensorimotor experience, an adult has compressed much of this learning into specific patterns of behavior. The information is integrated in cortical areas of the brain. Disruption of sensorimotor processes precludes learning in a child, but an adult with damage to sensorimotor areas of the brain may be able to use previously learned systems to organize raw data into meaningful concepts. In other words, when the sensorimotor system is altered, the patient will be able to rely on past experiences of sensorimotor information to draw new conclusions. Intact cortical structures may be used to compare current obstacles to past patterns of behaviors (Luria 1973).

Although the OT often thinks in terms of gross perceptual motor tasks when choosing activities, it must be remembered that even tasks performed at a table top can be multisensory. Although table-top activities are not recommended for lower-level patients and caution must be used to ensure relevance, they can be effectively used with patients at the high end of the cognitive and perceptual continuum. Functionally, an adult must be able to listen and remember, look and discriminate, or read and retain relevant information. When treating a patient who has the potential to return to work, school, or high-level home management tasks, it is important to provide opportunities for covert thinking. Using relevant paper-and-pencil tasks to begin the training process may be effective. The therapist must remember that the patient's ability to generalize learning from a paper-and-pencil task to real life is questionable (Schleuderer et al. 1988). The patient can be assisted to analyze problems or use memory strategies during table-top tasks that relate to daily living skills. The OT must always move one step further, however, and help the patient to apply these techniques in unstructured daily living tasks. He or she must be challenged to use what has been learned in activities that require integration of cognitive, perceptual, and motor skills. For example, the high-level patient who has learned to use the telephone in the clinic to seek information from the operator can be asked to use that skill while standing in a crowded restaurant.

Any therapeutic activity that is selected should have a clear purpose and be relevant to function. A great deal of time must be spent to make the patient aware of primary deficits and of the rationale for the chosen treatment methods. The patient who appreciates the reasons for performing a task is much more likely to participate to the best of his or her ability. When cognitive limitations prevent the patient from comprehending deficits,

the family or caregiver must be instructed to help him or her understand the patient's problems and the suggested treatment.

To improve comprehension and acceptance of an activity, familiar, functional objects should be used rather than unfamiliar items. It is more helpful to stack plastic cups of various sizes than to stack cones. It is better to sort coins, cards, utensils, laundry, pens, pencils, or small tools by color, shape, and/or size than to sort blocks. Care must be taken to provide activities that are age-appropriate as well as suitable to the patient's cognitive and perceptual level. Computers can be motivating to a young patient or a businessman, but they may be intimidating to patients who have not been exposed to them. Crafts and games can address a wide range of cognitive and perceptual skills and are appropriately used when the patient previously enjoyed these activities. It is inappropriate to force a person to engage in them, however, if he or she previously found them childish or frivolous. On the other hand, the therapist should not allow his or her own biases to stand in the way of using an activity that will address specific skills and capture the patient's interest.

Using Enjoyable Activities

Csikszentmihalyi (1975), in his book *Beyond Boredom and Anxiety*, studied the nature of enjoyable activities. He studied activities such as chess, rock climbing, dancing, surgery, music composition, and basketball and found that three factors consistently related to enjoyment: creative discovery, overcoming challenge, and resolving difficulty. Different activities are enjoyable to different people. The activity may demand motor skill or intellectual ability. It may be competitive, social, or solitary. In all enjoyment, however, the person's skills are matched to the challenge so that mastery of the environment is experienced. In addition, society has a role in defining challenge. Thus chess is a challenge because at least some segments of society see it in this way.

When a person enjoys an activity, he or she is described as being in a "flow state." In this state, the activity matches the person's skill, the person is focused on relevant aspects of the task, the goals are apparent, the person has the means to reach the goals, and feedback about performance is clear. When too few opportunities are present to use one's skills, boredom results; when too many opportunities for action present themselves, anxiety results.

Csikszentmihalyi believes that both work and play may produce this flow state. He feels that flow activities have relevance on three levels: an environmental adaptation level, a neurological level, and a personal level. On an environmental level, people use pleasurable activities to learn skills needed for adult tasks, to express inner needs, and to relieve the monotony of routine. Neurological stimulation necessary for optimal arousal can be achieved through play, and personal satisfaction is a strong motivator for engaging in pleasurable activity. Csikszentmihalyi suggests a simple formula for making learning enjoyable: know the person's skills and level of proficiency, then provide gradually increasing opportunities to use those skills.

Csikszentmihalyi provides theoretical information that supports the OT's use of purposeful behavior. He stresses the wide range of activities that can be enjoyable, based on the person's skills and social experience. In addition, he supports the OT's method of carefully grading activity to promote optimal challenge. His studies dealt with a healthy population, but it seems useful to apply the information to people who have had CVAs. Perhaps occupational therapy will undertake research similar to his in order to better define meaningful activity with disabled populations.

By using a broad definition of activity, the therapist can be more creative. When suitable objects are not available, he or she can work effectively without them. The OT can engage the patient in multisensory, goal-directed activity that is at least as meaningful and possibly less offensive than filling a pegboard by using his or her hand as a visual target, the voice as auditory input, and touch as tactile input. The patient can be asked to count, answer questions, solve problems, or describe an event while working. The therapist can use the environment or enlist the help of family members and other people in the clinic to provide cognitive and perceptual stimulation. The spontaneous events that arise during the treatment session can be used creatively to provide effective, less contrived therapy. For instance, when a patient drops a tissue, rather than pick it up the therapist can have the patient problem solve a method of obtaining it independently. As Csikszentmihalyi described, challenge is defined by both the individual and society. Some patients may be persuaded by the therapist of the challenge and value of working with a pegboard. Others may not be able to remove the valid stereotypes that classify this task as childish.

OTs have at times been unaware of the emotional connotations of some of the activities they choose and have created negative feelings in patients, families, and other professionals. It is a challenge to provide adult activities that are appropriate, meaningful, and confidence building for a patient with limited cognitive and perceptual skills. By adopting a more liberal definition of meaningful activity, the therapist might choose very

specific cognitive, motor, or perceptual motor tasks for treatment of component deficits. Not every activity used by an OT to treat component skill deficits needs to be functional or multisensory. Each activity does need to relate to a skill necessary for function, and, at some point during the session, the therapist should help the patient apply the skill to a functional task. For example, the OT might work on a scanning activity and a problem-solving task during motor retraining. Later in the session the therapist might have the patient integrate all of these skills by having him or her locate a glass, pick up the glass, and obtain a drink of water at the sink. The therapist can cue the patient ahead of time to use the scanning techniques and problem-solving strategies discussed earlier, and can discuss the outcome of the activity after performance. If the activity provides challenge and creates a sense of mastery, it will have been meaningful and enjoyable to the patient. As Neistdadt (1988) states, research from psychology indicates that the therapeutic relationship is a key factor in successful treatment and may be more important than the techniques used. It is important to study this issue further, but in the meantime we must be aware of how we approach activity and how we build therapeutic rapport with the patient.

EDUCATING THE ADULT LEARNER

An important factor in the success of therapeutic intervention is how well the patient and caregiver can carry out what they have learned. Mosey (1986) discusses the therapist's role in designing appropriate learning situations. She stresses that, although the client is free to choose whether or not he or she wishes to learn, the therapist must be sure that the environment and the presentation of the material were effective, given the skills and style of the patient or caregiver. A thorough knowledge of the patient gained through the evaluation helps us to determine our teaching style. When providing caregiver instruction, our approach initially may be selected on the basis of information from social work or psychology. As we begin interacting with that person, the approach can be modified according to his or her response and ability to carry through. Simpson (1980) identifies many principles drawn from various learning theories. Some that seem useful in patient/caregiver education are the following:

- Behavioristic Theory
  1. Provide positive reinforcement to promote desirable behavior.
  2. Although less effective than positive learning experiences, allowing the person to experience difficulty can sometimes help him or her under-

stand the need to learn new, more effective methods.

3. Analyze an activity and help the person to practice each component separately to avoid overwhelming him or her. Later provide opportunities to practice the task as an integrated whole.

4. Since positive role models facilitate performance, be sure to model desired behavior and arrange for the person to interact with others who are good role models.

5. Challenge the patient and caregivers by engaging them in activities that stimulate them to learn more.

- Cognitive Theory

  1. Provide opportunities to experience situations similar to those that will be encountered outside the hospital.

  2. Provide information that can help the patient organize his or her experiences: i.e., explain the purpose of activities and relate new skills to previously learned information.

- Psychoanalytical Theory

  1. Be aware that excessive stress will interfere with learning. Therefore, address the patient's or caregiver's anxieties before the training session begins.

  2. Be aware of the symbolic meanings a particular activity may hold for a patient. Culture and gender should be considered when choosing tasks.

- Self Theory

  1. Ensure that instruction is relevant to the patient and caregiver. If it is not, learning will be significantly decreased.

  2. Be aware that some patients and caregivers will resist learning a new technique because it will alter self-perception. For example, some spouses may feel that the nature of their relationship will be seriously compromised by assuming a caregiving role.

  3. Involve the patient or caregiver in selection of the activity or technique that he or she would like to learn.

  4. Provide opportunities for self-initiated participation in activities that promote positive emotions and stimulate thought.

These principles can be used to design teaching situations that are individualized for the patient or caregiver, reflect the goals and interests of the client, and promote practical learning in a step-by-step man-

ner. Whenever possible, both the caregiver and the patient should have multiple opportunities to practice the identified activities. When little time for teaching is available, goals should be limited, outpatient instruction arranged, or a home health therapist advised to monitor home carry-over.

Goals for home carry-over should be realistic for the time, skill level, and life style of the client. It is unfair for the therapist to expect an elderly spouse to care for his or her own needs, manage the household, perform the patient's basic care, and carry out an extensive exercise program. A younger family member may be burdened with work and care of children. The therapist must be aware of the ethical dilemmas experienced by the caregiver who is expected to care for the patient as well as himself or herself (Hasselkus 1991). If the therapist's expectations are too great, or do not take into account a particular home situation, the home program may be discarded and the caregiver may feel guilty. When the therapist works with the caregiver and patient, a compromise plan can be devised that includes the most important aspects of care and is more likely to be followed. Although prevention of deformity and preservation of maximal function is important, our instruction must be realistic and sensitive to the caregiver. A paid caretaker can be expected to carry out a more extensive program. He or she is encouraged to attend at least one day of therapy (more if possible) to learn all aspects of managing the patient.

Strategies that ease the care of cognitively impaired patients should be stressed when instructing caregivers. Some strategies recommended by Baum (1991) for home management of people with Alzheimer's disease may also be effective with confused stroke survivors. These include behavior modification techniques, organization of a schedule, organization of the environment, exercise, use of familiar activities, encouraging interpersonal relationships, and involvement in support groups. Several of these techniques will be explained more specifically in Chapter 7. When possible, the caregiver should be given opportunities to use these techniques followed by discussion about effectiveness with the therapist. Encouragement should be given for caretakers to attend support groups.

At times language barriers limit instruction. A translator should be obtained if possible. If not, demonstration and practice can convey some aspects of the program; however, they do not allow rationales or behavioral observations to be shared. A written program translated to the caregiver's language may be helpful. In general, written information should be kept simple, should be illustrated with pictures or diagrams when possible (Picariello 1986), should be presented in large type or clear handwriting, and should cover the most important aspects of the home program. While some people relish vast quantities of written information and explanatory materials, others become overwhelmed. Those who seem to be seeking more information can be given supplemental materials or referred to publications by the American Heart Association or the National Stroke Foundation for further reading.

ADAPTING THE ENVIRONMENT

It is well known that modifying an environment can promote function. Much research has been done to identify environmental factors that promote independence in the elderly. Some of these principles can be applied to those who have had a CVA. Since many stroke patients are elderly, the environmental concepts are applicable because of age alone. Cognitive and perceptual deficits caused by a stroke make safe environments even more important. As with other forms of intervention, it is important to consider the patient's cultural background, interests, and life style prior to initiating home modifications. Collaboration is important to ensure that changes are recognized as beneficial and are accepted by the patient (Levine and Gitlin 1990).

Visual limitations make clear lettering, large type, and distinct contrasts in color important. It is helpful to avoid materials with a patterned background because they make it harder to distinguish items in the foreground (Christenson 1990a). Lighting is also important. It is helpful to provide adequate light, but avoid glare. The use of matte surfaces and shades to shield light bulbs from direct vision is helpful. Light switches should be easily accessible and placed so that the room can be lighted before entering. Touch-activated lamps may be helpful to prevent fumbling with light switches (Christenson 1990b).

Auditory distraction can be minimized by using sound-absorbing materials. It should be recognized that many people who have had a CVA find excessive noise and confusion overwhelming. Initially they may be cautioned to avoid large gatherings or crowds. Gradually they can increase their exposure and ability to respond to multiple conversations or auditory input.

Because falls are common in the elderly, and stroke patients with cognitive, perceptual, and motor problems are more vulnerable, caution must be taken to ensure safety during mobility. Patterned floor coverings may be distracting for a person with visual perceptual loss coupled with motor impairment. Scatter rugs are dangerous because they may have raised edges that can cause tripping. Small rugs that do not contrast with the floor are even more dangerous because visually they do not stand out. Christenson recommends avoiding scatter rugs, using low-pile wall-to-wall carpeting, tacking or taping rugs at the edges if possible, and using nonskid backings. Floors can be polished with nonskid wax, and thresholds should be removed. Stairs should be well maintained, well lighted or accented with contrasting paint, and have plain-colored low-pile carpet or nonskid treads. Extension cords should not cross any pathways. In the bathroom, nonskid mats should be used inside and outside the tub. Grab bars and raised toilet or bath seats can improve mobility.

General safety can be improved by ensuring that the water heater is set below 130 degrees, that appliances have easy-to-read dials, and that items are stored to minimize bending and reaching. Potentially dangerous products such as cleaning supplies, medicines, and sharp objects should be stored separately so that they are not inadvertently mishandled. Telephones should be easily accessible in both the bedroom and the main living area. An enlarged number pad or an automatic dialer may be considered. An easy-to-read list of important numbers should be placed near the telephone. Emergency call systems may be considered when a person lives alone or has difficulty reaching the telephone. All rooms should be cleared of clutter and easy to move through. In the bedroom, the mattress should be firm and of a height that allows the person's feet to touch the floor when sitting. Closets and drawers should be arranged to minimize clutter and avoid reaching and bending.

Adaptive equipment or methods may help to compensate for cognitive, perceptual, and motor loss. Pill organizers can help to ensure that proper amounts of medication are taken routinely. Long hot-mitts can improve safety in the kitchen, as can the use of a microwave oven. Adapted cutting boards reduce slightly the amount of visual discrimination needed to cut food safely. Prepared foods reduce the cognitive and perceptual demands of meal preparation.

Adaptations to the environment often can promote increased safety and independence despite cognitive and perceptual deficits. A wide range of general principles helpful in planning treatment for the stroke survivor have been discussed. These should be kept in mind when specific activities are planned to remediate or compensate for particular cognitive and perceptual deficits.

Chapter 7

Cognitive and Perceptual Treatment Techniques

This chapter provides specific treatment ideas that may be used with patients demonstrating various cognitive and perceptual deficits. It is meant to be used in conjunction with Chapter 6, which discusses general treatment principles. It is important to evaluate each patient carefully, both initially and informally, as treatment progresses to ensure that activities are effective and are correctly graded on the basis of the patient's unique abilities. The topics in this chapter are arranged in a hierarchical manner just as in Chapters 4, 10, and 11.

COGNITIVE TREATMENT IDEAS

Arousal and Attention

Arousal

Arousal and attention are parts of the same continuum. Arousal is at the low end of the continuum, and alternating attention is at the high end. The area of the brain described by Luria (1973) as the first functional unit is primarily responsible for maintaining appropriate levels of arousal and attention. Patients who demonstrate low levels of arousal are likely to have damage to the reticular activating system, an area deep in the brain that is important in maintaining a state of wakefulness. Since this is a hard-wired system, it is less amenable to change than are other systems.

Treatment for decreased arousal should begin with stimulation of the vestibular system through movement. This movement should be controlled by the patient whenever possible and can be prompted by participation in functional activities or clinic tasks. The movement that occurs when moving in a wheelchair, rolling, bending, reaching, working in proprioceptive neuromuscular facilitation diagonals, or moving from sitting to standing stimulates the vestibular system (Figure 7-1). Spinning is not advocated; no benefit to adults from this activity has been documented, and it is not a normal adult activity. It is theorized that the numerous connections between functional unit one, or the reticular activating system, and the vestibular system promote arousal (Warren 1990). Whole-body movements, especially those that create some postural insecurity, also activate primitive protective responses

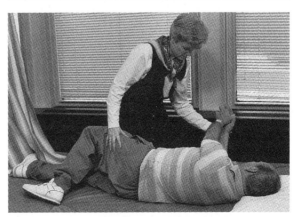

Figure 7-1 Rolling stimulates the vestibular system, promotes body awareness, and enhances arousal prior to participation in functional activities.

(Warren 1990). Moving the patient thus alerts the system and provides the attention necessary to engage in further activity. When the patient is unable to participate actively in treatment, the therapist may begin the session by moving the patient and providing sensory stimulation, but the therapist should work to enlist the patient's active participation as soon as he or she is alert.

Sensory stimulation increases alertness. When first presented, novel tactile, auditory, or visual information will activate the orienting response, a temporary reaction that allows the person to determine whether the information is worthy of further attention. The occupational therapist (OT) often can use the novel stimulation to initiate participation in a task, and thus can successfully transform the patient's orienting response to a goal-directed activity. For example, the patient's olfactory system can be stimulated with cologne. Once aroused, the patient can apply the cologne and then may be able to make the transition to another oral/facial hygiene activity. Similarly, an orienting response may be elicited through rubbing a warm washcloth on the patient's cheek or touching a sweet banana to the lips. Once arousal and attention to the stimulus have occurred, treatment can proceed with face washing and feeding, respectively. Meaningful activity is important to low-functioning patients as well as to those who are more intact. A patient may attend to a familiar voice longer than to a radio show that has no relevance, or may be motivated to attend visually to a picture of a family member rather than to an irrelevant item from a test kit. To initiate treatment with a patient showing low levels of arousal, activities should be chosen that are familiar and meaningful, incorporate movement, and provide a variety of controlled sensory stimuli.

Decreased arousal is a poor prognostic sign for functional recovery. If changes in arousal do not occur, goals should focus on caregiver teaching, and treatment sessions should include the caregiver when possible to ensure that he or she is able to carry out the recommended treatment techniques.

Attention

Attentional deficits also may respond to techniques such as vestibular stimulation and sensory input. Movement should be used to alert the patient and challenge him or her, but it should not cause fear. If the patient feels posturally threatened, he or she will be unable to attend selectively to another activity because all attention will be directed at maintaining balance.

Sustained Attention. When a very distractible patient focuses on a variety of stimuli irrelevant to the task, he

or she may have damage to the third functional unit, the frontal lobe. The patient is unable to inhibit the orienting response and therefore attends to any stimuli that draw his or her attention. This type of patient should begin by working on sustained attention. The ability to sustain attention varies according to level of arousal, the length of time attention is required, and the complexity of the information. When working to improve this level of attention, training should be carried out in a quiet environment.

The therapist should begin training with an activity that is judged to match the patient's skills and interests. The use of a simple, concrete activity that can be completed in a short amount of time is helpful when beginning to focus on increased attention (Figures 7-2 and 7-3). Specific directions can assist the patient to attend for the required amount of time. For instance, the OT may help the patient by saying, "I want you to finish eating your meal." A clock or timer can also be useful in directing a patient to an activity. Instructions such as "You can stop at half past ten" or "You must work for three more minutes" can be helpful to a person with a very limited attention span. Games such as "Simon" may be interesting and effective for increasing attention in some patients (Bolger 1982). Gradually, the OT will work to increase the length of time the patient attends and the complexity of the information. For example, more effort is required to sustain attention while balancing a checkbook than while sorting laundry (Figure 7-4). When sustained attention to a particular task is adequate, the person should be able to inhibit internal distractions such as preoccupation with eating, personal comfort, or the sensation of his or her clothing. The therapist then can work to improve attention in a distracting environment.

Selective Attention. To improve selective attention, three factors are relevant: the complexity of the mate-

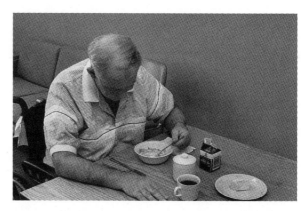

Figure 7-2 Eating in a quiet environment is a simple, motivating activity for building sustained attention.

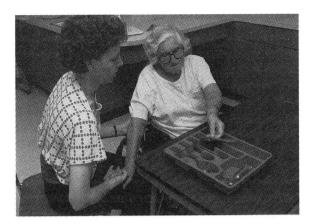

Figure 7-3 Sorting utensils encourages the patient to attend to a simple task through completion.

rial, the patient's motivation for the task, and the amount of distraction. A patient may be able to screen out irrelevant environmental information when working at a task that is interesting and is somewhat easy, or below his or her maximal capacity. When the task becomes more difficult, or approaches a patient's maximal cognitive capacity, he or she will continue to be able to screen out irrelevant information only if highly motivated to attend to the task. If the patient is unmotivated, distraction is likely. When the task exceeds a person's cognitive capacity, he or she will become frustrated and/or distracted by irrelevant information. Regardless of the patient's motivation and the appropriateness of the task, extreme levels of distraction will prevent participation. Distractions that are threatening (e.g., physical challenges to safety, a fire drill, or another patient's crying in pain) may prevent focus.

Alternating Attention. When selective attention is established, the patient may work on alternating attention. An activity can be selected that requires working on several steps simultaneously, or the patient may be

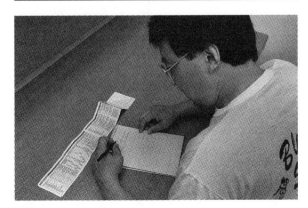

Figure 7-4 Sustained attention is challenged by tasks that require increased concentration, such as planning a bus trip.

asked to participate in two activities at once. For instance, a work simulation task that requires answering the telephone, taking messages, and tabulating columns of figures challenges alternating attention. The factors of motivation, duration, difficulty, and distraction continue to be relevant at this level of attention. Consequently the therapist may begin to work on alternating attention in a quiet environment, gradually increasing both the complexity of the task and the distractions.

Some tasks of alternating attention can be emphasized only when motor patterns have become reintegrated enough to work as spontaneous programs of action. When a person is first learning to walk, all of his or her attention is required to conduct that activity. As walking becomes more automatic, the person may be able to attend to surroundings and navigate in an unfamiliar area. Initially, a patient may need to focus attention on sitting to maintain an upright position on a mat. Later he or she may be able to play a card game while sitting unsupported. This type of attention is addressed when the patient is working to integrate movement programs sufficiently to allow simultaneous control of motor performance while engaged in another cognitive or perceptual task.

Webster and Scott (1983, 71) describe a specific technique to improve attention. Their method is based on the theory of Luria (1973) that higher cognitive processes can compensate for impaired functions. Their single case design shows the benefit of teaching a mildly impaired, highly motivated patient to use self-instructional training to overcome attentional deficits. The technique involved having the patient say statements aloud as follows:

1. "To really concentrate, I must look at the person speaking to me."
2. "I also must focus on what is being said, not on other thoughts which want to intrude."
3. "I must concentrate on what I am hearing at any moment by repeating each word in my head as the person speaks."
4. "Although it is not horrible if I lose track of the conversation, I must tell the person to repeat the information if I have not attended to it."

Training involved having the patient listen to, and repeat, short pieces of information from reading material that the patient had identified as interesting. Next, the patient was asked to whisper the phrases after they were presented. Finally, he was trained to repeat the information silently to himself. The amount of time he was given to repeat the information was gradually reduced from five seconds to zero seconds after each sentence. The patient felt that this technique was helpful.

He reported improvements at work and with sexuality, possibly due to increased attention to the relevant aspects of the activity.

Results of this case study were positive, and although such a systematic training approach has not been used by OTs at the Rehabilitation Institute of Chicago (RIC), it appears feasible for high-level motivated patients. Obviously, a language-based method of intervention would be effective only with those who have retained adequate language skills. As used by OTs, this technique would be applied to activities and would not be applied primarily to written material. Similar rehearsal strategies might be used to help a patient attend to visual and kinesthetic information.

A kinesthetic approach has been used effectively with our patients to help them attend to and learn a movement pattern or posture. The therapist begins by directing the patient's attention to a passive movement; the therapist then asks the patient to repeat it with the noninvolved extremity, focus again on passive movement of the affected extremity, and then try to carry out the movement independently. This forced attention appears helpful in retraining motor skills. As the patient progresses, he or she is able to attend independently to the quality of movement on the affected side, compare it to movement on the nonaffected extremity, and initiate changes to improve motion. Visual information has also been rehearsed by having patients verbalize what they see in a room, on a tray, or in a drawer. They are assisted to scan the information systematically in a logical manner. After they are able to verbalize what they see, they are encouraged to use these strategies to scan the environment independently. The therapist periodically checks the patients' use of this strategy by asking them to recall what they have seen.

Orientation

Problems with orientation may result from difficulty in attending to environmental cues that help distinguish people, places, and time. Poor memory may also interfere with recalling orientation information. Techniques designed to improve memory and attention therefore will be useful when working with patients who demonstrate orientation problems.

Orientation is important for normal function in any self-care skill. Profound deficits will affect ability to dress appropriately for the weather, ability to anticipate meals or other events correctly, and ability to relate to caregivers. Mild deficits may interfere with recalling dates, or remaining aware of the passage of time.

A patient who demonstrates severe disorientation will benefit from environmental structure and frequent verbal orientation to the surroundings. Provision of col-

ored room markers, calendars, and large-faced clocks; adherence to routine schedules; consistency of caregivers; and avoidance of changes in the location of the patient's room, meals, therapy, or other activities are helpful. In addition, caregivers routinely should introduce themselves and state the purpose of their visit.

A conversational tone can help present orientation information in a natural manner. Patients often become frustrated as, hour after hour, each caregiver fires a list of questions at them, such as "Where are you now?" "What is the date?" "Who am I?" It is more effective to greet the patient naturally and to introduce the therapy and the activities that are planned. You may then ask if the patient remembers your name, or what he or she had worked on previously in occupational therapy, reassuring the patient that it is difficult to remember so many new people and activities. During the session, conversation can touch on the weather: "Have you heard what the weather is like today?" If the patient is unable to answer, he or she can look out the window or look at the paper. Holidays, sports, and news events also provide natural leads for discussion.

When written work or a project is done, the patient can be asked to label the work with name and date. The patient can use a calendar if this is difficult. Alternately, the OT can ask in an offhanded way whether the patient knows the date as a form is filled in or an activity is labeled. This can become part of the daily treatment session by creating a record of exercises or a list of the time spent on activities of daily living (ADL) that is tabulated and dated each day. Time can also be spent during each session to mark the correct date on a calendar that the patient carries. This calendar might be mounted in plastic on a lapboard or an armboard, or placed in a storage pocket in the wheelchair.

It is also possible for the OT to refer to the time of day during the session. "It is ten o'clock now. Please let me know when it is five after ten so that we can use the kitchen," or "Check the clock; should we clean up now?" It is also helpful to refer to the patient's daily schedule and ask him or her to identify the next session. While it is important to use orientation information frequently during an occupational therapy session, structuring situations in which the information is logically needed is much more helpful than bombarding the patient with questions at the start or end of every session. Just as in other areas of treatment, the information must be used in a functional, meaningful way.

Patients who have more subtle orientation problems and are motivated to change may agree to practice specific techniques. They can be encouraged to use a memory book to summarize events, list relevant names, and note important dates. A schedule book with space in which to write key events each day may be helpful for a student or worker who would like an inconspicuous method of maintaining orientation information. High-level patients who have difficulty in monitoring the passage of time may practice estimating various lengths of time, first without any distractions and later during an activity. For example, the therapist can ask a patient to indicate when he or she has exercised for approximately one minute. A stopwatch or timer can be used to compare the actual amount of elapsed time with the estimated time (Figure 7-5).

Topographical Orientation

Topographical orientation requires visual spatial skills to process the relationship of one key landmark to another. In addition, memory is necessary to recall these relationships. The patient can practice locating various items in his or her room, on the nursing floor, and throughout the hospital. Initially, the therapist can begin by helping the patient to identify and organize important landmarks that will assist in navigation. The patient can then be asked to bring the OT to a particular place. As skill improves, the patient can be asked to meet the therapist at a particular place. By observing progress from a distance, the therapist can ensure that the patient does not get lost. Finally, the therapist can ask the patient to provide directions to a known location within the facility. These directions can then be followed to assess their accuracy.

When topographical orientation is demonstrated indoors, community trips can challenge the patient further. The process described above can be used. In addition, maps can be introduced (Figure 7-6). A simple walking route may be used first. Later the patient can be asked to determine complex car or public transportation routes from one point to another. A functional test of this skill may involve planning an excursion to a local attraction, or asking the patient to provide directions

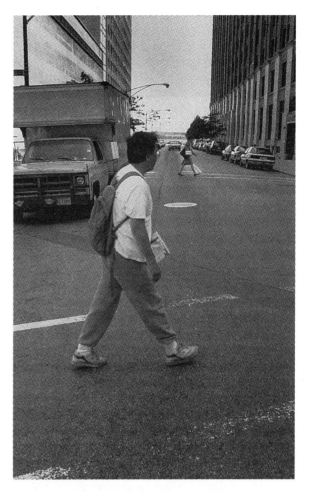

Figure 7-6 Navigating in the community by using a map is a high-level topographical orientation challenge.

and navigate during a trip for a home visit. Naturally, the OT must confirm all instructions and have an alternate plan in case the patient becomes confused.

Memory

Just as there are many types of memory deficits, there are many interventions. A review of some of the mechanisms of memory seems useful for understanding treatment concepts. Information processing theorists describe the first level of memory as sensory memory (Kimble 1985). Luria (1980) describes it as direct impression of traces, and Higbee (1988) describes it as encoding or acquisition. During this phase, large amounts of information enter through sensory receptors. This information is then imprinted in the brain for up to 30 seconds (Luria 1980).

The information that is attended to is moved to short-term memory (STM). This type of memory is also termed *working memory* or *temporary storage*. At this

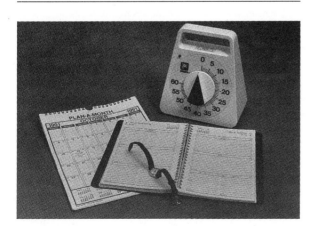

Figure 7-5 A timer, a watch, a calendar, and a schedule book can be used to promote improved orientation.

stage the individual can generally retain seven pieces of information, plus or minus two (Kimble 1985). Information is stored for less than a minute in STM (Siev et al. 1986) and is vulnerable to interference from competing information. Short-term memory allows us to do such things as maintain an updated awareness of our surroundings, follow a conversation, and remember the goal that we are currently working toward (Higbee 1988).

If the information is important and is rehearsed, it is moved to long-term memory (LTM), where it can be recalled or retrieved as needed. Information in LTM can remain for years, but it is gradually forgotten. The process of forgetting actually allows learning to occur. If we were unable to forget old information, our behavior would remain biased by patterns and memories from long ago. By ensuring that unused information is gradually forgotten, newer information can serve as a foundation for our decisions. Forgetting is therefore adaptive (Moore 1990).

Treatment of Memory Deficits

Difficulties in imprinting sensory traces can arise from deficits in the brain areas described by Luria (1973) as functional units one and two (see Chapter 6). When arousal is severely limited due to a lesion in brain unit one, sensory traces will not reach the brain and therefore cannot be recorded. If a particular receptor site in the parietal, temporal, or occipital region of functional unit two is damaged, sensory traces may also remain unrecorded. Although deficits in the first unit affect all sensory modalities equally, damage to the second unit affects certain types of memory more than others (Luria 1973).

Memory deficits arising from poor arousal or attention to stimuli due to lesions in unit one can be treated as described previously. Memory deficits arising from an inability to code specific sensory information due to lesions in unit two may respond to treatment designed to make use of intact systems or enhance damaged areas (Schwartz et al. 1979). For instance, when visual memory is limited, the patient may use verbal descriptions or manual exploration of an object to enhance registration. Techniques described in the visual perception portion of this chapter also may improve registration of information. Patients with this type of memory loss retain the ability to organize information for learning (Luria 1973) and therefore can profit from compensation techniques.

Another type of memory loss is related to interference from other (irrelevant) information. This type of loss, which is not modality specific, may arise from le-

sions in the first or the third functional unit. Lesions in the first unit can cause a person to lose a thought completely once a new thought is introduced. These lesions also can cause a patient to mix parts of a new idea with the original thought. Mild modality-nonspecific memory loss can be improved by providing organized information (Luria 1973) to improve coding and storage. Severe memory loss of this type is frequently accompanied by a decreased level of consciousness and is not amenable to cognitive strategies for learning. For these patients, it is important to maintain a consistent routine and provide structure or cuing. Caregiver instruction about the effects of the deficits on function and strategies for minimizing them are also an important treatment focus.

Lesions in the third functional unit affect the patient's ability to use strategies to organize and categorize information. Since information has not been stored properly, it is very vulnerable to interfering information. Once new information is presented, it may over-ride previously learned information (Luria 1973). The therapist can work to eliminate distractions that interfere with coding information and can help the patient attend to and organize information in meaningful ways. A person with a severe frontal lobe deficit, however, may be unable to incorporate these strategies.

If the patient is able to learn strategies, there are many techniques that can be used by patients with third functional unit damage. The rehearsal technique described in the attention section may be helpful. In addition, asking the person to describe what has just been said or to pick out the main points can help him or her to focus on and organize the material to improve input. Butler et al. (1983) found that providing meaningful verbal descriptions of a visual scene enhanced memory in patients with right hemisphere lesions. The use of a computer for retraining memory functions was studied by Towle et al. (1988). The software emphasized visual and verbal material, such as recall of faces, pictures, words, and maps. They found little significant improvement in memory in their group of 11 patients. Despite limited objective gains, they felt that the ability to provide graded levels of difficulty, immediate and correct feedback, and time limits were positive aspects of most computer games. The patients generally required assistance during computer activities; therefore, direct treatment time was not reduced. Like other authors (Ross 1992; Robertson 1990) who have studied computer use with cognitively and perceptually impaired people, they recommended further evaluation of effectiveness.

Since STM can manage approximately seven pieces of information, grouping words, thoughts, or images into chunks can increase the amount of data processed. For example, when attempting to remember *bread, butter,* and *pickle,* an image of all three words as a sandwich will create one chunk from three separate items. Siev et al. (1986) suggest providing short memory-training sessions that emphasize strategies that can be applied to various situations. For example, relating new information to facts the patient already knows can enhance memory. Various mnemonic devices can be taught to improve a high-level patient's ability to learn lists or names.

Use of Mnemonic Devices. Popular literature describes many mnemonic devices that occasionally may be helpful to patients who have had a cerebrovascular accident (CVA). The use of peg words is one such device. Peg words are rhyming words that can evoke a visual image. They are paired with a number or a letter, for example, 1—*bun,* 2—*shoe,* 3—*bee*; or A—*tray,* B—*bee,* C—*sea.* These words are memorized. When a person must learn a list, he or she can pair the words in the list to the peg words. For example, a patient is asked to remember to bring glasses, his crossword puzzle book, and his wife's office telephone number to therapy. He could memorize the list using the number peg system by imagining a bun on his glasses, his crossword puzzle book in a shoe, and a bee flying near his wife's telephone. A similar system involves selecting various familiar places in the home or neighborhood and then pairing words in a list with each location. For example, the patient would envision his glasses near the front door, his puzzle book on the kitchen counter, and his wife's telephone number on the dining room table. Names and faces can be recalled by associating a feature of the face with the name. For example, to remember a woman with blue eyes named Ms. Fox, the patient might imagine a fox with blue eyes (Higbee 1988). Although it is helpful to be familiar with these strategies, it must be emphasized that they require a very high level of thought processing and are successful only with a few highly motivated patients who show minimal language or cognitive deficits.

Strategies To Enhance Declarative, Procedural, and Episodic Memory. When treating memory deficits, it is helpful to consider not only the area of the brain damage but also the type of memory involved. Declarative memory is the ability to remember factual data (Moore 1990); procedural memory is the ability to remember repetitive motor activities or habits through practice (Saint-Cyr et al. 1988); episodic memory is the ability to recall events; and prospective memory is the ability to remember to do something in the future. While learning theorists and the popular literature deal primarily with declarative memory, OTs must address all forms of memory. Many of the mnemonic techniques deal specifically with declarative memory. Chaining may be used to improve procedural memory. The therapist systematically increases the number of steps the patient must perform either at the beginning or end of the sequence (Figures 7-7 and 7-8). Consistency and repetition are necessary for improving procedural memory. Episodic memory is influenced by emotion. A pleasant, fulfilling event is more likely to be remembered than a distasteful activity. The therapist can use this information to provide a pleasant, but challenging, atmosphere to enhance event memory.

Techniques To Enhance Prospective Memory. Prospective memory is probably related to the regulatory functions and the ability to sustain effort which is mediated by the frontal lobe. To help the patient remember to remember, the therapist can reinforce strategies such as reviewing and rehearsing important dates, or periodically stopping an activity to reflect on the day's schedule. The use of compensation techniques can also be reinforced. The patient can be encouraged to place notes in prominent places, use a timer to signal a change of activities, use a schedule book, or refer to a calendar.

Techniques To Enhance Retrieval. When information has been meaningfully recorded in LTM or STM, the person must be able to retrieve it for use. Free recall requires retrieving the information from memory through a process of active searching without external cues. Techniques such as linking a word with a mental image or pairing a name with an event can help assist free recall. Context is also helpful for recall. Encouraging a patient to return to or imagine the location where

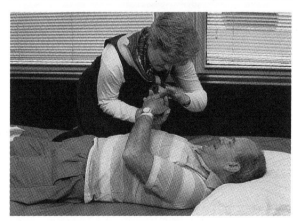

Figure 7-7 Learning to correctly perform self-range of motion exercises requires attention, bilateral integration, awareness of the affected side, motor planning, and procedural memory.

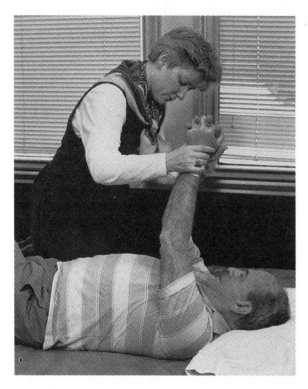

Figure 7-8 The therapist uses demonstration, repetition, and consistent motor patterns to enhance procedural memory.

learning occurred can facilitate retrieval of information. At times the necessary information has entered LTM; however, the person is unable to gain access to it. In these cases, aided recall may be used to help the patient retrieve the information. Cues, such as "My name begins with the letter *K*," may be provided. When cues are provided to remember the steps of an activity, they should be given close to when the action is needed (Siev et al. 1986). If free recall proves too difficult, the patient can be challenged to recognize the correct information from several choices. For instance, recognizing a therapist's name on a list is easier than recalling the name without cues. For recognition to occur, the person merely must match the information with his or her memory.

Techniques for Compensation

Since remediation of memory storage and retrieval problems is a slow process at best, the use of memory aids is often more practical. Devices such as memory books, calendars, clocks, and landmarks can be used as described in the orientation section. Glasgow et al. (1977), in a single case report, describe a brain injured patient who improved his ability to remember names by writing them on a 3 × 5 card. This technique may be helpful to stroke patients who have adequate language

skills. Training in the use of a memory book is detailed by Dougherty and Radomski (1993) in *The Cognitive Rehabilitation Workbook, Second Edition.* They suggest a six-step process. Initially the patient must want to use the book to assist with memory. The contents of the book should be organized, and a routine for using the book, first in the clinic and then outside of therapy, must be established. Assignments should be written in the book to facilitate reliance on it, and the patient should be taught to write clearly to ensure that notes can be used later. Finally, use of the book should be practiced and reinforced to ensure long-term use.

Memory deficits challenge the creativity of the therapist, since encoding, organizing, and retrieving information is a very involved process that demands integration throughout all levels of the brain. Damage to any part of this complex structure will diminish memory (Luria 1973). Treatment will vary, depending on the area of the brain affected and the type of problem seen.

Problem Solving

Problem solving is a complex activity that relies on a foundation of more basic cognitive and perceptual skills. Treatment of problem-solving deficits therefore requires the therapist to analyze the cause of the patient's difficulty. The CVA patient frequently has trouble with various components of problem solving. For instance, difficulty in retaining new information will impair the patient's ability to learn from mistakes, and poor alternating attention will interfere with awareness of relevant factors in the environment. When a component skill deficit limits problem solving, it must be addressed separately. Therapy for many patients will concentrate on the component skills that are prerequisites for problem solving. Other patients may benefit from focusing on one or more steps of the problem-solving continuum. For the purposes of this protocol, the steps are: problem identification, generating solutions, planning, implementation, self-monitoring, and outcome.

Novices and experts solve problems in different ways. Our patients are novices in dealing with disability. They may tend to view problems in simplistic terms, unaware of underlying factors that affect performance. Experimentally, novices tend to use simple formulas to deal with a problem, rather than trying to understand its unique nature and its interrelationship with the environment (Slater and Cohen 1991; Resnick 1985). Patients, too, often relate all their problems to a single factor, such as an inability to walk. They may attempt to solve problems through ineffective, but simple, solutions. It seems reasonable that, by providing information, helping patients understand the nature of their problems, and teaching various methods for solving problems, these skills might improve.

The activities that are used for problem solving can range from solving self-care difficulties, such as how to open a box (Figure 7-9); to solving difficulties in the clinic, such as how to pick up a dropped item; to solving high-level problems, such as how to obtain food items and prepare meals from a wheelchair. Problem solving can be encouraged during routine ADL tasks, complex ADL tasks, and finally during work or school activities. For patients who enjoy them, games and computer activities can challenge problem-solving and planning skills (Figures 7-10 and 7-11). Worksheets that deal with financial or transportation problems can also be useful when applied to real-life situations.

Problem Identification

Since identification of a problem is the first step in the problem-solving continuum, patients who are unaware of the nature of their deficits may benefit from being allowed to make mistakes. The therapist who is too quick to intervene may deny the patient valuable opportunities to learn how deficits affect performance. When difficulties are experienced, the therapist can ask the patient to define the problem. Reasons for the problem and possible solutions might then be discussed. In this way information necessary for problem solving is provided, and problem-solving strategies are modeled. Selection of a solution and its implementation may then be facilitated. The therapist should carefully choose and grade activities to challenge the patient without overwhelming him or her.

When a patient has had an opportunity to experience difficulties but persists in being unable to identify a problem when it occurs, he or she may need to work on

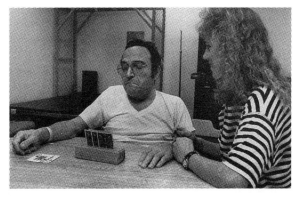

Figure 7-10 Playing cards is an enjoyable way of challenging problem-solving, perceptual, attentional, and memory skills.

more basic sensory awareness skills. For example, a patient who repeatedly falls to the left during functional tasks and does not recognize this difficulty is not ready to address problem solving. He or she should be provided with sensory and motor experiences that allow more accurate perception of the body in space.

Generating Solutions

Some patients may recognize problems when they occur, but be unable to anticipate them. Similarly, they may be able to generate a solution through a trial-and-error approach, but be unable to plan ahead. Whether or not this behavior is a problem is debatable. It may be argued that the ability to anticipate and avoid problems is a more adaptive way to handle difficulties. There are people in the nondisabled population, however, who use trial-and-error approaches effectively in daily life. They are able to learn from and avoid mistakes. The trial-and-error approach may be helpful when first learning about the effect of the CVA on performance. It must be realized that cognitive limitations may pre-

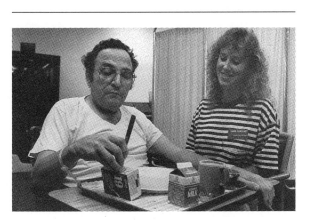

Figure 7-9 Opening a box with one hand presents a problem-solving opportunity.

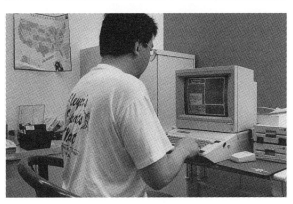

Figure 7-11 This patient enjoys playing high-level computer games that require memory and problem solving.

clude anticipatory problem solving. If a goal of anticipatory problem solving is being considered, be sure that the patient is capable of abstract reasoning and that he or she was able to use this technique prior to the stroke. Methods such as minimizing distractions to allow the patient to focus on relevant aspects of a task can facilitate problem solving. Cuing the patient to slow performance in order to think about alternatives and the consequences of intended actions may also prove helpful. Eventually, the patient should be taught to monitor behavior independently, to slow the pace of a task, and to think before acting.

The patient should be encouraged to generate several solutions to each problem. If he or she is capable of covert problem solving, these solutions can be generated ahead of time. If the patient is at a trial-and-error level, various solutions should be tried during actual problem situations (Figure 7-12). The patient should be encouraged to evaluate the effectiveness of the various solutions.

Planning

Planning skills can be promoted by offering opportunities to plan and carry out multistep tasks. The amount of material, number of steps, and complexity of the task can be graded to increase challenge. Planning a short activity, such as a simple meal, should precede planning a longer task, such as a community trip (Figure 7-13). The use of work-simplification techniques should be encouraged. Time constraints can challenge planning skills further. For example, it is more difficult to prepare a simple lunch in 10 minutes than to use an entire hour. The therapist initially should use a mutual problem-solving approach. By solving problems with the patient, the OT can prompt consideration of a variety of factors relevant to task performance after a CVA.

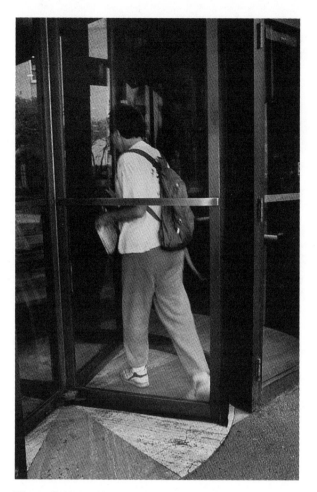

Figure 7-13 Multistep community activities require a wide range of problem-solving skills.

Once a plan has been devised, the patient with adequate language skills can write down the sequence of the activity to facilitate orderly task completion. Pictorial cues can sometimes assist the aphasic patient's ability to organize a task. Gradually the patient should be given more responsibility to plan and carry out tasks without intervention.

Implementation

Poor problem-solving skills frequently result in decreased safety. When safety is compromised, the OT might suggest structuring the environment to minimize distractions and obstacles. For example, the patient who persistently attempts to stand and step over wheel chair foot plates might be better served by removing them. The therapist can provide graded structure and cuing to gradually allow the patient to make some decisions. The safety implications of an action should also be discussed with the patient. Alternative actions that would promote increased safety can be suggested. Un-

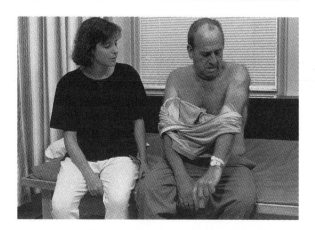

Figure 7-12 Encouragement is given to generate solutions to problems encountered during upper extremity dressing.

like other areas of problem solving, goals for safety are frequently written for patients at all levels of function. Safety is of primary importance to the patient, the family, and reimbursers. Although problem solving as a whole is a high-level skill, the importance of safety makes it an appropriate goal area for many patients. Safety may be addressed through use of compensation devices, environmental modification, remediation of component skill deficits such as visual attention or body awareness, and improvement of problem-solving skills.

Self-Monitoring

The patient must learn to evaluate his or her performance independently as the activity is occurring. Judgment is required to analyze how the task is proceeding and whether changes should be made. To promote this skill, the therapist can encourage the patient to evaluate his or her actions and can provide cues to attend to relevant information in the environment. Gradually the difficulty of the tasks should increase. Eventually the patient should be required to analyze subtle features of a problem and make quick decisions. Ongoing decision making and alteration of plans based on environmental factors should be encouraged. This requires rapid integration of various environmental features.

Outcome

The final outcome should be reviewed with the patient. Was the task completed safely and efficiently? Were the goals met? Problems should be discussed and alternative actions considered. By modeling effective problem solving and by assisting the patient to consider all facets of a situation, function can be improved. Gradually the high-level patient should be able to analyze problems without help. At this point, he or she will have achieved true independence.

PERCEPTUAL TREATMENT IDEAS

Visual Perception

Sensory Registration

When deficits in primary visual processes are revealed through screening or are suspected through observation, referral to an optometrist is recommended. The optometrist can define problem areas more specifically and can provide corrective lenses, or in some cases may prescribe vision therapy (Cohen and Soden 1981; Gianutsos et al. 1988, 1989). Visual field defects, which may occur in combination with or independently of unilateral visual inattention, can be treated as described under unilateral visual inattention. Although visual retraining techniques are beyond the scope of this book, occupational therapists in rehabilitation settings are working with optometrists to provide specialized visual therapy. Advanced training through consultation, workshops, and reading is advised before offering this type of treatment.

Unilateral Visual Inattention

Unilateral visual inattention is one of the most frequently encountered visual perceptual deficits. Its severity may range from total neglect of one half of visual space to subtle deficits only with rapidly presented or complex visual information. Although it is common, research is unclear about the underlying mechanisms of the deficit. Some authors believe that attention is the underlying problem, while others point to a deficiency in visual motor scanning. Probably the most accurate explanations are those that point to various factors, any combination of which can lead to neglect.

Description of Unilateral Visual Inattention. Mesulam (1981) describes an integrated network consisting of four brain regions that work together to direct attention to extrapersonal space. The posterior parietal component provides an internal sensory map and may best be tested through bilateral simultaneous stimulation. In this area, the ability to attend to visual stimuli contralateral to the lesion is regulated. When a lesion affects the posterior parietal area, the patient may be able to focus on visual information presented on the affected side only if there are no distracting stimuli on the unaffected side. When relevant visual information is presented in both visual fields, the intact side takes precedence and information in the impaired field is extinguished. In mild cases this may be seen only when two equally relevant stimuli are presented in the extreme visual fields. A patient with severe deficits, however, may be distracted by any environmental stimuli.

The frontal component regulates movement of the eyes and limbs into contralateral space. Patients with lesions in this area may have marked difficulty moving the eyes past midline. More theoretically, Mesulam (1981) proposes that the cingulate area enhances awareness of events of biological importance, and that the reticular component regulates general arousal. Deficits in one area may lead to mild neglect, whereas deficits in many areas will lead to more severe problems. The author stresses the interconnections of various areas in the brain and suggests that improper internal representation on the sensory map will lead to faulty movement and, conversely, that faulty movement will lead to improper sensory input.

Treatment of Severe Deficits. Because severe deficits in visual attention most likely affect older, deeper, brain structures, treatment strategies that emphasize whole-body movements, multisensory stimulation, and concrete activities will be most effective. When the deficits are severe, it may appear that the patient is unable to process even unilateral visual stimuli on the affected side. Mesulam (1981) recommends darkening the room to diminish environmental stimuli and then using a penlight to test each visual field unilaterally and bilaterally.

For severely involved patients, the types of stimuli are important in eliciting attention to the neglected side. The therapist should experiment to determine the best activities for promoting visual attention. For many patients, self-care skills provide a relevant task that can stimulate improved awareness of the affected side. Searching for a favorite food, soap, or a sweater when chilled can be very motivating. Frequently, severely affected patients also show marked unilateral tactile neglect. Activities such as oral/facial hygiene, bathing, and dressing promote tactile and visual awareness. A patient who is frustrated by a severe deficit and resistive to ADL performance may respond if he or she is expected to participate in only a small portion of the task. For instance, once a washcloth is prepared, the patient can be asked to take it and wash his or her face.

Increasing Awareness of the Deficit. Since patients frequently are not cognizant of unilateral visual inattention, therapy should first be directed at increasing their awareness of how the deficit affects function. Many self-care activities provide feedback about whether a task was performed correctly. For example, use of a telephone requires a patient to search for the numbers (Figure 7-14). If they are not correctly identified, a wrong number is reached. The patient receives immedi-

ate feedback about the effectiveness of his or her actions. For a lower-level patient, assistance in locating needed items during ADL tasks or help in becoming aware of obstacles during wheelchair mobility will concretely point out the necessity of scanning the affected visual field. When the patient has adequate cognitive skills to recognize the problem, the therapist should help the patient identify instances when visual inattention caused difficulties. Self-cuing or asking the caregiver to give verbal reminders or tactile cues to turn the head and eyes to the affected side can be helpful.

Some severely affected patients will be unable to recognize the impact of unilateral visual inattention even in concrete activities. Caregiver teaching should then be a priority. The caregiver should observe ADL tasks and be shown tests that clearly demonstrate the neglect. It is not enough to describe the deficit. Showing the caregiver how the problem affects the patient's performance and then teaching strategies for cuing or compensation will improve understanding and carryover. When a caregiver is learning to cue a patient, he or she should be given opportunities to practice, with the therapist offering feedback.

Multisensory Stimulation. Warren (1990) states that providing multisensory stimulation through a single activity is most effective in treating unilateral visual inattention because it promotes increased arousal and attention. In contrast, sensory information coming from a variety of sources can cause the brain to tune out what is interpreted as extraneous information. Multisensory stimulation can be added to an activity by integrating movement, tactile qualities such as weight or texture, and auditory cues into a single goal-directed task. When auditory cues are being used, the therapist should be positioned close to the target object. Otherwise, the auditory input may be distracting and result in decreased attention to the task. Olfactory properties can be incorporated into feeding or hygiene tasks by using the smells of certain foods or the scents of lotions and colognes to help encourage the patient's visual search.

Many traditional occupational therapy activities combine several sensory properties. Searching for items on a tray, on a counter, or in a drawer requires a moderate degree of attention to the affected side. For some patients, craft activities can be motivating. Materials can be placed in the affected visual field while the activity is positioned at midline to promote awareness of the entire space. Finding items in the clinic, in a cupboard, or in the community requires attention to a larger visual area.

In the clinic, large boards can be used to play checkers, and reaching activities can be set up to promote

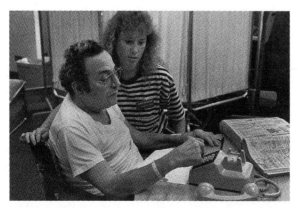

Figure 7-14 Using a telephone requires visual attention to the affected side.

awareness of an affected visual field. Warren (1990) suggests activities such as erasing letters from a blackboard; matching playing cards, baseball cards, or visual illusion cards; playing dominoes; or performing letter cancellation tasks with large sheets of paper (Figure 7-15). Large Velcro boards can be constructed on which shapes, letters, cards, or numbers for scanning or matching can be arranged (Figure 7-16). These activities first should be organized in a structured way, in columns and rows, for example. As scanning improves, the items can be scattered randomly to increase the challenge. The distance between items and the sizes of the stimuli can be varied to grade the challenge. Visual mazes or trails of objects that must be followed visually from one point to another can be provided to further increase the level of difficulty. Proprioceptive neuromuscular facilitation (PNF) diagonals can be used with reaching activities or in isolation. The patient is asked to keep his or her eyes on the hand, thus promoting visual and tactile attention in combination with vestibular stimulation (Figures 7-17 and 7-18).

The Eyespan device from ATHCO gives multisensory stimulation by requiring that the patient respond to a light by pointing. An auditory signal provides feedback when the correct light is touched. Warren (1990) reports successful clinical use of this product; however, Robertson and his associates (1990) cite a study in which light board training was not found to have significant carry-over to other types of scanning tasks. It is important, therefore, to use caution when training visual attention with clinical activities. Training activities must be followed with functional tasks that use the same skills in order to improve the likelihood of carry-over.

The items used in these activities should always appeal to the patient. As discussed in Chapter 6, the thera-

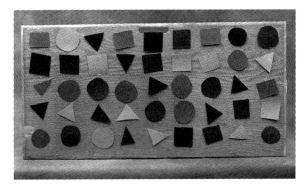

Figure 7-16 The patient can be asked to remove specific shapes on this board to encourage visual scanning and visual attention.

pist must consider the emotional tones that an activity might elicit, and choose carefully those that promote maximal involvement from the patient. In some cases the patient may be willing to participate in a task if sufficient rationale is given. The therapist should be aware of unspoken feelings, however, and realize that at times feelings may not be divulged for fear of offending the therapist. Since almost all tasks require visual scanning, the creative therapist with a good understanding of the patient should be able to provide a variety of activities that are effective and motivating.

While multisensory stimulation is generally helpful, the therapist must be careful not to overload the patient. Herman (1992) provides an excellent description of three theories of spatial neglect and proposes various treatment approaches based on these theories. She suggests the use of shapes and forms that stimulate the right brain while limiting the use of letters and numbers that stimulate the left brain. Manipulation of objects in the left visual field with the left hand can further stimulate right brain functions. Cuing to turn the head and providing advanced warning that information will be provided in the affected field can be helpful. Use of excessive verbal stimulation should be avoided because it will activate the dominant hemisphere, thus making attention to the left more difficult. Limiting the amount of stimuli in the right visual field will help the patient attend to the left. As in all treatment approaches, careful thought will help the therapist grade the type and amount of stimulation and challenge based on the patient's unique skills and goals.

Vestibular Stimulation. Pizzamiglio et al. (1990) describe studies of caloric stimulation of the vestibular system with resulting improvements in visual attention to the affected side. They propose that vestibular stimulation increases the attentional bias toward the affected

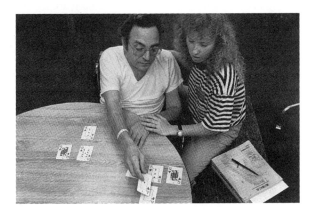

Figure 7-15 Attention to the affected side is required for this card game.

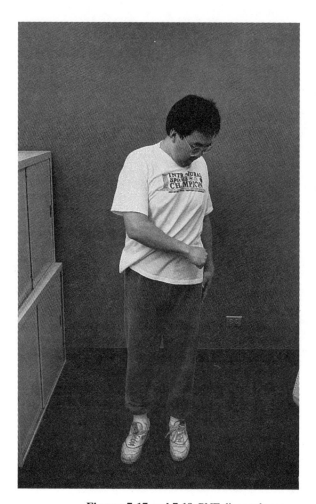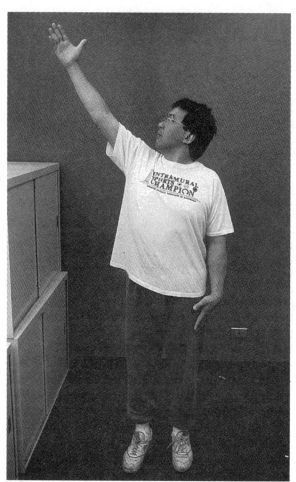

Figures 7-17 and 7-18 PNF diagonals encourage visual and tactile attention to the affected side.

body side. They conducted an experiment in which moving stimuli were presented to 33 patients with left visual inattention. The moving stimuli were presented in either a leftward or rightward direction until nystagmus was observed; the patient was then asked to bisect a line. Significant displacement of the perception of center was induced by both the rightward and leftward movement. For left hemiplegic patients, they propose that stimulating the optokinetic reflex through moving visual stimuli can be useful in treating visual spatial inattention especially during the early stages of therapy. Furthermore, based on other research, they believe that spatial awareness can be stimulated by vestibular, optokinetic, and/or vibratory information. Depending on the location of the lesion, they feel that one or more of these systems can be helpful in temporarily reducing spatial bias toward the unaffected side.

Farber and Zoltan (1989) describe various visual-vestibular interactions. Although they found little documented research on the benefits of using vestibular

stimulation with brain injured adults, they propose that, based on research with children and normal adults, this form of treatment may be useful. Treatment implications extrapolated from the literature indicate that providing stimulation immediately prior to a learning activity may be most effective, that stimulation may improve the ability to organize environmental stimuli, and that vestibular stimulation may increase visual exploratory behavior.

Visual Scanning Training. For patients with failure to orient the eyes to the affected side, or for those with unsystematic scanning patterns, organized patterns must be taught. The patient can be cued always to begin the scanning pattern in the affected field to improve integration, to view reading material from left to right and top to bottom, and to use a clockwise scanning pattern for less structured visual scanning such as when attempting to locate a razor on a night stand. Initially, head movements may accompany all attempts to compensate for the visual neglect. The goal, however, should be to use eye movements toward the affected side without head movement (Bouska et al. 1985).

Tactile Exploration To Enhance Visual Scanning. Controversy exists in the literature about the effects of using tactile exploration with visual scanning to improve performance. Weinberg and his associates (1977) classified neglect based on the patient's execution of cancellation tasks and the presence of visual field deficits on confrontation. They found that systematic visual scanning training improved performance in academic tasks. Their training program used the principles of

- anchoring, in which a cue is provided to initiate scanning in the impaired visual field
- pacing, in which the patient is encouraged to delay a response in order to minimize impulsive answers
- density, in which the distance between target stimuli is increased to improve responses
- feedback, in which the patient is given information about performance.

In a later study of 53 patients (Weinberg et al. 1979), they found that adding sensory awareness and spatial organization training further improved visual awareness. They suggest encouraging the patient to look to the left and then asking him or her to tactiley explore that area to confirm what was seen. These authors did not specifically relate improvements in test scores to improved function; however, they proposed that improvements would occur.

Chedru (1976) studied 91 right-side and left-side hemiplegics both with and without clinical signs of visual neglect. He defined neglect that affected daily activities as major neglect, and neglect seen only in drawing or writing as minor neglect. He asked each group of patients to tap keys on a keyboard with their eyes occluded and with their eyes open. In contrast to other authors, he found that most of the patients with visual neglect performed the task more symmetrically when vision was occluded.

It is possible that the patients Chedru selected, on the basis of functional signs, were different from those selected by researchers who based their selection on performance of paper-and-pencil tasks or confrontational testing. It is also possible that neglect of visual information and bodily sensations are different. Some patients may show both types of neglect and others may only show one type. Chedru concludes that for patients with primarily a visual neglect, exploration with eyes closed and then with eyes open may improve awareness of the affected side. This technique would be suitable for

some clinical activities; however, it would have limited application when the task involves messy or potentially dangerous items. While eating, for instance, it would usually be too messy to ask the patient to explore the tray manually with eyes closed.

Use of Paper-and-Pencil Tasks. The use of paper-and-pencil tasks for training visual awareness is frequently reported in the literature (Carter et al. 1988; Anderson and Choy 1970). Most of the studies, however, show improvements in academic skills or other paper-and-pencil tasks similar to the training material (Robertson et al. 1990). Poor carry-over to other types of functional tasks has been found. Therefore, when paper-and-pencil activities are used, they should relate to a functional task relevant to the patient. For instance, when a patient desires to read or write for work or pleasure, paper-and-pencil scanning tasks may have value. When used as part of a carefully graded program designed to enhance skill transfer (Toglia 1991), they also may have value. When the patient does not routinely engage in paper-and-pencil activities, however, other tasks related to his or her interests and roles are usually more appropriate.

Upgrading Speed and Complexity of Tasks. As awareness of the affected visual field improves, objects can be placed farther from midline, the complexity of the task can be increased, and a faster response speed can be required. Increasing the complexity of the task forces the patient to handle effectively the visual attention aspects, the motor aspects, and the cognitive aspects of the task simultaneously. When a patient begins to master a task, the therapist must carefully upgrade the skill requirement to maintain challenge without creating frustration.

For instance, consider a patient who is able to sit on the edge of a mat, reach for functional objects placed at waist height in the left visual field, and place them on the floor to the right. The activity can be upgraded in many ways. The position of the patient can be changed. He or she can be assisted to a kneel-standing position or perhaps is able to work in a standing position. He or she can remain in the sitting position, but can be asked to sort cards by color, suit, or numerical order, thus increasing the cognitive demands of the task (Figure 7-19). Finally, the response speed could be increased by requiring the patient to quickly pick up an object that was touched briefly by the therapist.

When visual attention is adequate for static activities, speed can be introduced by playing games such as catch or balloon volleyball; by working on mobility in a busy clinic or in the community (Figure 7-20); or by taking a high-level patient on a bus or car trip, during

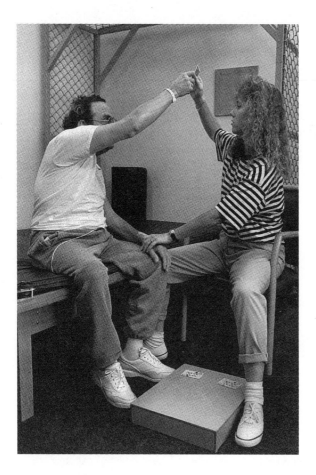

Figure 7-19 This card-sorting task is made more difficult by increasing the motoric demands.

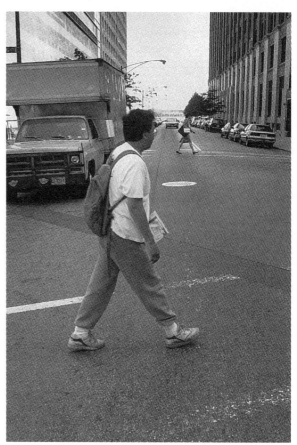

Figure 7-20 Visual attention is challenged in the community because the environment is less predictable, the area to be monitored is large, and fast response speeds are required.

which he or she must observe for landmarks and street signs.

Use of Computers. Computer games or programs designed to promote visual attention, such as SEARCH by Life Science Associates, may also be effective for introducing speed to visual attention tasks; however, support for using computer activities to improve visual scanning training is limited (Herman 1992). In a well-designed study, Robertson and his associates (1990) studied 36 patients with neglect, 33 of whom had had a CVA. A mean number of 15.5 hours of intensive computerized visual scanning and attention training was provided to the 20 patients in the treatment group. In contrast to single-case studies that are cited, they found no significant improvement in the treatment versus the control group. Although the computer may be valuable in treating other cognitive and perceptual deficits, Robertson et al. recommend treating visual scanning deficits during functional tasks.

Ross (1992) offers a comprehensive review of the literature about the use of computers for visual scanning training and describes a study of computer training with three head injured patients. Her study revealed that software intervention for visual scanning did not result in improved functional performance. Despite the results of her research, she believes that computer intervention can be one tool for addressing particular cognitive or perceptual problems, but that its use should always be combined with functional activities. The therapist's ability to select appropriate software based on the targeted cognitive problem, his or her ability to grade computerized and noncomputerized activities, and the ability to assist the patient in translating computer learning to functional experiences all influence the usefulness of the tool.

It is believed that a computer should be used for treatment of visual inattention only after careful consideration of the patient's interests and goals. In most cases functional activities would be more appropriate for treatment. When selected as an activity, it should be complemented by numerous functional activities in which the same skills are practiced. Awareness of the patient's ability to generalize information can help the therapist determine whether this modality is appropriate. For patients who will use a computer at home, for leisure, or in work activities, it may be a very appropriate and meaningful activity. For other high-level patients who are able to generalize learning, the computer can provide graded activities, repetition, and immediate feedback.

Bed Positioning. Positioning a patient's bed to promote sensory stimulation to the involved side is often suggested as a method of improving visual awareness. Interestingly, a study by Loverro and Reding (1988) found no difference in outcome for rehabilitation patients whose beds were oriented to provide visual stimulation to the neglected side versus those whose bed positions provided stimulation to the unaffected side. Possibly this is due to the fact that the active multisensory stimulation occurring during the bulk of the day influenced improvement more than did the passive positioning of the patient in bed.

Compensation Techniques. Compensation methods might include the use of brightly colored markers to call attention to the neglected side of a page. Use of a finger or a blank sheet of paper as a guide for reading can also help improve anchoring and organization (Figure 7-21). Numbers can be placed on the lines of an activity to ensure that the correct sequence is followed and that the entire line is reviewed. A patient's pace can be slowed by asking him or her to name or point to each item in the sequence. All compensation techniques should be practiced first during a simple activity. Gradually the complexity and motor demands can be increased while decreasing the number of cues provided. Many of these compensation methods can be used as training techniques by gradually withdrawing them as improvements are seen.

Task Modification. When the patient is unable to use compensation strategies independently and caregivers are not available to provide cues, it may be necessary to place self-care objects, the call light, and meals in the unaffected visual field. As a practical measure, placing items where they can be seen may increase independence. When improvement in visual awareness occurs, functional items can be moved gradually to a midline position and eventually can be used to facilitate visual searching in the affected field. Likewise, if the patient is unable to attend to any information presented on the affected side, the therapist and the activity should be positioned on the unaffected side to ensure that stimulation is provided. Gradually the OT will move toward the affected visual field to facilitate bilateral awareness.

Visual Spatial Awareness

Because table-top activities such as copying peg designs for visual spatial awareness are generally not advocated and all activities involve a motor component, treatment techniques are discussed under visual construction. If the patient's poor awareness of his or her body in space is believed to be the cause of deficits in visual spatial awareness, the treatment listed under body awareness would be used. Activities that combine body awareness and visual spatial skills provide the highest level of challenge. Propelling the wheelchair in the clinic requires adequate awareness of visual information as well as knowledge of the position of one's body relative to the environment. Higher level patients can be asked to push a grocery cart in a busy store or to maneuver with a cane in a crowd. Frequent opportunities to combine movement with visual awareness should be provided.

Visual Analysis and Synthesis

Both Benton (1985) and Bouska et al. (1985) use visual analysis and synthesis to describe visual perceptual activities that require integration of visual perceptual and cognitive skills. Tasks such as recognizing fine distinctions between objects, discriminating foreground from background, and combining parts to form a whole are included. These authors suggest that this skill is qualitatively different from other types of cognitive skills, since a patient may show good verbal analytical and synthetic abilities but be unable to perform visually. Like all perceptual skills, visual analysis and synthesis require correct processing at various levels in the brain. Adequate sensory registration, the ability to

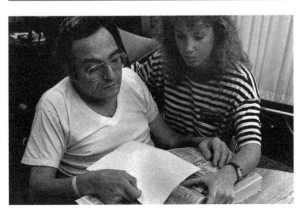

Figure 7-21 A sheet of paper used as a guide helps this patient attend to the relevant information.

detect spatial differences, sufficient attention, the ability to organize information, and memory are required.

The treatment of this type of deficit is poorly documented compared with treatment techniques for unilateral visual neglect. When the problems are due to deficits in attention, spatial perception, or sensory awareness, those skills should be addressed specifically. When integration at a more complex level is affected, several strategies may be used. Bouska et al. (1985) advocate helping patients with visual analysis difficulties to distinguish finer and finer details when they view an object or picture. This may be done by gradually introducing materials with smaller details, more subtle characteristics, or a more distracting background. They suggest asking the patient to highlight distinctive details by using colored markers. Drawing can also enhance awareness of visual details. Writing or discussion also can be encouraged to enhance awareness of visual information.

In our department most visual processing activities are presented in the context of functional therapeutic tasks. Table-top visual analysis and synthesis activities are rarely used. A very-high-level patient with clearly identified problems in this area who has a strong motivation to improve skills might be given structured table-top visual analysis activities of graded difficulty. The skills that are emphasized in these structured tasks would then be applied to functional activities.

Functionally, finding items in the clinic, on shelves, or in drawers requires visual analysis and synthesis. Sorting items such as laundry, cards, or coins requires varying degrees of visual analysis. Many of the visual scanning activities that are listed under unilateral visual inattention require visual analysis and synthesis.

As skills improve, more challenge can be introduced by obscuring part of the item, placing very similar objects together, or scattering the items in a random way. A clinic cabinet can provide high-level challenges. Computer programs can present simple or complex visual information at a variety of speeds. By increasing complexity and speed, the demands on visual analysis and synthesis skills increase. Community activities such as buying spices at a grocery story, choosing a birthday card at a drugstore, finding a book in the library, locating an item on a menu, or following sports figures on a playing field present high-level challenges. Adequate attention to these more complex forms of visual perception is important. Tobis et al. (1990) find that elderly people rely more on visual perception to prevent falls and maintain balance than do younger subjects. The influence of visual perception on safe mobility may be even greater for stroke patients who generally have impaired motor skills and balance re-

sponses. If visual perception is compromised, safety precautions must be emphasized to both patients and caregivers.

When improvements are slow and visual analysis and synthesis are interfering with function, compensation methods might be taught to the caregiver. The caregiver can observe the patient, while the therapist points out how the deficits interfere with function and provides suggestions to enhance independence. Good lighting for tasks and organized drawers, closets, and shelves are important. Extraneous items should be removed, and those that lack contrast, such as medicine bottles, should be kept in separate locations or should be clearly marked. Hazardous items should be removed. Items should be arranged so that features and colors contrast and so that the most used items are in the foreground. During meals, food should be presented one or two items at a time to minimize clutter (Siev et al. 1986). Objects can be marked to emphasize relevant features such as an on/off switch. When a patient has difficulty in locating the nurse call light, a red cover or colored tape can make it more distinctive. Similarly, brakes on the wheelchair can be highlighted with colored tape, or a shirt can be marked to distinguish the front from the back.

Visual Construction

Visual construction requires foundation skills of sensory registration, attention, scanning, visual spatial awareness, and visual analysis and synthesis; in addition, motor activity is required. It is the most complex of the visual perceptual skills. When any one of the component skills is impaired, treatment should address that area. In most cases, occupational therapy treatment will focus on visual perceptual and motor-planning skills. Complex constructional activities, which require the integration of various skills, can best be addressed during function.

Making a bed, preparing a sandwich, getting dressed, wrapping a gift, arranging flowers, folding a letter, stuffing an envelope, folding clothes, organizing dishes on a shelf, and placing cards on a bulletin board are examples of visual construction tasks that integrate various levels of visual processing and motor performance. Even a task such as pouring cereal into a bowl requires visual spatial awareness, coupled with motor control. Because the cereal must be poured into the bowl in a fairly precise way, it can be considered a simple construction task (Figure 7-22). Grading the complexity, amount of distraction, motoric challenge, and type of cuing can change the task demands.

Putting on a shirt is often a very complex task for patients with visual perceptual problems. Even though

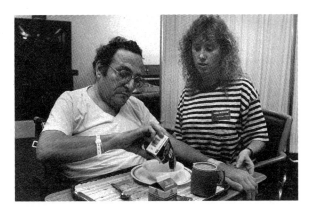

Figure 7-22 Pouring cereal into a bowl requires visual spatial awareness coupled with motor control, and can be considered a simple construction task.

lower extremity dressing requires more mobility, it seems to be perceptually less challenging, possibly because the activity takes place within full view. To improve performance in upper extremity dressing, the patient can be encouraged to look for distinctive features, such as a collar or a label, in order to orient the shirt correctly. When buttoning is difficult, pullover or zipper shirts can be suggested, or buttoned shirts can be left partially buttoned and worn as pullover shirts (Figure 7-23). Alternately, the patient can be cued to always start at the bottom of the shirt, where buttons and buttonholes are more easily aligned. To make a sleeve more visible and prevent tangling, it can be dangled between the knees. Tips such as "make sure the armhole is past the elbow" before the patient attempts to insert the other arm can help keep the shirt from becoming twisted. When possible, the therapist should help the patient use familiar methods of dressing.

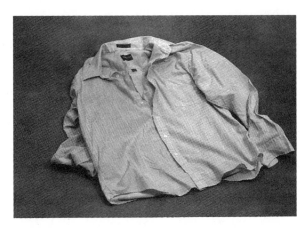

Figure 7-23 Partially buttoning a shirt can make putting it on easier.

For those who have an interest in handicrafts or home repairs, these make excellent visual construction activities. They can be made simple or complex; can be graded by providing assistance; and can be taught by using demonstrated, written, verbal, or pictorial instructions. In addition, they provide multisensory stimulation.

Caution must be used when choosing clinic activities for treatment of constructional deficits. In a study of treatment for constructional deficits in head injured patients, Neistadt (1992) found that functional skills training was more effective than perceptual training (although the difference was not statistically significant) in improving functional test scores. Task specific learning was shown, and patients who participated in perceptual tasks improved on tests that measured that particular activity. Her results suggested that these patients did not learn any general strategies that could be transferred to other activities. Although some attempts were made to use techniques described by Toglia (1991) to promote transfer of learning, Neistadt (1992) speculates that perhaps there was not enough variation in treatment activities to promote generalization. She recommends emphasis on a functional training approach when treating this population. Although the results of her research with head injured patients cannot be applied specifically to patients with strokes, it can be conjectured that perhaps CVA patients may have similar difficulties in transferring learning. Experience suggests that patients who show more significant cognitive and perceptual deficits learn best in a task specific manner. Those with mild cognitive and perceptual limitations appear to be more able to generalize information.

While a few patients may enjoy puzzles, those that are basic enough for people with constructional deficits are often demeaning. Simple animal or face puzzles designed from photographs or a series of graded outdoor-scene puzzles are available and may be interesting to some adults. Peg designs or parquetry designs might appeal to some patients when they are incorporated into motor activities. They should not be used as a static table-top task. Neistadt (1989) stresses the need for carefully graded tasks and suggests that parquetry tasks can be graded as follows: colored patterns with full detail, black and white patterns with full detail, colored patterns with partial detail, and black and white patterns with partial detail. She found that when given a clear explanation of the relationship to function, sufficient challenge, and feedback about speed of performance, clients experienced more satisfaction with the activity. If a person enjoys drawing, he or she can be asked to copy simple designs of figures. To increase tactile and kinesthetic properties, drawing in powder, in sand, or on a clay board may be introduced. The game "Pictionary" incorporates drawing in a competitive, time-limited activity.

Body Awareness

Since body awareness is defined in this book as the integration of sensory and perceptual components allowing accurate visualization of the body, treatment is generally directed at the interfering component parts. Thus, sensory input will be provided if that is thought to be the basis of the problem, whereas emphasis on midline orientation, bilateral integration, or tactile discrimination might be appropriate for another patient. Each of these categories is discussed below.

Tactile Sensory Loss

There is little literature to support treatment of primary tactile sensory loss in brain-damaged individuals. It may be hypothesized that sensory retraining can provide some benefit due to brain plasticity. Treatment of tactile inattention or impaired tactile discrimination may be more effective. Refer to those sections for ideas to improve awareness of tactile sensation.

In some low-functioning patients, the protective tactile system may be working while the discriminative system is not. These patients may be tactilely defensive. Deep stroking in the direction of hair growth, weight bearing, and proprioceptive input can be calming (Chapparo and Ranka 1987).

Compensation for sensory loss is important for safety. The patient can be taught to test water temperature by using the unaffected extremity prior to bathing or washing. The patient must visually monitor the affected side near hot items such as radiators, stoves, or lighted cigarettes. Likewise, the extremity must be monitored during mobility or when using sharp objects, to prevent bumps, bruises, and cuts. Armboards,

lapboards, or slings might be used when the patient is unable to monitor the upper extremity effectively (see also "Safely Managing the Affected Extremity").

Unilateral Tactile Inattention

Unilateral tactile inattention may be seen in affected limbs as well as in more central aspects of the body. Since unilateral tactile inattention appears to be related to unilateral visual inattention, treatment of both deficits can be more effective than treating only one. Weinberg et al. (1979) found that combining sensory awareness and spatial organization tasks with visual scanning was highly successful, especially with more severely involved patients. Patients who demonstrate difficulty with unilateral tactile awareness and decreased awareness of double simultaneous stimuli should be given cues and graded opportunities to experience sensory input on the affected side. Neglect of one side of the face is sometimes seen during oral/facial hygiene. Patients can be encouraged to attend to the sensations that occur when they are washing, shaving, applying makeup, brushing their teeth, or combing their hair (Figure 7-24).

Stimulation should be applied in a quiet environment, and the patient should be encouraged to attend to, and describe, the sensation. A wide range of Bobath techniques and other neurorehabilitation procedures lend themselves to increasing awareness and control of the affected body side. As attention increases, the patient can be challenged to focus on more complex tactile sensations in a more stimulating environment.

Tactile awareness may be enhanced by providing stimulation during clinic and self-care activities. Rough textures, such as Velcro, can be applied to self-care objects to increase sensory input. The textures of items such as a washcloth, shirt, water, and lotion can be pointed out and the patient can be encouraged to attend to these properties as the items are being used (Figure

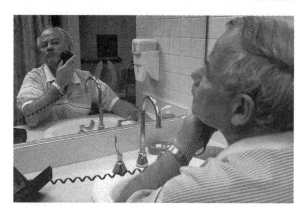

Figure 7-24 Shaving provides sensory input to the affected side of the face.

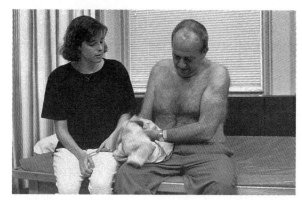

Figure 7-25 Upper extremity dressing promotes awareness of the affected arm.

7-25). During motor retraining and range of motion (ROM) exercises, proprioceptive, kinesthetic, and tactile input provides sensory stimulation. The patient can be given cues to watch the extremity as stimulation is applied (Anderson and Choy 1970), to attend to the sensations and can be asked to compare feelings on the affected side with those on the unaffected side.

Although some therapists advocate bilateral activities, their use is controversial because they do not promote normal movement and because, when two limbs are used together, extinction of sensation in the affected extremity may occur. Patients who show extinction on unilateral tactile attention tests, therefore, should not work bilaterally. First, the patient will need to be aware of sensory input directed primarily to the affected side. Once attention to unilateral sensation is reliable, bilateral or more challenging activities can be introduced gradually. At this stage, incorporation of the affected arm as a stabilizer or as an active assistant during dressing or hygiene can be useful. Just as the therapist working on unilateral visual attention would not begin training in a highly distracting, unfamiliar environment, the OT working on unilateral tactile attention would not begin with multisensory, bilateral movements.

When motor recovery is slow, the use of guiding techniques can be helpful to provide more normal tactile, kinesthetic, and functional input to the affected limb (Figure 7-26). The technique of guiding—which was developed by Affolter (1987), a speech pathologist, to aid voice production—is useful for providing meaningful sensory input. To perform this technique as described by Davis (1988), the therapist places his or her hand over the patient's affected hand and guides the hand through the task. Contact with a surface is maintained throughout the movement to increase the patient's ability to process the tactile information. The therapist must be sensitive to direct the patient's hand in a way that is natural, so that normal movement patterns are experienced and the rhythm of performance is not interrupted (Davis 1988).

As the patient becomes more aware of the affected extremity and unilateral control improves, tasks that involve bilateral simultaneous attention can be introduced. For instance, the patient may be able to attend to the affected arm when engaged in unilateral therapeutic activities. When he or she begins working with the unaffected arm and the affected arm simultaneously, however, attention is lost. This is also seen when a patient is asked to carry an item while walking. The patient's focus on the mechanics of ambulation may cause him or her to forget the object in the affected hand. Although good upper extremity control might be seen in more static tasks, it is lost as the number of distractors increases (Figures 7-27 and 7-28).

Patients with this type of problem might benefit from bilateral activities such as screwing a lid on a jar, wringing a cloth, washing dishes, stabilizing a package or envelope while opening it, stabilizing a bowl while mixing, hanging clothes on a line, folding clothes, preparing vegetables, zipping, buttoning, rolling hair, catching a large ball or balloon, tying shoes, or cutting paper. Many clinic activities, such as dowel rod exercises, towel exercises, active ROM exercises, and a wide range of other gross or fine motor activities, can be used to promote bilateral integration and awareness. These activities must be customized to match the motoric and attentional capabilities of each patient.

Safely Managing the Affected Extremity. To ensure safety, it is often necessary for the therapist to cue and assist the patient with upper extremity management. When the patient is turning in bed, PNF or Bobath techniques can be used to ensure safe movement of the arm. Generally, when the affected arm will be used as a passive stabilizer during a table-top activity, the therapist must be present to ensure proper positioning. A piece of Dycem under the forearm can help maintain the desired position. When supervision is not available and the patient has difficulty with self-monitoring, it may be best to position the affected arm at his or her side to prevent the arm from touching a hot plate or inadvertently sliding off the table.

In the wheelchair, a transparent lapboard can be used to position the arm in the visual field without blocking vision of the lower body. Lapboards are confining and may limit mobility; therefore, a more functional patient may benefit from an armboard. A supportive sling might be indicated for patients whose neglect is severe and damage to the extremity may result. These devices can position the arm safely and prevent injuries; however, the therapist must keep in mind their limitations. They promote static positioning, which can further in-

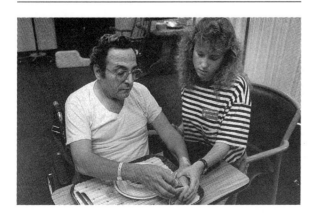

Figure 7-26 Guiding techniques provide sensory input during meaningful activities.

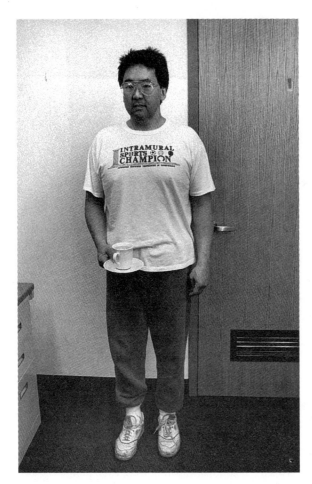

Figure 7-27 Good control is seen as the patient holds a cup and saucer while standing.

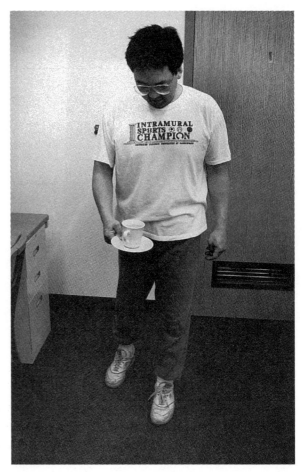

Figure 7-28 As the patient begins to walk, his attention is drawn to the task of mobility, and upper extremity control decreases.

hibit awareness, decrease spontaneous use, and increase tone. Alternative positioning devices such as an axilla roll or a humeral cuff sling may be appropriate for some patients, however, they do not protect the forearm and hand from injury. There are no solutions that work for all; therefore, the therapist must weigh the advantages and disadvantages for each patient.

Tactile Discrimination

Tactile discrimination requires refined sensory awareness. The patient who shows good attention to tactile stimulation during bilateral and challenging activities may benefit from improving tactile discrimination.

Specific techniques developed for retraining sensation after peripheral nerve injury can be used with a motivated and alert patient who has the potential to use his or her affected arm. A stimulus is applied to the hand, first with the patient's eyes open, then with the eyes closed. For example, a patient may be asked to feel sandpaper, first with the eyes open, then with them closed. He or she should be cued to attend to the sensations that are experienced. The patient may then be asked to discriminate between two textures. The task can be made more difficult by choosing textures or shapes that are very similar. Another activity requiring tactile discrimination involves finding objects hidden in a container of rice or beans through the sense of touch (Figures 7-29 and 7-30). This technique has been helpful in making patients more aware of the altered sensations that have resulted from the CVA.

Fox (1963) researched a technique for enhancing tactile discrimination. She found that a procedure of alternately rubbing the dorsum of the affected arm with a rough cloth for 30 seconds and then asking or assisting the patient to grasp the hard surface of a cup tightly for 30 seconds was effective (Figures 7-31 and 7-32). This procedure was to be carried out for at least four min-

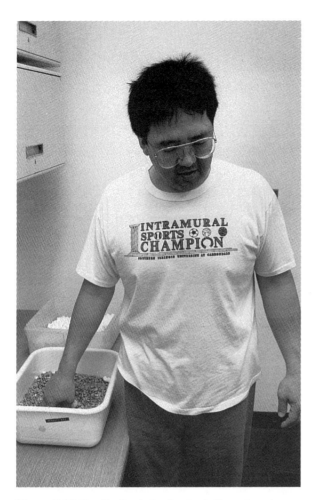

Figure 7-29 Tactile discrimination is challenged as the patient searches for an object with his hand.

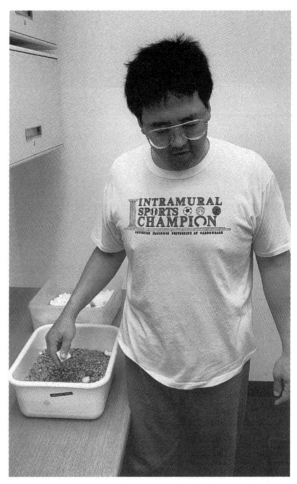

Figure 7-30 The patient is encouraged to attend to the sensation of the object in his hand.

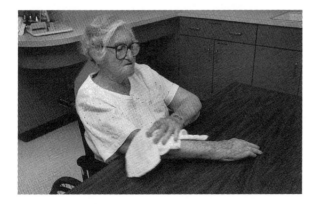

Figure 7-31 Rubbing the dorsum of the arm and . . .

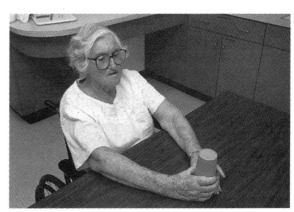

Figure 7-32 Grasping a cup is useful for enhancing tactile discrimination.

utes. The therapist must be alert for signs of discomfort or withdrawal and should change the area that is stimulated if such signs are noticed (Zoltan et al. 1986). Dannenbaum and Dykes (1990) suggest that sustained touch pressure should be considered when assessing functional tactile sensation. They point to clinical observations that patients are often aware of a sensation when the stimulus occurs, for example, when picking up an item; however, perception of the stimulus decreases as an item is being held. Dannenbaum and Dykes developed a device for measuring sustained touch pressure and, based on a small sample of patients, advocate retraining awareness of this type of sensation. Occupational therapists should be alert to further research in this area. While the techniques described in this book do not address sustained touch pressure specifically, the importance of helping the patient maintain sustained awareness of the affected extremity is emphasized.

Combining movement with tactile discrimination activities is thought to be helpful because the vestibular and tactile systems share many neurological links. Movement enhances participation in tactile tasks that require the discrimination of gross differences between objects. It also helps to integrate tactile and motor responses at a subcortical level. For example, asking the patient to describe tactile sensations experienced during a reaching activity may help improve discrimination. It must be realized, however, that when a person is asked to make fine distinctions, the body should be stable, allowing concentration on the sensory input. A person with no sensory limitations would have difficulty feeling the difference between a penny and a dime while being jostled in a crowd. Thus a patient should not be expected to attend to subtle distinctions while involved in a challenging motor task. As in all activities, motor, cognitive, and perceptual factors must be balanced to promote success. Eventually, as components of an integrated skill improve, they can be combined into more complex actions.

Body Parts Identification

To assist with labeling and organizing parts of the body, the therapist can use names of body parts during exercise, dressing, or grooming; can give directions using these names (e.g., shave your chin, touch your toes); and can ask the patient to name the part as activities are performed. Specific drills in which the patient is asked to point to or name a long series of body parts are not advocated.

Right-Left Identification

Because the use of right and left labels can be incorporated naturally into mobility, dressing, and exercise, it is thought that drilling the patient on the location of right and left is inappropriate. The therapist can use situations that arise spontaneously to teach and reinforce right-left concepts. A cue such as a watch, a ring, or a weight on one limb may help the patient to follow directions or to use these terms appropriately. If language or body awareness difficulties continue to limit the patient's ability to follow right-left instructions, the caregiver can be instructed to avoid the use of these terms. Rather, the caregiver can point to or describe the direction of movement (Zoltan et al. 1986).

Midline Orientation

When patients are unable to appreciate midline and cannot perceive when they are properly aligned, the therapist should provide opportunities to experience functional total body movements. These may include rolling, moving from supine to sitting, moving from sitting to standing, or other developmental positions, depending on the patient's motor skills. Since transitional movements are a functional necessity and should be in-

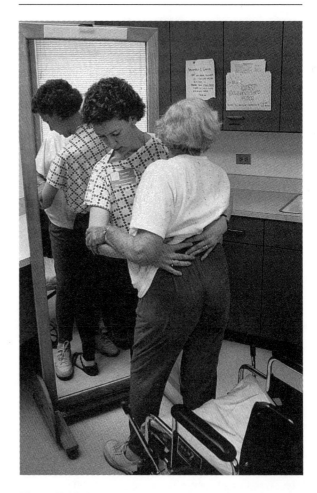

Figure 7-33 This patient pushes to the affected right side when standing.

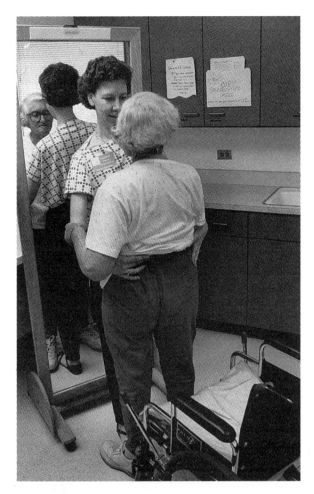

Figure 7-34 Facilitating and cuing . . .

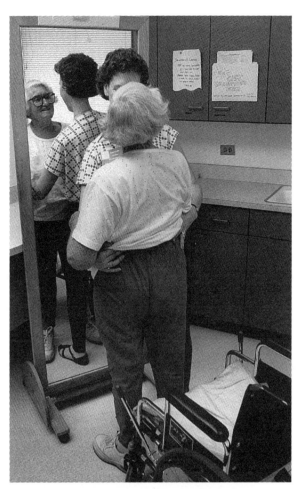

Figure 7-35 Promotes improved midline orientation.

troduced early in treatment, the therapist should facilitate body awareness when helping the patient move into various positions. Midline awareness is promoted through the use of Bobath techniques that encourage symmetrical postures, incorporation of the affected side, and equal weight bearing during movement. Techniques such as placing both hands on the affected knee when moving from sitting to standing can be helpful.

Because symmetrical short sitting is initially the posture that will be used in most functional tasks, it should be emphasized. Some patients may be fearful when in this position. The therapist can sit close to the patient's side with an arm around the patient's back to help promote anterior pelvic tilt. The patient's forearm may be placed on the therapist's thigh for weight bearing. The patient's feet should be supported so that the knees are slightly below the hips. A beanbag, bolster, or wedge can be placed behind the patient to provide added security. Alternatively, the therapist can sit or kneel behind the patient with his or her arms providing lateral security. In some cases, the patient may be so fearful of

movement that two therapists are needed to provide security and control. This would be an excellent opportunity for co-treatment with the physical therapist.

At times, a patient with poor midline orientation will push toward the affected side (Figure 7-33). If the patient is sitting, the therapist can sit on the sound side and encourage the patient to "keep your shoulder next to mine." When the patient is standing, the therapist may use his or her hand as a cue, e.g., "touch your shoulder to my hand." Standing the patient with his or her sound side near a wall or another solid surface can be helpful. The patient is then cued to maintain contact with the supporting surface. The aim is to position the patient correctly and securely so that normal posture can be experienced without fear (Figures 7-34 and 7-35).

If there is no history of significant degenerative joint disease, gentle joint approximation through the head and neck or through the shoulders can be provided to enhance sensory input and promote stability. Rhythmic stabilization techniques advocated by PNF theorists can be helpful for promoting stability in any position

(Figure 7-36). The patient should be encouraged to visualize his or her position and attend to the sensations of upright posture. As the patient improves in sitting, higher developmental positions, appropriate to the activities the patient will perform, can be introduced. For some patients these positions will include kneeling and half-kneeling; however, most patients will focus more on standing (Figure 7-37). In some cases a mirror or a vertical landmark can help patients orient themselves. Those who have severe visual perceptual problems, however, will have difficulty using visual cues.

Once the patient is able to tolerate static positions, slight movements away from midline can be introduced. It may be easiest to move toward the sound side first and then back to midline. As confidence is gained, the patient can be facilitated, using Bobath methods for adult hemiplegics, to move toward the affected side. Weight bearing can be incorporated into these movements. At first the movements will be small and the therapist will provide a lot of support. Reaching activi-

ties that promote more dynamic movement can then be added gradually. The therapist can decrease hands-on control by using a bolster, a wooden box, or a table to promote weight bearing on the affected arm and provide support on the patient's affected side. PNF patterns can be useful to challenge the patient further.

Forward and backward movements are also functional, and the patient must learn to move to and from a stable midline position in these directions. When asking the patient to move forward, the therapist should be positioned in front of the patient and can gently guide from the scapulae while supporting the patient's arms. A table or a ball placed in front may provide additional security (Figure 7-38). The patient can be asked to slide his or her arms forward on the table while the therapist facilitates symmetrical weight bearing and guides the movement. Gradually, the surface can be lowered. For example, a bench might be used next, with the patient eventually reaching to the floor. When midline orientation is sufficient to allow the patient to move easily into

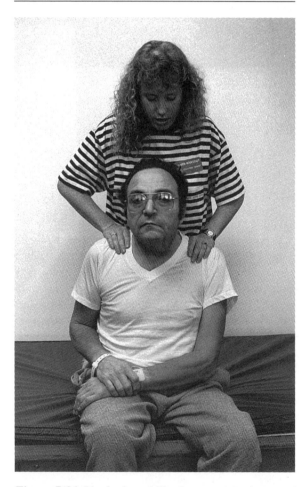

Figure 7-36 Rhythmic stabilization promotes improved midline awareness.

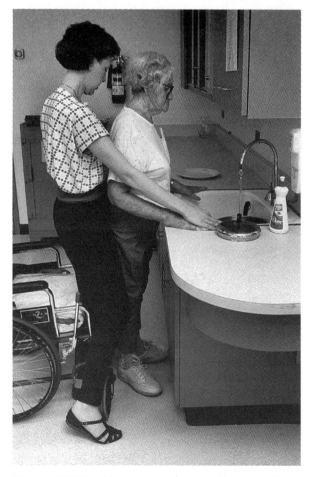

Figure 7-37 Working at a counter encourages midline awareness in standing during a functional activity.

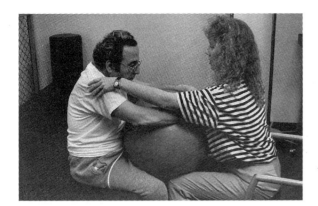

Figure 7-38 Symmetrical forward movement can be facilitated by using a ball.

and out of a variety of positions, speed can be added by playing catch or a balloon game. The patient who has gained control in sitting can work in standing or in an intermediate developmental position that corresponds to postures he or she will need for function.

Another approach to treating poor midline awareness is drawn from the work of Lackner (1988). He describes experiments in which vibratory stimuli applied under specified conditions causes people to experience changes in body orientation. He finds that the perceptual representation of the shape of the body is quite unstable. He speculates that the limbs may maintain accurate position sense through their interaction with the environment. The body, which does not interact to the same degree with the external environment, may maintain its somatosensory representation by contact with the mobile limbs (Lackner 1988). To speculate further on his theory, it can be imagined that a patient who loses mobility on one side of the body may experience changes in central body awareness, which in turn may lead to poor midline orientation. As therapists, we must therefore provide appropriate sensory motor stimulation to the limbs when addressing midline orientation. Aware of the powerful role that sensation has in influencing body perception, occupational therapists should take care to provide controlled and meaningful input. Guiding techniques (Affolter 1987) or neuro-reeducation activities may improve midline awareness by providing the central body with information about position in space through the limbs. Movement of the affected body side may help balance the input given by the nonaffected limbs and provide more accurate information about the body.

In a study of control subjects and patients with neglect, Mark and Heilman (1990) asked participants to locate the point at which their midline intersected a slit on a board placed in front of them. The subjects partici-

pated in various test conditions (i.e., vision of body occluded; vision of body not occluded; test slit positioned to the right, left, or center). Mark and Heilman found that the ability to see their body during the activity did not improve awareness of midline in patients with neglect. Although normal subjects showed a rightward bias during the vision occluded condition, their performance improved when able to see their body. A leftward slit led to leftward errors and a rightward slit led to rightward errors. The position of the slit influenced both normal and neglect subjects, however, those with neglect showed far greater inaccuracies. The authors described the phenomenon as a stimulus-bound overattraction to extrapersonal visual stimuli. Although the stimulus varied, Mark and Heilman's findings were similar to findings by Pizzamiglia et al. (1990) who studied exposure to a moving stimulus that induced optokinetic nystagmus. When the stimulus was not moving, they also found rightward displacement in both neglect and control subjects. Moving stimuli to the left led to leftward displacement and movement to the right led to rightward displacement. These studies indicate that visual stimulation in the left visual field can enhance both midline orientation and visual attention.

Motor Planning

Skilled motor planning relies on the integration of all cognitive and perceptual motor skills. When any subcomponents of motor planning are identified as faulty, treatment should be directed at their remediation. Treatment must also address the holistic activities that are required for function. Although the presence of aphasia does not ensure the presence of apraxia, or vice versa, the two deficits are closely associated. It is believed that language skills are closely tied to the conceptual aspects of motor planning. Through language, a person codes actions, rehearses movements, and sequences activities.

Role of Language in Treating Motor-Planning Deficits

In therapy, language can affect motor planning. It is thought that helping a patient state the steps of an activity vocally and eventually subvocally is beneficial. If the patient is unable to use language effectively, the therapist can provide verbal cues, pictorial cues, demonstration, and assistance. These cues should relate directly to the action of the activity, since too many unrelated words can be distracting. When a patient uses inappropriate words to guide motor actions, verbalizations should be stopped. Visual and kinesthetic cues should be used instead. Rhythm also may help sequence a task when words fail. When initiation and sequencing of speech is affected, as in Broca's aphasia, tactile cues can be used to initiate a motor action. Simple action words also may help give meaning to the movement (Chapparo and Ranka 1987).

For those with global aphasia, learning will be limited. Repetition of simple, familiar tasks in their usual context and at their usual times is beneficial. Soothing voice tones may help regulate the level of arousal. The patient should be assisted to manipulate objects, and hand-over-hand guidance can be given to increase his or her understanding of the action (Chapparo and Ranka 1987). If practice occurs regularly and in the same manner, it may be possible for the patient to code the information so that it becomes more automatic and no longer relies as heavily on verbal mediation. Providing encouragement and a motivating task can go a long way toward facilitating optimal performance.

When the execution stage of an activity is affected, excessive speech may confuse the patient. Reliance on prelearned sequences of movements is more beneficial. To illustrate the conceptual and execution stages of an activity, one can consider learning to type. At first, each key must be learned, and conscious attention is required to locate the correct letter. Drills are conducted in which letters are called out and typed. Language and conscious thought are very important in these initial stages of learning the task. When a person has learned to type well, he or she no longer thinks about each movement when touching a key. In fact, the more the person thinks about hand placement, the more difficult the task becomes. The activity is now carried out through the execution of a preprogrammed motor sequence. When the task features change, for instance, if the person moves from a manual to an electric keyboard, more conscious thought may again be required until the motor program is modified.

Treating Adults versus Children

Much of the occupational therapy literature dealing with apraxia focuses on children. Ayres (1978) studied adult-onset apraxia extensively. She recognized fundamental differences in adult-onset apraxia and developmental dyspraxia; however, she used research on adult brain injury to draw conclusions specific to children. It appears that some therapists have taken her work with children and applied it to adults, ignoring the differences that she described.

Adults presumably have learned the specific patterns of movement required for performance of their life roles. The problems resulting from adult brain damage are therefore different from the problems that arise when a child, who has not yet learned skilled motor se-

quences, suffers brain injury. Adults will show more specific types of problems based on the area of the lesion, whereas a child will show diffuse motor-planning deficits resulting from poor integration of damaged sensory systems. Since adults may retain previously learned patterns of motor behavior, an extensive storehouse of previously learned motor skills can be adapted to a new situation. Thus, treatment for adults can sometimes utilize cognitive strategies and skill-specific training. However, when severe motor-planning deficits exist and new movement patterns must be learned, treatment will need to emphasize sensory processing, vestibular input, and skill practice.

Treating Conceptualization Problems

When a patient loses the knowledge of an object's purpose, no longer understands the qualities of that object, or cannot conceptualize how to perform a task, he or she can benefit from verbal or perceptual input (Figure 7-39). Familiar objects can be presented to help the patient learn the action and qualities of an object. A more severely involved patient may require the use of backward chaining. The therapist might wet and lather a washcloth, and then begin to wash the patient's face. The patient then can be cued or assisted to continue the activity. For eating, this technique may be used by scooping the food with a spoon and placing the spoon in the patient's mouth. The patient is allowed to remove the spoon and hopefully will initiate the next bite. The most severely involved patients may require hand-over-hand assistance throughout a task. In general, patients with conceptualization problems will work on simple, familiar tasks, in environments as familiar as possible. Abstract, unfamiliar activities should not be used, since they promote confusion. Treatment emphasizing basic mobility, feeding, and possibly toileting or oral/facial hygiene will prove most beneficial.

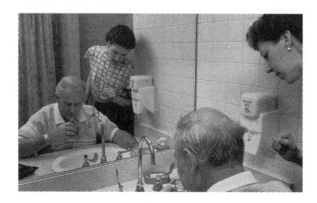

Figure 7-39 Because of motor-planning deficits, the patient attempts to bring lotion to his mouth.

Treating Production Problems

Learning the steps of a task and the sequence of an activity may best be facilitated by using familiar activities that encourage automatic responses. For a mildly affected patient, it may be enough to present the items needed for a task. For instance, bringing the patient to the sink and opening the medicine cabinet can initiate the oral/facial hygiene routine. The perceptual cues given by the objects and the situational context promote the desired action (Figure 7-40). Other patients may need to have each piece of equipment presented sequentially in the correct order. The therapist might bring a patient to the sink, cue him or her to turn on the water, present a washcloth, wait for the patient to wet it, and then provide the soap. Hand-over-hand assistance may be needed when incorrect motor patterns are used (Figure 7-41).

When working on self-care skills with a patient who has motor-planning deficits, the therapist should attempt to use techniques and sequences that are familiar to the patient whenever possible. If these techniques are not successful, and the patient has shown some potential to learn unfamiliar tasks, alternative methods may be introduced. The patient should be instructed by using verbal or tactile cues and demonstration or assistance as needed (Figure 7-42). Gradually the therapist should withdraw assistance and note the patient's ability to carry the task over. Caution is advised when providing adaptive equipment unless the patient has demonstrated the ability to use it independently and spontaneously.

Improving Skilled Movement Sequences

When skilled movement sequences are affected, motor control must be developed. Although decreased strength and abnormal tone make motor execution more difficult, they are distinct problems. There are pa-

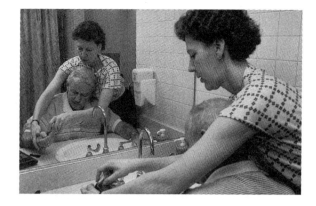

Figure 7-41 Hand-over-hand assistance and demonstration are required to apply shaving lotion.

tients who can spontaneously perform fine finger motions or skilled wrist movements with the affected hand; yet when they attempt an activity, the appropriate movement cannot be produced.

Generally, motor-planning difficulties are seen with the unaffected side as well as with the affected side. There may be more than normal difficulty in using the nondominant extremity for fine motor tasks, perseverative movements may be seen, and objects may not be placed in the proper spatial alignment. The motor-planning deficits often are more pronounced with the affected side, however, since previously programmed actions are no longer operating. In a sense, all movement with the affected side becomes unfamiliar. If motor function can be improved, the patient can use old ways of performing familiar tasks, and independence will be increased. Patients who show difficulty in using the movement patterns they have, or who have difficulty in learning new movement sequences, can benefit from motor execution training. In practice, the techniques used to remedy motor execution problems

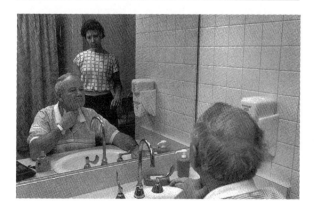

Figure 7-40 Objects on the counter provide contextual cues that aid sequencing of the task.

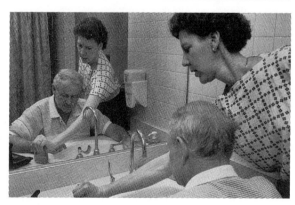

Figure 7-42 A one-handed method of applying lotion is demonstrated.

and pure motor problems are very similar. It is the underlying cause that is different.

For remediation of motor execution problems, the therapist must analyze functional movement and define the missing components. For instance, when the patient is bringing a spoon to the mouth, forearm supination may be lacking. When he or she is drinking, there may be slight radial deviation at the wrist, and forearm pronation may be absent as the glass is brought to the lips. Any movement can be analyzed by carefully observing normal performance, being aware of the variations from normal that exist, and then observing the patient's performance for the missing components. A motivated and cognitively aware patient can be taught to analyze his or her own motion by observing normal movement patterns and noting differences in performance.

Functional analysis should precede any treatment session focusing on motor control. The cognitively aware patient can be made cognizant of the part of per-

formance that is problematical. Therapeutic techniques can be used to enhance performance, and then the functional movement pattern can be attempted again. Successful treatment should result in improvements within the therapy session. Obviously, the movement patterns selected should be within the patient's capabilities. For some, the emphasis might be on using the unaffected hand and leg together when propelling the wheelchair, shifting the weight forward while transferring or learning how to pull a refrigerator door and step backward simultaneously; for others, the focus might be on fine control of the affected extremity.

When components that interfere with optimal movement have been identified, the patient can be assisted to perform them through cuing, manual guidance and facilitation, or inhibition techniques. After the patient can perform the movement in isolation, it should be incorporated into a variety of tasks demanding varied degrees of sequencing, postural adaptation, fine and gross motor control, excursion, and force. When a movement

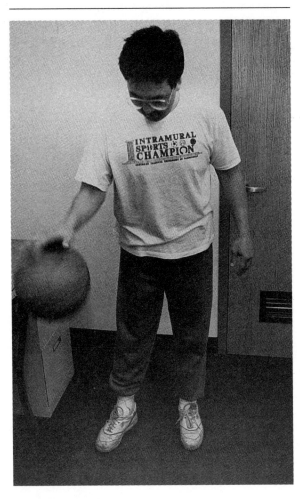

Figure 7-43 Bouncing a ball introduces speed into a motor-planning activity.

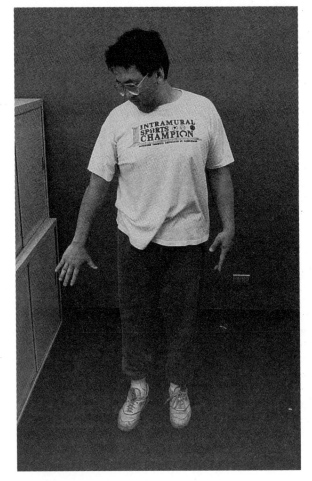

Figure 7-44 PNF diagonals require sequencing and execution of an unfamiliar motor pattern.

sequence has become routine, subcortical integration should be facilitated. At this level, language is no longer as valuable and, as described in the typing example, may be an interference. Providing many opportunities for the patient to practice a sequence in various settings can be helpful.

For instance, once the patient is able to supinate the forearm independently of activity, various tasks to promote use of this skill in a variety of contexts can be devised. He or she can be asked to supinate against resistance, to turn cards over, remove cups or boxes of various weights and sizes from a shelf, screw in a light bulb, comb his or her hair, brush his or her teeth, or eat ice cream with a spoon. The therapist can correct a movement through tactile or judiciously used verbal cues and can facilitate correct posture. When needed, the task can be stopped and the isolated movement or background posture practiced, inhibition or facilitation techniques used, or normal movement observed. This practice then can be incorporated into the activity. In addition to clinic practice, the capable patient should be given assignments to carry out in the evening on the ward or at home.

Exercises to music, or activities that require the organization of several steps, can be used when the sequencing or rhythm of performance is defective. For instance, the patient may be asked to bounce, then roll, and then throw a ball to the therapist in a repetitive sequence. The patient can be asked to bounce a ball with alternate hands, or to walk while bouncing a ball (Figure 7-43). PNF diagonals provide excellent high-level motor execution challenges (Figure 7-44). Modified aerobics, dowel rod, or ROM exercises also provide opportunities for practicing sequences of movement.

Caregiver Instruction

Caregiver instruction is particularly important because motor-planning difficulties are difficult to com-

prehend. The caregiver should observe functional performance, and deficits should be pointed out. Methods of cuing or providing assistance should be taught. The caregiver should then have the opportunity to practice them under the supervision of the therapist. Ineffective use of cuing by the caregiver can be more detrimental than helpful; therefore, training is critical. A demanding, overly verbal, or very solicitous caregiver may interfere with performance and elicit negative responses from the patient. When efforts to modify the caregiver's techniques are not successful, the therapist may decide that allowing the caregiver to do more for the patient will reduce frustration and result in a more effective outcome.

Motor planning deficits are frequently seen in the right-sided hemiplegic patient. The severity of the deficit may vary from difficulty conceptualizing the use of objects, to difficulty initiating or sequencing motor patterns, to subtle problems with refined movements. The therapist must be able to define the underlying causes of the problem, analyze activities carefully, and provide opportunities for the patient to learn and practice correct movement patterns. The activities must be carefully graded to provide challenge without undue frustration.

CONCLUSION

In this chapter, techniques that may be helpful for specific problems are described. In actual treatment situations, the patient will demonstrate a variety of problem areas, strengths, and interests. Treatment techniques must be chosen that address a variety of problem areas and are motivating to the patient. The therapist's creativity, knowledge of the patient, awareness of general treatment principles and understanding of the interplay of various problems will assist him or her in selecting appropriate therapeutic activities.

Chapter 8

Driver Rehabilitation after Stroke

Roseann Cumbo-Misheck

Occupational therapists, acting as advocates for their patients, should encourage survivors of a cerebrovascular accident (CVA) to maintain independence in driving as well as in other high-level activities of daily living (ADL). However, many have been left with residual cognitive and perceptual deficits that may impede their ability to operate a motor vehicle safely. For example, Wilson and Smith (1983) noted poor awareness of other vehicles, difficulty with complex decision making, difficulty maintaining the car in the proper lane, and difficulty negotiating traffic. Although patients who have suffered a mild CVA may resume driving regardless of their cognitive or perceptual limitations, it has been reported that 58% of CVA patients who drove before their strokes do not resume driving thereafter (Legh-Smith et al. 1986). Both groups of patients can benefit from participation in a comprehensive driver rehabilitation program. Such a program can evaluate driving skill and teach techniques that will allow all capable patients to resume safe driving.

Driver rehabilitation programs typically consist of a referral process, an inpatient or outpatient clinical evaluation, a behind-the-wheel (BTW) evaluation, and, finally, training/modifications or recommendations. This chapter provides information about cognitive and perceptual factors relevant to driving. For additional information related to the physical challenges that stroke survivors face when returning to driving, refer to the local chapter of the Association of Driver Educators for the Disabled for suggestions and treatment strategies.

REFERRAL PROCESS

Often, therapists or physicians have questions regarding "appropriate" referrals. For optimal benefit, a patient with the diagnosis of CVA should show no evidence of diplopia, severe neglect, or severe hemianopia. Patients with mild neglect or hemianopia have the potential to be trained to compensate for these deficits pending sufficient cognitive skills and ability to meet minimal requirements for visual fields. The patient must be able to participate in community tasks without needing supervision, should be able to follow simple verbal or written instructions without assistance, and should have the ability or potential to transfer into and out of the vehicle/wheelchair without assistance.

An example of a group of patients who may not meet the criteria above, yet who may be appropriate for a driving evaluation, are those who are aphasic. Aphasia is defined as a loss in the ability to understand or use the symbols of language (Golper et al. 1980). Despite this loss, aphasic patients may retain relatively good judgment and the ability to perform tasks not requiring language facility, including driving. The degree of aphasia and the extent of brain injury should be evaluated thoroughly before a BTW evaluation.

In her paper, "Drivers with Brain Damage," Simms has provided suggestions to assess the extent of communication impairment: Can the patient follow simple verbal instructions (e.g., signal left, check mirror)? Are gestures needed to clarify verbal instruction? Can the patient follow two-step directions (e.g., check your mirror and pull out when the road is clear)? Does the patient understand words relating to position and direction? Can the patient read road signs? If an aphasic patient is unable to participate in the assessments outlined in this chapter, the driving evaluation should focus on functional performance behind the wheel. At the Rehabilitation Institute of Chicago, patients who present with aphasia and pass the driver rehabilitation evaluation are issued an "aphasia card." This is a driver's license-sized card that gives the patient's name, address, and telephone number; the physician's name and telephone number; and a brief explanation of the diagnosis and problem with expression. Patients show this card to law-enforcement officials or personnel at the department of motor vehicles as needed.

Some physicians may refer patients who do not meet the usual criteria for safe driving. The physician may desire specific documentation of the patient's deficits in relation to driving or may hope to demonstrate to a risky patient the need to refrain from driving. Consultation with the physician prior to the evaluation will ensure that the evaluator is informed of the physician's goals.

Thorough information gathering prior to evaluation helps to determine whether a patient is ready to participate in the evaluation and training process. Involving the patient's physician, family, occupational therapist, physical therapist, and speech pathologist in the referral process helps the driving evaluator gather pertinent information. This information may be gathered through referral forms or direct contact. The information should include the following:

- diagnoses and prognoses (if applicable)
- family hopes/concerns related to patient's resuming driving
- visual status, including acuity and presence of diplopia or amblyopia
- perceptual status, including visual perception, body awareness, and motor planning
- cognitive status, including high-level attention skills, memory, decision making, problem solving, and safety awareness
- verbal skills or presence of aphasia
- ability to perform high-level ADL tasks (e.g., meal preparation, work skills, community tasks, or leisure skills)
- medications and their side effects, if any
- presence of seizures, dizziness, fatigue

- functional mobility, including use of affected extremities, ambulation, wheelchair propulsion, and transfer ability
- driving record (i.e., traffic violations, suspensions)

After the necessary background information has been gathered, the clinical evaluation can begin.

CLINICAL EVALUATION

The clinical evaluation is used to gather pertinent background information, including the patient's goals for driving, and to screen for visual, perceptual, cognitive, or motor deficits that may be potential risk factors once the patient is behind the wheel. Facilities vary with regard to the time allotted and the types of standardized testing performed during the clinical evaluation. A review of the literature shows that there is a lack of consensus regarding which tools are the best predictors of BTW performance (Hopewell and Price 1985; Galski et al. 1990; Gouvier et al. 1989; Van Zomeren et al. 1987; Sivak et al. 1980, 1981; Quigley and DeLisa 1983; Jones et al. 1983). When determining which formal tests will be used to detect perceptual or cognitive deficits, it is important to keep in mind the following:

- When evaluating an inpatient, which test results can be obtained from the patient's primary therapists, to prevent duplicating services?
- With what tests and information regarding perception and cognition are the physicians concerned? While many physicians are interested in results of formal tests, others are concerned with how the deficits affect functional performance.
- Which tests give the results that are needed with the least time and expense?
- What research is available to promote the use of a specific tool in predicting driver performance?

Suggested clinical evaluation tools for vision, perception, and cognition are described later in this chapter. Selective use of these tests can help guide observations and help plan treatment if skill deficits are found.

Testing the patient with a simulator is very helpful during the clinical evaluation to assess driving skills before the BTW evaluation. Although the simulator has been traditionally useful in training defensive driving techniques and emergency procedures, it is also an important tool for observing scanning skills, perception, directionality, ability to follow commands, sequencing, and ability to learn new behaviors (Quigley and DeLisa 1983). The Rehabilitation Institute of Chicago currently utilizes a simulator provided by Doron Precision Systems, Inc. The patient is observed transferring into the driver seat, turning the key in the ignition, operating the turn signal and gear selector, and completing full hand-over-hand turns (when appropriate) in both directions. Sequencing and motor-planning deficits may be noted while the patient performs these tasks. Next, if needed, the patient is instructed in the use of adaptive equipment while the evaluator assesses potential motor-planning deficits and new learning.

The evaluation continues with a brake reaction-time test. The patient watches a series of flashing red, green, and yellow lights as they are displayed across the dashboard. The patient is instructed to take his or her foot from a depressed accelerator and place it as quickly as possible on a brake pedal when two red lights are seen to come on simultaneously (Miller 1989). The average score, based on 10 trials, is computed and compared with the norm.

Next, the patient is asked to remain sitting in the simulator while viewing a film projected on a screen. The film presents a series of international road symbols that appear on the screen and change locations thereon every 2.5 seconds (Miller 1989). The patient is shown one to four symbols at one time while watching for the stimulus that requires a reaction. The stimulus is presented in various positions on the screen, requiring the patient to use scanning skills. This film is therefore useful in determining visual neglect. Once the patient identifies the stimulus, a decision must be made regarding which action to perform: turn left, turn right, or stop.

The final examination provided by the simulator is a test for threat recognition. The patient is asked to drive the simulator while 10 scenes are projected onto the screen. Each scene shows a potentially threatening situation in which the patient must react. The evaluator can observe skills of scanning, attention, judgment, decision making, reaction time, and motor planning when the patient is faced with a threatening situation (Figure 8-1).

Following the clinical evaluations, a recommendation can be made about whether to continue with the BTW evaluation or to focus on additional skill training. Information about specific deficit areas can be provided to the primary therapist so that treatment can focus on improving these skills. When a BTW evaluation is indicated, the therapist can observe the patient's ability to use a variety of skills in this complex task.

BEHIND-THE-WHEEL EVALUATION

The BTW evaluation is used to give the evaluator the opportunity to obtain functional observations of the patient's actual driving performance, to determine how the clinical assessments affect BTW performance, and to serve as the basis for further treatment and training. As with the clinical evaluation, the length of time allotted for the BTW evaluation varies from facility to facility. Some facilities put together a standard route and base their recommendations for further training or discontinued driving on specific performance guidelines that they have established. This is generally a pass/fail situation. Some facilities may use performance from the evaluation route as a baseline with which to compare results of a re-evaluation after driver training. Other facilities utilize a standard route as well, but base recommendations on observation of functional performance and the patient's ability to carry over newly learned techniques or adjust driving performance following constructive feedback. At the Rehabilitation Institute of Chicago, an hourly guideline is set for the BTW evaluation. For example, the BTW evaluation may last for two hours without an established route. Driving may begin in a structured environment and progress to more complex traffic situations as appropriate. Again, recommendations are then based on observation of functional performance and the patient's ability to carry over newly learned techniques or to adjust driving performance following constructive feedback. Examples of observations noted during BTW evaluation for vision are given in Table 8-1; for perception, in Table 8-2; and for cognition, in Table 8-3.

DRIVER TRAINING

Once the evaluation is complete, the results and recommendations about the type and length of training

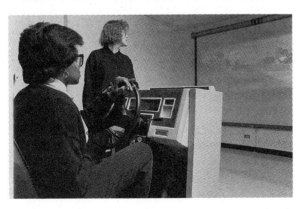

Figure 8-1 A threat recognition film is beneficial for assessing scanning, attention, judgment, motor planning, and reaction.

Table 8-1 Vision Evaluation Chart

Deficit	Clinical Observation and Evaluation Results	Observation of Performance Behind the Wheel
Poor visual acuity	• Does not meet state's requirement for far vision	• Unable to see far enough ahead to plan course of action • Drives slowly to allow more time to read signs (Cassin 1984)
Loss of vision in one eye	• Decrease in visual field to affected side • Loss of depth perception	• Decreased ability to identify objects and vehicles on affected side • Poor judgment in maintaining appropriate following or stopping distances • Difficulty driving at night • Difficulty driving in curbside lanes, where cars or pedestrians may be obscured (Milkie 1974)
Visual field loss	• Field score less than 140 degrees • Poor score on cancellation test	• Inability to identify vehicles, pedestrians, or obstacles on affected side
Poor glare vision, night vision, or glare recovery	• Poor score on glare tests	• Drives more slowly at night to allow more time to identify and react to other vehicles and signs • Increased time needed for eyes to recover from headlight glare of oncoming vehicles • Poor ability to see with consistent headlight glare of oncoming traffic
Poor contrast to sensitivity	• Poor score related to norm on contrast sensitivity test • Complains of "washed-out" vision	• Unable to identify large objects or signs at dusk, during night-time, or on cloudy days • Drives more slowly at above times to allow more time to identify and react to other vehicles, pedestrians, and signs
Poor ocular motor skills	• Poor performance on tracking, fixation, and saccade tests • Slow performance on Trail Making Test A and B and Symbol Digit Modalities Test • Poor eye-hand coordination during gross motor activities	• Difficulty in following moving objects • Poor ability to note all aspects of road scene • Poor ability to move eyes to read signs, then back to traffic ahead • Difficulty detecting traffic flow patterns • Performance deteriorates as speed increases or length of driving time increases

should be shared with the physician. If the physician is in agreement, training may begin. The evaluator should also discuss the results of the evaluation and recommendations with the patient prior to beginning training. This is to ensure that the patient has an understanding of deficit areas that need to be addressed as well as potential modifications that may be needed. The focus of training should be on the specific deficit area and its importance in safe driving performance. For example, a patient who showed poor visual spatial skills (e.g., difficulty in maneuvering around stopped vehicles or inability to interpret available space for merging into traffic) should be given the opportunity to improve performance first in a structured environment (e.g., a parking lot) and then in increasingly unstructured environments (e.g., two-lane highways, crowded city streets).

Patients who will require modifications to their vehicles will use the training sessions to become familiar with the equipment and to improve performance while using modifications in all types of traffic and maneuvers. Occasionally, patients who need modifications may require numerous training sessions because of the preserved automatic acts of driving. In some cases these very automatisms may interfere with a learning program when the latter requires a drastic change in motor patterns (Van Zomeren et al. 1987). For example, a patient learning to use hand controls may find it difficult to over-ride the impulse to operate the vehicle by using the foot pedals. In addition, the flexibility that is required for new learning may be absent or reduced.

Oftentimes during the course of training, recommendations regarding the number of hours required may

Table 8-2 Perception Evaluation Chart

Deficit	Clinical Observation and Evaluation Results	Observation of Performance Behind the Wheel
Poor color discrimination	• Unable to score within norms of stereoscopic instrument • Difficulty identifying signs based on color only	• Unable to identify colors in stoplights • Difficulty identifying colors of signs or street markings • Difficulty identifying deeper red color of railroad signals
Unilateral visual neglect	• Low score on formal testing • Poor scanning skills to right or left side noted during paper-and-pencil testing, functional activities, and simulator films • Disregard of relevant objects or people in right or left visual field during community activities • Increased disregard of affected side when task becomes more difficult, environment is distracting, or activity requires speedy performance	• Disregard of street signs, pedestrians, traffic signs, or potential hazards to right or left side • Hugs one side of road or curb
Poor depth perception	• Below standards on stereoscopic instruments • Poor score on threat recognition film	• Stops too close to or too far from vehicle ahead at stop sign • Stops in crosswalk or too far behind crosswalk • Drives too close to other vehicles when passing • Difficulty judging speed of approaching vehicles • Difficulty identifying when vehicle ahead is slowing down
Poor visual spatial skills	• Poor score on formal testing • Poor score on threat recognition film • Difficulty positioning an object in relation to self or another object (e.g., positions clothing incorrectly during dressing)	• Inability to interpret available space for merging into traffic flow • Difficulty maneuvering around stopped vehicles or other obstructions • Difficulty parking • Difficulty operating car in reverse
Poor body awareness	• Unilateral neglect of upper or lower extremity while engaged in a task • Inability to use both upper extremities in a coordinated manner while in simulator • Loss of control of steering wheel of simulator with affected upper extremity despite adequate sensation and motor control	• Unable to follow instructions with right-left component • Difficulty controlling steering wheel while following verbal or visual instruction • Inability to use both upper extremities in a coordinated manner while driving (e.g., hand-over-hand turns, lifting one hand from wheel to turn radio on/off)
Decreased motor-planning skills	• Difficulty using familiar objects • Poor ability to learn new or complex motor sequences (e.g., wheelchair propulsion, range of motion exercises) • Poor performance on screening tests • Uncoordinated use of a limb despite adequate motor control and sensation	• Misuse of primary controls (e.g., ignition key, gear selector) • Misuse of secondary controls (radio, lighter, temperature selector) • Difficulty using adaptive driving aids • Difficulty executing sequences of movement for starting car, changing lanes, parking • May perform maneuvers slowly (turning, parking, backing) • Difficulty coordinating upper extremity movements for steering with lower extremity control of gas/brake
Poor visual analysis and synthesis skills (i.e., decreased figure-ground, visual closure, visual form discrimination)	• Low score on formal screening or testing • Difficulty finding items in drawers or on shelves • Difficulty distinguishing subtle differences between objects • Difficulty recognizing object when part is covered or obscured	• Inability to distinguish important information, such as road signs or traffic lights, from insignificant background • Inability to identify a car pulling out from a side street • Inability to recognize a partially hidden road sign • Inability to distinguish pedestrians in busy location

Table 8-3 Cognition Evaluation Chart

Deficit	Clinical Observation and Evaluation Results	Observation of Performance behind the Wheel
Poor attention skills (sustained, selective, divided)	• Poor score on clinical assessments • Unable to concentrate while performing stereoscopic or simulator tasks • Poor attention to visual stimuli on brake reaction tests, resulting in low score • Score below norm on AAA brake reaction-time test or simulator reaction test	• Inability to perform tasks simultaneously (e.g., drive and listen to instructions, drive and operate secondary controls) • Inability to shift focus of attention to signs and back to road ahead • Errors in following directions or noticing traffic signs increase as evaluation proceeds • Inability to attend in increasing traffic conditions • Difficulty performing maneuvers in distracting environment (traffic, radio on, thunder/rain) • Increased time noted when braking for potential emergency situations
Poor topographical orientation	• Difficulty finding way around nursing unit, hospital • Difficulty pathfinding outside the hospital • Difficulty orienting self to map	• Difficulty navigating in familiar areas • Difficulty recalling a route previously traveled
Poor problem-solving skills, including poor judgment, decision making, and reasoning	• Poor performance on clinical assessments • Inability to generate solutions to problems encountered in self-care, meal preparation, and community tasks • Inability to generate solutions to potential problematical driving situations • Low score on driver performance test • Poor responses to questions posing potential problematical driving situations • Inability to make a timely, appropriate decision on clinical assessments	• Inability to generate solution(s) to problems encountered on the road (e.g., roadblock, detour, slow vehicle ahead) • Inability to generate solutions to problems encountered while performing maneuvers (e.g., not enough space to parallel park) • Inability to choose most appropriate solution to problems encountered on the road • Poor safety noted when generating solutions and carrying out actions • Inability to make a timely decision during unexpected situations (ball rolls into street, detour sign)
Deficits in memory	• Inability to recall instructions given prior to testing • Inability to recall driver knowledge or to recognize traffic signs	• Failure to retain instructions given by the evaluator • Failure to recall speed limits and other traffic information (e.g., construction ahead, merge ahead) • Inability to recall rules of road or to recognize traffic signs

change. In some instances, patients will show improvements in driving performance sooner than expected. In other instances, additional hours may be recommended because of poor carry-over, poor ability to respond to constructive feedback, or lack of improvement in the deficit area(s). Any changes in the training recommendations should be discussed with the physician, and in severe cases the physician may cancel training until further notice.

POOR CLINICAL OR DRIVING PERFORMANCE

Each driver rehabilitation facility should become familiar with its state's rules regarding reporting changes in medical status and reporting "impaired" drivers. In Illinois, "any member of the judiciary may submit information to either the Department or the Secretary of State relative to the physical condition of a person . . . if such condition interferes with the person's ability to operate a motor vehicle safely" (Illinois Vehicle Code 1990). Therefore, when a patient shows impairments in vision, perception, cognition, or motor skills that warrant concern regarding driving performance, the physician must be contacted. The physician may then send a medical report to the secretary of state, describing diagnoses, medications, opinion regarding driving safety, or restriction requests. Under the Illinois Vehicle Code, no physician "shall be liable or subject to criminal or civil action for any opinions, findings or recommendations, or for any information supplied to the Board of the Department regarding persons under review . . ." (Illinois Vehicle Code 1990, 506-12). Illinois has established a medical advisory board, which reviews medical reports submitted by physicians. In the event that a physician feels that a patient is unsafe to drive, the medical advisory board will contact the patient by mail regarding revocation of the driver's license.

In some cases, a patient may be referred to a driver rehabilitation program as a result of improvements in functioning, yet the patient's license is no longer valid because of an earlier medical report issued to the secretary of state. The physician must then send an updated medical report to the state, indicating the medical changes and the need for the patient to undergo a driving evaluation with an instructor at a driver rehabilitation facility. The secretary of state will then contact the patient by mail, requesting that the patient present an authorization to the department of motor vehicles. At that time, the patient will be required to pass a vision test and a written examination in order to receive an instruction permit. A medical card is also issued with the permit, authorizing the patient to drive only with an instructor from the specified facility. Upon completion of driver training, a final medical report must be sent to the state by the physician, stating successful completion of the driver training and requesting that the license be reissued to the patient. The medical advisory board will then review the report and contact the patient regarding reissuance of the driver's license.

It is clear that the procedure in Illinois is quite complicated and can become even more so if there are license issues (e.g., a poor driving record). Therefore, it is imperative that each facility become knowledgeable regarding its state codes in order to assist the physician and the patient in licensing procedures.

The remainder of this chapter contains information about evaluation and treatment of vision, perception, and cognition for CVA patients participating in a driver rehabilitation program. Specific suggestions for testing vision, perception, and cognition are given. It is felt that a comprehensive program should be equipped to test a wide range of skills and that, once specific evaluation tools are chosen, each patient who comes to the program be tested with each tool. This ensures a thorough evaluation for all and may eventually assist in potential research projects.

EVALUATION OF DEFICITS

Acuity

Every state has established minimal requirements for visual acuity and visual fields. Some states may require examinations of color discrimination and depth perception, but licensing is not determined or denied on the basis of these skills. According to Strano (1989), the rehabilitation driver evaluator must first determine

whether the patient meets the state's vision requirements, and then determine whether additional visual problems exist and whether they affect the patient's driving performance.

Visual acuity is defined as a measurement of the eye's ability to distinguish objects, details, and shapes (Cassin 1990). For driving, far-point acuity (the ability to distinguish objects, details, and shapes in the distance) is more important than near-point acuity. Each driver's rehabilitation program should contact its department of motor vehicles to determine the state's requirements for far-point acuity. For example, in Illinois, drivers must meet a standard of 20/40 in order to drive at night. Drivers with less than 20/40 acuity must meet a standard of 20/70 to drive during the daytime only. Visual acuity of less than 20/70 does not meet the Illinois state requirement.

Visual acuity can be tested by using Snellen charts as well as a variety of stereoscopic instruments (e.g., Titmus Vision Tester, Optec 2000, Keystone View). Most instruments are similar to those used at the department of motor vehicles, and test for color discrimination, depth perception, phoria, and visual fields as well. (*Phoria* is defined as the relative directions assumed by the eyes during binocular fixation of a given object in the absence of an adequate fusion stimulus [Stedman's Medical Dictionary 1990].) Although a patient's score on any of the above instruments is directly correlated with a Snellen equivalent, the evaluator is advised to document merely whether or not the patient was within the state requirements. At the Rehabilitation Institute of Chicago, patients who score below the state requirement for night-time driving are often advised to return to a vision specialist to be evaluated further.

Most states permit drivers with a loss of vision in one eye to operate a motor vehicle with the addition of extra mirrors, restrictions for daytime driving only, or speed limit restrictions (Strano 1989). During the evaluation, a patient with a loss of vision in one eye will show a decrease in the visual field to the affected side and a decrease in depth perception. When evaluating a patient with a loss of vision in one eye with a stereoscopic instrument, do not attempt to give the phoria test, because it is for those with binocular vision only.

Visual Field

The American Medical Association's Committee on Medical Aspects of Automotive Safety has recommended that driving candidates must have the ability to identify an object throughout a visual arc of at least 140 degrees (Committee on Medical Aspects of Automotive Safety 1969). Therefore, patients with suspected hemianopia or those who score poorly on confrontational or other visual field tests should be referred to an ophthalmologist for more specific field tests. Some driver rehabilitation facilities own and are trained to operate their own automated perimeter. Automated perimeters (e.g., Kowa, BioRad, Humphrey) can measure the sensitivity of the retina for each area of the visual field (Cambridge Automated Perimeter 1990). The instruments are simple to operate, and test each eye in approximately six minutes. A printout is produced once the test is completed, enabling the evaluator to compare left and right hemifields and quadrants. Again, evaluators are advised to report whether or not a patient meets the state requirements. Patients scoring below requirements should be referred to an ophthalmologist for verification and treatment suggestions.

Night Vision, Glare Vision, Glare Recovery

The American Automobile Association (AAA) offers the Night Sight Meter, which evaluates night vision, glare vision, and glare recovery. (For other vendors, see Appendix 8-A.) It is important to screen these three areas in addition to acuity and visual fields, especially if BTW evaluations do not occur at night. The Night Sight Meter comes with suggested norms. According to the test results, the clinician will be able to give recommendations to the patient and the physician regarding the patient's potential inability to (1) see on the road at night, (2) see in the face of glare from headlights, and (3) recover normal vision after glare has passed. Evaluators with concern regarding a patient's ability to perform in these three situations should consult with the patient's physician. The physician may feel that it is necessary to send a medical report to the secretary of state's medical review board requesting that a daytime restriction be put on the license.

Contrast Sensitivity

The Snellen chart evaluates how well a patient can see details under high contrast (e.g., dark letters on a white background); but when driving at dusk, nighttime, or on cloudy days, patients need to be able to identify large objects against a low-contrast background. Therefore, many driver rehabilitation facilities are finding the need to assess contrast sensitivity in addition to acuity. Contrast sensitivity testing provides a look at high and low contrast (Bosse and Lederer 1988). Contrast sensitivity tests can reveal problems with vision, even if visual acuity appears to be normal. This is especially important in CVA patients who also have glaucoma or cataracts. These patients may com-

plain of "washed-out" vision or inability to see at night, yet their acuity is good.

Contrast sensitivity tests present patterns of light and dark bars. The bars are presented in varying spatial frequencies and contrasts. Spatial frequency is defined as the number of bars on the pattern (Bosse and Lederer 1988). A low spatial frequency will have a few wide bars, whereas a high spatial frequency will have many thin bars. Contrast, then, is the difference between the dark and light bars. When the bars are at the darkest and brightest, contrast is high. When the bars appear gray, and therefore similar, contrast is low. The evaluator first presents low-contrast patterns to the patient, then slowly increases the contrast until the patient can see a bar pattern. At that time, the evaluator notes the measurement. After several repetitions, a curve can be plotted and compared with a curve of normal results. As with glare testing, the evaluator can use the test results to decide whether further testing should be performed by a vision specialist and to notify the physician regarding concerns about the patient's ability to drive under low-contrast situations. Contrast sensitivity testing is available in a wall unit or on slides for stereoscopic instruments (e.g., the Optic 2000).

Ocular Mobility

Although ocular mobility problems occur more often in patients who have had severe head injuries than in patients who have had a CVA, an evaluation of fixation (the microeye movements that help to maintain one or both foveas directed at a target [Abreu 1990]), pursuits (the tracking eye movements that help maintain the image of a moving object on the fovea [Abreu 1990]), and saccades (rapid eye movements that accomplish transfer of gaze from one fixation point to another [Abreu 1990]) should still be performed. Failure of the eye muscles to focus on the same object during tracking or saccades may result in double vision, blurred vision, and suppression of vision in one eye, as well as fatigue (Milkie 1974). Any of these problems could adversely affect driving performance. Again, concerns regarding ocular motor skills should be reported to the physician (Figure 8-2).

Perception

There are many formal tests and clinical observations described in other chapters of this book. The driving evaluator should obtain as much information as possible regarding these areas of function from the primary therapist. When complete information is not available, the driving evaluator should select tests designed to challenge the patient in areas that are poten-

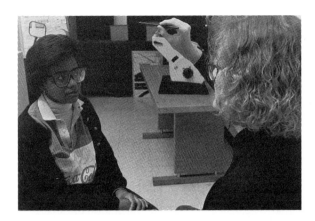

Figure 8-2 Tests of ocular motor skills are an important part of the clinical evaluation. Here, the therapist uses a pen to evaluate pursuits.

tially disrupted. Suggested high-level tests for each critical area of perceptual function follow. The therapist may choose one or two tests based on his or her facility's protocol and the patient's presentation.

- Unilateral visual neglect (given when high-level neglect is suspected)
  1. Rey Complex Figure Test (copying) (Rey 1941)
  2. Albert's Test (cancellation) (Fullerton et al. 1986)
  3. Letter Cancellation Test (Diller et al. 1974)
  4. Reaction Time Measure of Visual Fields (Gianutsos and Klitzner 1981)

- Visual spatial awareness (given when judging distances is difficult)
  1. Judgment of Line Orientation (Benton 1983a)

- Visual analysis and synthesis (given when distinguishing items in the environment or reading signs is a problem)
  1. Visual Form Discrimination (Benton 1983b)
  2. Figure-Ground Test (Ayres 1966)
  3. Hooper Visual Organization Test (Hooper 1983)

- Body awareness (given when following right-left directions or operating a vehicle is difficult)
  1. right-left discrimination
  2. Bilateral Integration (Roach and Kephart 1966)
  3. bilateral simultaneous stimulation

- Motor planning (given when using equipment or sequencing activity are difficult)
  1. observation during function
  2. imitation of postures

In addition to the formal tests listed, it is important to screen depth perception and color discrimination. Depth perception is the ability to determine relative distance of one object to another (Strano 1989). Depth perception is important for determining stopping distances, estimating appropriate space gaps for passing, and positioning one's vehicle in relation to other vehicles on the road. The stereoscopic instruments mentioned earlier utilize various pictures to test for depth perception.

Color discrimination is important to evaluate, although with standard location of colors in traffic lights, those with difficulty in this area are able to learn to compensate easily. Stereoscopic instruments provide test screens for color discrimination. In addition, Lezak (1983) lists "coloring of pictures" or "wrongly colored pictures" as effective tools by which to test color perception.

Cognition

As for the perception evaluation, when complete information is not available regarding the patient's cognitive skills, the driving evaluator should select tests designed to challenge the patient in areas that are potentially disrupted. Suggested high-level tests for each area of cognitive function follow. Again, the therapist may choose one or two tests based on his or her facility's protocol and the patient's presentation.

- Attention (given when sustained, selective, or divided attention is difficult)
  1. Visual Vigilance Test (Abreu 1987)
  2. Letter Cancellation Test
  3. Random Letter Test (Strub and Black 1985)
  4. Trail Making Test
  5. Symbol Digit Modalities Test (Smith 1982)

- Topographical orientation (given when problems with pathfinding in familiar and unfamiliar environments are suspected)
  1. functional observation of pathfinding performance inside and outside the hospital
  2. map reading

- Problem solving (given when identification of a problem, generating and carrying out solutions, judgment, reasoning, or decision making are difficult)
  1. functional observation of performance during self-care, meal preparation, community tasks, and work simulation

2. block design and Rey Complex Figure Test (Rey 1941)
3. block arrangement problem
4. driver problem-solving questions (see below)
5. driver performance test (see below)

- Memory (given when deficits in long- or short-term memory are suspected)

1. Digit Repetition (Strub and Black 1985)
2. Visual Memory Test (adapted from Abreu 1987)
3. driver knowledge examination (see below)
4. sign recognition examination (see below)

At the Rehabilitation Institute of Chicago, the evaluator asks the patient questions related to potential problematical situations that may occur on the road (driver problem-solving questions); for example, What would you do if the vehicle behind you was following too closely? What would you do if your vehicle began to slide on an icy street? The questions can also involve potential emergency situations; e.g., What would you do if you ran out of gas on the highway? The patient is to answer the question as thoroughly as possible, while the evaluator looks for the following: Does the patient use sound judgment when verbalizing his or her course of action? For example, would he or she move into the right-hand lane to let a vehicle pass, rather than driving more slowly to enrage the other driver? Does the patient take into account safety issues related to potential actions? Is the patient able to generate a number of appropriate solutions and choose the best one for a particular situation? Is the patient able to back up responses with appropriate reasoning skills? When the evaluator finds that a patient is having difficulty with judgment, reasoning, or decision-making skills, the patient's actual driving performance may need to be evaluated first in a structured, nondistracting environment to assess further whether these deficits will interfere with safe driving performance.

Knowledge of the rules of the road and the ability to recognize and react to signs are important areas to assess in the clinic as well. Although van Zomeren et al. (1987) have found that examinations of traffic laws are poor predictors of driving performance, these examinations may be useful in determining the extent of memory loss. In addition, these tests give the evaluator an idea of how much time will be needed to teach the rules of the road. Multiple-choice questions can also give the evaluator an opportunity to assess the client's ability to make an appropriate selection, given choices. The Rehabilitation Institute of Chicago assesses the patient's driving knowledge through a 10- to 20-question examination, using both true/false and multiple-choice questions (Exhibit 8-1). Sign recognition may be evaluated by using a driving manual or the study booklet provided by the department of motor vehicles. The Rehabilitation Institute uses a work sheet provided by Louisiana Technical University Center for Rehabilitation Science and Biomedical Engineering. The work sheet consists of 21 signs in black and white, with 21 choices listed. The patient is to match the sign with the appropriate name or action. Again, a low score will give the evaluator an idea of how much education may be needed.

Knowledge of driving and problem-solving skills can also be tested through administration of the driver performance test. This test uses a series of videotaped scenes of potentially dangerous driving situations (Gouvier et al. 1989). Patients view each scene and are presented with four choices for ways to respond safely to the threat in the scene (Figure 8-3). Each of the 40 scenes requires one subskill of problem solving: search, identify, predict, decide, or execute. Patients are then given an overall score as well as a score for each subskill, with the rating of excellent, above average, average, below average, or poor. Although the driver performance test is a comprehensive evaluation of driving knowledge, problem solving, and safety, it is also a difficult test even for cognitively intact persons because of the time limit constraints placed on each scene. Variance is noted among individuals regarding their thoughts on the most appropriate answer. Scores may reflect some inconsistencies in the test design. It is thought that the test is valuable for observing problem-solving approaches, but that scores should not be interpreted rigidly.

In addition to formal screening and tests of attention, topographical orientation, memory, and problem solving, it is important to assess the patient's skills in the ability to follow verbal or visual directions and reaction time.

The ability to follow directions can be assessed by providing verbal instructions for completing a test. The evaluator will be able to identify any difficulty following simple or more complex verbal instructions. The ability to follow written directions can be assessed in a similar manner by using written instructions for completion of assessments. For aphasic patients it may be helpful to ask a family member or a speech pathologist for advice regarding the best way to communicate. When the patient has difficulty following verbal commands, does he or she respond better to gestures or to simple written words or symbols? Does he or she need demonstration to perform more complex commands? How does the patient perform following gestures or demonstration?

Exhibit 8-1 Rehabilitation Institute of Chicago Driver Knowledge Test

1. Motorcycles are entitled to use the full width of a traffic lane, the same as a vehicle. Therefore, when you are driving a vehicle and want to pass a motorcycle, you should:
   (   ) Cautiously pass the motorcycle, sharing the same lane that it is using
   (   ) Follow the motorcycle without passing it
   (   ) Do not pass the motorcycle in the same lane that it is using, but change lanes and pass the way you would pass another vehicle
2. Your driving privileges will be revoked in the state of Illinois if you are convicted of:
   (   ) Leaving the scene of an accident in which you are involved as a driver, if the accident results in death or personal injury
   (   ) Drag racing
   (   ) Driving or being in actual physical control of a vehicle while under the influence of alcohol or other drugs (including prescription drugs that may impair driving ability) and/or combinations, thereof
   (   ) All of the above
   (   ) None of the above
3. You are waiting at an intersection and the traffic light changes to green. You may then go ahead:
   (   ) Immediately
   (   ) When you think it is safe to do so
   (   ) After first yielding the right-of-way to any persons or vehicles that are within the intersection
4. When driving on a slippery road and the rear end of your vehicle starts to skid, you should:
   (   ) Turn the front wheels in the direction of the skid
   (   ) Hold the wheel firmly and steer straight ahead, braking gradually
   (   ) Apply the brakes quickly
5. Each driver and front-seat passenger of a motor vehicle (age 6 and up) is required to wear seat safety belts while driving on Illinois roadways. Violators are subject to:
   (   ) Suspension of their driver's licenses
   (   ) A $50 fine plus court costs
   (   ) A $25 fine plus court costs
   (   ) None of the above
6. When a school bus is stopped on a two-lane highway and its red warning lights are flashing and its stop signal arm is extended, you must:
   (   ) Slow down, sound horn, and pass the bus with caution
   (   ) Pass the bus on the left if there are no vehicles approaching
   (   ) Stop your vehicle before reaching the bus
7. When you come to a stop sign, you must stop your vehicle:
   (   ) As close to the stop sign as possible
   (   ) At a marked stop line, before entering the crosswalk, or before entering the intersection if there is no crosswalk
   (   ) At a place near the intersection, providing you come to a full stop
8. When an authorized emergency vehicle that is using its siren and flashing it lights approaches your vehicle, you should:
   (   ) Increase your speed
   (   ) Continue at the same speed
   (   ) Pull over to the right-hand side of the road and stop, if possible
9. After consuming alcohol, time is the only effective way to remove alcohol from the body
   (   ) True
   (   ) False
10. The "2-Second Rule" works like this: When the vehicle ahead of you passes a fixed object such as a tree, if you begin counting "one thousand one, one thousand two" and you reach the same tree before saying "one thousand two," you are following too closely.
   (   ) True
   (   ) False

Source: Adapted from the Community Driving School, Inc., sample permit test.

Reaction time may be tested by using a driver simulator or by using simulated car foot pedals connected to an electronic reaction timer (Figure 8-3). Simple accelerator-to-brake reaction times are measured in response to random illumination of a red light (Jones et al. 1983). The AAA offers the automatic brake reaction timer, which includes norms for comparing the patient's speed with that of unimpaired people of his or her age.

These tests can help detect specific deficits that affect driving performance. The patient, physician, and primary therapist can then be given information about areas of concern and skills that will require treatment. Treatment of visual, perceptual, and cognitive deficits may occur in the driving clinic, with the primary occupational therapist, or with another professional, depending on the type and severity of the problem.

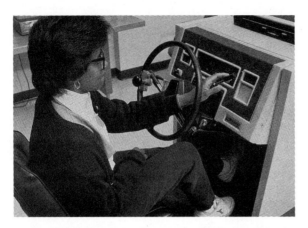

Figure 8-3 Performing a simulator evaluation provides the therapist with the opportunity to observe the patient's ability to problem solve and motor plan. (This patient identifies a solution to moving the gear selector.)

TREATMENT SUGGESTIONS

Treatment of Visual Deficits

When the patient demonstrates a deficit in acuity, glare vision, or contrast sensitivity, the best course of action may be to contact the physician or a vision specialist. He or she can provide information regarding vision status, potential for improvement, and driving restriction recommendations. For example, the evaluator may note that a patient scored poorly on the contrast sensitivity test in the clinic and was unable to identify large objects or signs when driving at dusk. The patient appeared to drive more slowly at dusk to allow more time to identify signs. The evaluator recommends that the patient schedule an ophthalmology appointment. After the eye appointment, the evaluator discusses the patient's status with the physician, who states that the patient's visual status will not likely improve and recommends restricting driving to daytime hours only. The evaluator then can assist the physician in discussing these recommendations with the patient in addition to filing the necessary paper work with the secretary of state to request a restricted license.

In another example, the evaluator may notice that the patient had difficulty with acuity throughout the evaluation and, on discussing the results with the vision specialist, finds that the patient required a new prescription for glasses. The patient can then be re-evaluated to assess driving skills.

Patients who present with loss of vision in one eye or a visual field deficit, yet appear to be good candidates for completion of a driver training program, can be trained behind the wheel to compensate for their deficit. Many hours may be spent reviewing the importance of turning the head toward the affected side in order to view objects, vehicles, and pedestrians that they are otherwise unable to see. Patients with loss of vision in one eye will need to be trained in judging the appropriate stopping distances. Suggestions may be given to the occupational therapist to incorporate visual compensation training into treatment sessions. Performing community tasks such as grocery shopping and pathfinding encourage the patient to utilize the compensation techniques. Repetition in a variety of activities may result in carry-over to driving tasks.

Patients with ocular motor deficits are usually referred to a developmental optometrist for oculomotor therapy or visual retraining prior to BTW training. Recommendations can also be given to the occupational therapist for exercises to be performed in the therapy session. An example of an exercise to improve visual fixation is wall fixation (Maino 1986). The therapist uses six three- by five-inch index cards, each with a two-inch numeral ranging from one through six written on it. Cards 1 and 2 are placed one foot from the ceiling and six feet apart. Cards 5 and 6 are placed in the center of the wall directly under the first two cards. Finally, cards 3 and 4 are placed one foot from the floor, directly under the others. Thus, two columns are created, the left column containing numbers 1, 5, and 3 and the right column containing numbers 2, 6, and 4. The patient is then positioned about six feet from the wall, centered between the rows of numbers. The therapist should stand facing the patient so that fixational movements can be observed. The patient is asked to look at the numbers in the following sequence: 1, 2, 3, 4, 5, 6, 1, 2, 3, 4, 5, 6, etc. The patient is directed to change his or her fixation point when the therapist claps or when the next number is called out, depending on the patient's cognitive level. This exercise should be performed first with the right eye, then with the left eye, then with both eyes for a duration of five minutes.

Oculomotor exercises that require less equipment can be performed by using a light pen or a large pencil for pursuit exercises. The patient follows the object, which is being moved slowly by the therapist in all visual ranges, first with the left eye, then with the right eye, then with both eyes.

Visual motor skills can be incorporated into scanning exercises by positioning the patient in front of a large chalkboard. The therapist writes the numbers one through ten on the chalkboard, but spreads them out across the length and width of the board. The patient is then asked to connect the numbers in order, while the therapist observes scanning and visual motor skills.

Finally, functional activities such as locating items on a shelf or clinic cabinet can also be incorporated into treatment sessions. The therapist is encouraged to use creativity and motivating treatment activities to maximize the patient's visual skills.

Treatment of Perceptual Deficits

Difficulty with color discrimination may be addressed during driver training sessions. Assisting the patient in learning the sequence of colors of traffic lights, identification of warning signs or signals, and identification of the deep-red color of railroad signals should be the primary focus. The primary occupational therapist may reinforce the patient's learning while he or she is performing community tasks.

Patients with unilateral visual neglect can be trained to compensate in the same way as those with loss of vision in one eye or visual field deficits. Driver training should focus on cuing the patient to turn his or her head to the affected side in order to observe signs, pedestrians, and vehicles that might otherwise go unnoticed. Again, recommendations may be given to the occupational therapist for incorporation of this compensation technique into treatment sessions. Activities described in Chapter 7 can be used during treatment sessions and may aid in carry-over to driving tasks.

Patients showing difficulty with depth perception or visual spatial skills typically are retrained in these skills behind the wheel. The evaluator may assist the occupational therapist in generating creative treatment activities to address these areas. For example, pushing a shopping cart or wheelchair in a crowded grocery store will provide the patient with opportunities to improve stopping distance from other shoppers, improve maneuvering ability through crowded aisles, and improve judgment for interpreting available space.

Meal preparation or avocational activities may be used by the occupational therapist during treatment sessions to address the patient's difficulty with body awareness. Woodworking, gross motor activities, and wheelchair propulsion activities that incorporate the use of both upper extremities while following verbal or visual instruction can be challenging, as can stirring or chopping tasks in the kitchen. Repetition of activities requiring the use of both upper extremities in a coordinated manner hopefully will result in improved body awareness behind the wheel.

Poor motor-planning skill is another deficit area that may be addressed in therapy sessions using techniques suggested in Chapter 7 with the hope of improved skills in driving. The driver evaluator may use the simulator or facility vehicle to practice repetitions of transfers, use of primary or secondary controls, or use of adaptive equipment. In addition, motor activities that require coordinating the upper and lower extremities (e.g., rowing, bicycling) or activities that require maneuvers (e.g., pushing a grocery cart) may be addressed in individual therapy.

Visual analysis and synthesis deficits can be addressed during driver training by cuing the patient to be more attentive in busy intersections or while passing side roads, where cars may pull out or be partially hidden. Periodically the patient can be asked to describe briefly the car behind him or her, to describe each traffic sign he or she passes, or to identify other items in the environment. Again, creativity and motivating treatment activities will help to facilitate improvement in perceptual skills.

Treatment of Cognitive Deficits

In 1981, Sivak et al. noted improvement in driving skills following training sessions using cognitive paper-and-pencil tasks. Cancellation tasks, which require sustained visual attention, were used along with other visual activities. In addition to paper-and-pencil tasks, attention skills can be improved through challenging functional activities provided in occupational therapy. Sustained attention may be addressed through participation in an activity for an increasing length of time (e.g., sorting mail, making photocopies). Selective and divided attention may be addressed in the community during pathfinding activities. Requiring the patient to attend to specific landmarks or to locate a certain item in a hardware store will also provide challenge. Preparing a multistep hot meal is one way to address the patient's ability to attend to more than one task at a time.

Pathfinding tasks are also a useful part of driver training to assist in improving topographical orientation and the ability to follow directions. Patients may be asked to follow verbal or written directions and identify specific landmarks or street signs in order to reach a destination. Incorporating verbal directions of left, right, north, south, east, and west may be attempted as well.

Difficulty with problem solving, decision making, judgment, and reasoning can be addressed during driver training as problematical situations present themselves. The occupational therapist may also use treatment sessions to discuss potential problematical situations with the patient. The topics can range from emergency situations, to driving situations, to basic problems of self-care (e.g., What would you do if your washing machine broke down?). The patient may be asked to provide his or her reasoning behind making certain decisions and to generate additional solutions.

These skills also should be addressed during actual performance of community tasks, meal preparation, avocational tasks, or work simulations. When presented with a problematical situation, the therapist can structure the problem-solving procedure according to the patient's needs.

The driving evaluator may find it helpful to discuss specific memory deficits with the occupational therapist to aid in treatment planning. If the patient is having difficulty retaining verbal instructions given while he or she is driving, the therapist can plan treatment tasks incorporating retention of two- and three-step commands, especially while the patient is performing community tasks. If the patient is unable to recall speed limits or other traffic information, the therapist may plan pathfinding activities requiring the patient to observe and recall specific landmarks or street signs. Difficulty with long-term retrieval of rules of the road or sign recognition may be improved by reviewing and testing these areas. Finally, teaching compensation techniques may be helpful. The use of clearly printed directions or a map can assist the patient if visual or verbal memory fails.

CONCLUSION

It is important that we, as occupational therapists, encourage our patients to return to their previous life styles. Yet it is also important for stroke survivors to participate first in a driver rehabilitation program to evaluate safe return to driving. The driver's rehabilitation program at the Rehabilitation Institute of Chicago consists of a referral, patient interview, and comprehensive evaluation of visual, perceptual, cognitive, and motor skills (range of motion, manual muscle testing, sensation). Behind-the-wheel evaluations are provided to those appropriate, as well as driver training. When possible, a patient may be referred to additional therapy in hopes of further improving specific skills required for driving.

Stereo-Optical
3539 N. Kenton Avenue
Chicago, IL 60641-3879
1-800-344-9500
(312) 777-2869
(vision testing equipment)

BIO-RAD
237 Putnam Avenue
Cambridge, MA 02139
1-800-628-5227
(visual field)

Vistech Consultants, Inc.
1372 N. Fairfield Road
Dayton, OH 45432-2644
1-800-Vistech
(contrast sensitivity)

Simulator Systems International, Inc.
11130 E. 56th Street
Tulsa, OK 74146
1-800-843-4764

Doron Precision Systems, Inc.
P.O. Box 400
Binghamton, NY 13902
1-800-847-1303

Chicago Motor Club
999 East Touhy Avenue
Des Plaines, IL 60018
(708) 390-9000
or

AAA Traffic Safety Department
American Automobile Association
1000 AAA Drive
Heathrow, FL 32746-5063

Midwest Ophthalmic Instruments, Inc.
1303 Marquette Drive
Marquette Industrial Park
Romeoville, IL 60441
(708) 759-7666
1-800-831-1194
(vision testing equipment)

Chapter 9

Case Example Illustrating Evaluation and Treatment Principles

The following case example has been written to clarify the way in which evaluation and treatment techniques can be used with a specific patient. This example illustrates the use of selected tests based on the patient's presentation during functional activities that are relevant to his goals. The integration of the patient's preferences and anticipated discharge roles during treatment is described.

MEDICAL AND SOCIAL HISTORY

Mr. Jackson is a 58-year-old left-handed man who was a partner in a lucrative law firm. He liked all sports, but particularly enjoyed tennis, and played it often. He also enjoyed reading, listening to classical music, and playing board games such as chess. Although he was predominantly left-handed, as a child he had learned to use his right hand for writing. He lived with his wife and two of his five children, aged 18 and 21, in an affluent suburban neighborhood. He was not responsible for homemaking or cooking tasks, although he occasionally made a sandwich or fixed a snack. His children performed routine heavy home maintenance tasks, such as taking out the garbage, shoveling snow, and mowing the lawn. Other big jobs, such as painting, were done by hired professionals.

Approximately one week prior to admission to the rehabilitation hospital, Mr. Jackson suffered a right parietal cerebrovascular accident (CVA) with cortical damage and left-sided weakness, mild dysarthria, and decreased sensation on the left side. Cranial nerves 2 to 12 were affected, with resulting left-central facial droop. The right internal carotid artery was almost completely blocked, and the left carotid artery was 40 to 50 percent occluded. He had a history of kidney stones, but no other medical problems.

INITIAL EVALUATION

During the initial evaluation, Mr. Jackson was polite, compliant with all requests, and seemed pleased with the therapy process. His daughter was present during the first evaluation sessions. He stated that his primary goals were to "improve my left hand function, drive again, and return to work."

The initial self-care evaluation showed that Mr. Jackson required moderate assistance for grooming while standing at the sink and minimal assistance for feeding, primarily for cutting food. Minimal assistance was required for balance and shoe tying during lower extremity dressing. Toileting and taking a shower also required minimal assistance for balance when standing. He was independent with setup for sponge bathing. Mr. Jackson was able to use the telephone independently; however, he was slow when looking up an unfamiliar number in the telephone book. He could balance a checkbook and handle money up to $50.00, but he had difficulty with mental arithmetic calculations. Community skills, work activities, and cold meal preparation were to be evaluated once basic self-care skills had improved.

Prior to the stroke, Mr. Jackson had used his right hand for writing and his left hand for all other skilled activities. Consequently, he remained able to write his name clearly. The speech and language pathologist noted decreased organization and incomplete thoughts when writing paragraph-length material.

Observation of basic self-care activities and clinical tasks revealed difficulties in safety awareness, problem solving, high-level attention, and error awareness. He was occasionally impulsive, and required minimal cues to identify solutions to problems that arose during activities of daily living (ADL). Although attention was sufficient for completing basic self-care, the therapist wanted to check higher-level skills, since Mr. Jackson hoped to return to work and community-level tasks. Difficulties with sustained visual and auditory attention were seen when he was given the Visual Vigilance Test and the Digit Repetition Test. In addition, he showed difficulty when he was required to attend selectively to difficult material in a distracting environment and showed performance below norms on both the Trail Making Test and the Symbol Digit Modalities Test. Memory was adequate for remembering instructions from day to day.

Subtle deficits in estimating the passage of time were noted, as he frequently became preoccupied with the current task and unaware of his obligation to get ready for another class. When asked to estimate the time that a task required, he generally misjudged significantly. On a more formal task in which he was asked to estimate when a minute had passed, he erred by 30 seconds, which demonstrates significant impairment.

Although visual saccade and pursuits were within normal limits, visual perceptual problems were noted in self-care tasks. Moderate deficits were noted in his awareness of the left visual field and left extremities. At times he bumped into objects on the left and required cues to position his left upper extremity properly to avoid injury. Occasionally he showed incorrect orientation of his shirt. He also showed slight difficulty with the visual analysis and synthesis required to pick an object out of a cluttered drawer or recognize an object when part of it was hidden.

To define the extent and nature of these problems further, high-level standardized visual spatial, visual analysis and synthesis, and visual construction tests were used. Minimal distortion was seen when Mr. Jackson was asked to draw a person and a clock from memory. Poor spatial organization and mild neglect were evident when he was copying the Rey Complex Figure (1964) and when completing the Benton's Three-Dimensional Block Construction Test (1983e). Spatial awareness deficits were corroborated further through low scores on Benton's Judgment of Line Orientation Test (1983b). He performed within norms on the Hooper Visual Organization Test (1983) and the Benton Visual Form Discrimination Test (1983f) but showed mild deficits on Ayres Figure-Ground Test (1978), which measures high-level visual attention and organizational abilities. It appeared that when the information was cluttered, as it is in figure-ground activities, Mr. Jackson had difficulty picking out the relevant details.

Deficits in all sensory modalities in the left upper extremity were noted. In addition, unilateral tactile inattention was present. He could identify touch unilaterally on both the right and left hands; however, when given bilateral simultaneous stimulation, he extinguished the sensation on the left side. Despite these sensory deficits, Mr. Jackson was intent on using his left upper extremity and attempted to incorporate it in all bilateral activities. Midline orientation was adequate in sitting; however, in standing, poor left-sided awareness and bilateral integration interfered with equal weight bearing and a symmetrical posture.

Left upper extremity movement was shown in all joints, but control, refined distal motion, and overhead placement was inhibited by increased flexor tone throughout. Mr. Jackson was able independently to assume a sitting position from supine, engage in dynamic sitting balance activities, and reach in moderate ranges while standing with contact guard. In all mobility activities, cuing and facilitation enhanced the quality of movement, since Mr. Jackson tended to avoid weight bearing on the left side. He required minimal assistance with transfers, stair climbing, and ambulation using a wide-based quad cane.

Mr. Jackson's ability to communicate was slightly impaired by reduced sustained attention, problem solving, and eye contact. In addition, mild dysarthria caused by decreased left oral/facial strength diminished the intelligibility of his speech slightly. In general, his communication skills were adequate for day-to-day conversation, but they appeared insufficient for the high-level performance required in his law practice.

GOALS

Mr. Jackson, his family, and the therapist worked together to set self-care goals as follows:

- Mr. Jackson will be completely independent in all basic self-care while standing, as appropriate.
- Toileting and showering will be accomplished independently with equipment. In addition, cold meal preparation and community and work skills would be evaluated and appropriate goals set.

To reach these self-care goals, the following component skill goals were also collaboratively established:

Mr. Jackson would

- demonstrate attention, problem solving, and safety awareness sufficient to complete all basic self-care without cues
- show left-hand awareness and coordination adequate for tying shoes and manipulating fasteners such as buttons and zippers
- independently use one or two compensation techniques for visual perceptual deficits in functional tasks
- independently monitor left upper extremity tone and use appropriate tone-reduction techniques
- demonstrate equal weight bearing on both lower extremities during grooming tasks
- demonstrate standing balance sufficient to wash feet while showering and manage pants independently for dressing and toileting

To accomplish these goals, Mr. Jackson and the therapist agreed on the following plan: basic self-care practice four times weekly, community evaluation, work skills evaluation, cold meal preparation evaluation, upper extremity coordination activities, standing balance activities, instruction in upper extremity tone management methods, practicing techniques to improve/compensate for visual perceptual problems and sensory deficits, and participation in graded activities to enhance attention and problem-solving skills.

TREATMENT

Morning ADL sessions initially emphasized controlled use of the left upper extremity in bilateral tasks, but as improvements were seen, the focus changed to use of the left upper extremity as the dominant hand for reaching needed items, utensil use, and operating fasteners. Sustained attention and problem solving were required as Mr. Jackson learned to use inhibition and facilitation techniques prior to and during functional reach and grasp activities. To improve sensory motor awareness, he was encouraged to try a movement with his nonaffected extremity and then attempt to duplicate it with his left arm.

Tactile awareness was addressed by asking Mr. Jackson to attend consciously to various temperatures, textures, and sensations encountered during self-care tasks. As awareness of primary sensory modalities improved, simultaneous tactile sensation was addressed by asking him to perform bilateral activities. For example, when holding the toothbrush in one hand and the toothpaste in the other, he was asked to stop, look at each object, close his eyes and attend to the sensations,

and then open his eyes again. Initially, he was unable to perform bilateral manipulative tasks because sensory input on the right over-rode sensory input on the left. He was unable to maintain control unless he was visually guiding left-hand movement. With improved tactile attention, however, he could perform gross tactile manipulations without visual guidance and could perform coordinated movements with visual assistance.

Body awareness and standing balance during functional tasks were also emphasized, and Mr. Jackson was encouraged to ambulate in his room, obtain his clothes from the closet, reach for objects in drawers at various heights, and stand during oral/facial hygiene. Neurodevelopmental treatment techniques and motor relearning concepts were used to encourage equal weight bearing when sitting, moving from sit to stand, and while standing. These techniques enhanced awareness of sensory input and required attention as he focused on the subtle sensations and control necessary to improve movement.

Perceptual compensation techniques, such as consciously turning the head and eyes to the left, organizing drawers to reduce clutter, using his finger as a visual guide when scanning written material, and looking for boundaries and borders to ensure that the left side of an object was seen, were reinforced. As skill improved, he was challenged to use the same skills in more distracting environments, for example, while obtaining and eating a meal in the cafeteria.

As basic self-care became easier, community-level skills were evaluated. It was found that minimal assistance was required to attend to relevant visual details (especially on the left), recognize hazards, navigate in an unfamiliar location, solve problems, and maintain time awareness. Mr. Jackson found community-level tasks challenging and beneficial from an emotional and physical perspective. More speed was required in making decisions, more attention was required because of the vast amount of rapidly changing environmental information, and more balance and control were required to manage uneven surfaces and unexpected obstacles. Compensation techniques that were previously used within the hospital were now used to identify hazards, to locate important signs, and to differentiate specific items in a cluttered display. For example, on one trip in the community, following a map provided visual spatial challenge; locating a specific package of Lifesavers on a crowded rack used visual analysis skills; and maintaining awareness of street signs, hazards, and other people required left-side attention.

The idea of cold meal preparation was reintroduced; however, Mr. Jackson stated that he felt capable of performing this task and did not want to participate. Although he had previously agreed to make a sandwich, he now seemed resistive. The therapist decided to respect his preference, since she wished to maintain a collaborative relationship. She had seen him reach to high and low shelves during basic self-care and community tasks and felt that his constructional skills were sufficient to perform the task.

As performance continued to improve, Mr. Jackson identified several concrete job tasks on which he would like to concentrate. He experienced difficulty holding a telephone with the left hand while taking messages with the right. Several alternatives such as use of a speaker phone or a shoulder cradle were discussed; however, he was not interested in these adaptations. Instead, the focus was on maintaining simultaneous attention to the task of holding the telephone while listening and writing a message. This type of rapid alternating attention task was quite challenging and would be necessary for other job activities.

In the clinic, the component skills that limited optimal self-care performance were often practiced in isolation and their use in function was then discussed or applied as appropriate. Mr. Jackson's relatively intact cognitive status made it possible for him to transfer skills learned in the clinic to a variety of functional situations. The therapist encouraged independent problem solving during ADL tasks, but pointed out situations in which a perceptual compensation principle, inhibition procedure, or weight-shifting technique was appropriate if he did not spontaneously use the desired method.

Although paper-and-pencil tasks often are not appropriate for addressing cognitive and perceptual limitations, Mr. Jackson relied on paper-and-pencil tasks to perform his job. Various work sheet activities thus proved relevant, interesting, and challenging. He performed activities such as calling various airlines for flight information and choosing the most cost-effective trip that met the imposed time restrictions. He used maps to determine the fastest route between two points. With his therapist, he used the nearby library to locate journals and books. He balanced a checkbook, calculated tips, and scanned the classified advertisements for a deal on a used sports car. These challenging tasks were first carried out in a quiet environment, but later he was asked to perform in the noisy clinic in order to work on his ability to screen out distractions.

Learning inhibition techniques for upper extremity tone management and how to analyze his movement patterns challenged memory and attention to the left side of his body. Problem-solving skills were used to apply these techniques during functional tasks. As he learned more about how his body responded during gross motor, fine motor, and balance activities, he be-

came better able to judge which activities would be safe for him to engage in alone and which would require assistance. Thus problem solving improved as self-awareness was increased.

Inpatient hospitalization was relatively short because of his high level of function. When basic self-care goals were met, he returned home. He required Velcro shoe closures to speed dressing, a tub bench, and a grab bar near the toilet and tub for safety. It was anticipated that this equipment would become less necessary as further improvements were made; however, both Mr. Jackson and his wife wished to purchase the equipment in order to maximize independence. Outpatient follow-up sessions in speech, occupational therapy, and physical therapy were scheduled. In occupational therapy he hoped to focus on further improvements in upper extremity functional use as well as independence in community skills, work, and driving.

He continued to make motoric, perceptual, tactile awareness, and cognitive gains. Because of Mr. Jackson's desire to return to work, a complete neuropsychiatric test battery, a visit with the vocational counselor, and an occupational therapy work skills evaluation that included a half-day of simulated tasks were scheduled. The psychologist was provided with the results of the standardized perceptual tests administered by the occupational therapy department. Mild deficits in selective attention, high-level problem solving, rapid left visual and tactile attention, and motor skill remained, which could negatively influence work performance. A person engaged in a more concrete job may have benefited from intensive work training in a therapy environment, but the abstract and specialized nature of legal work is difficult to simulate. More easily simulated skills, such as telephone use, use of reference books, dictating, and writing reports, were carried out adequately. Mr. Jackson felt that he was ready to work part time, and since he was a partner in the firm, this plan was not resisted by his co-workers. The therapist, the vocational counselor, and the psychologist discussed limitations with Mr. Jackson, his wife, and one of his legal partners. It was agreed that he would initially return to work four hours a day, three times per week. The amount of work would gradually increase. Routine assignments would be given initially, and all work would be monitored carefully by the partner to ensure accuracy.

Because Mr. Jackson had shown markedly improved attention, safety consciousness, and left-side awareness in the community and was insisting that he intended to drive, a driving evaluation was scheduled even though the neuropsychiatric evaluation revealed continued difficulty with visual spatial skills and visual motor speed.

The importance of refraining from driving until he was tested was emphasized. His safety, the safety of others, and the lack of insurance coverage due to his altered physical and cognitive status were stressed. He agreed to wait until formal testing was completed.

During the driving evaluation, difficulty was shown with reaction time measures, visual fields, and visual-motor speed as evidenced by parts A and B of the Trail Making Test. He had difficulty with the simulator. During practice sessions in a parking lot, he hit several cones when navigating in tight spaces. Faced with this concrete evidence, he agreed to wait several months before re-evaluating his driving skill.

OUTCOME

Currently, Mr. Jackson works part time with no reported difficulties, although it is suspected that unfamiliar and highly complex material may cause problems. He and his family do not feel a need for further therapy at this time. He recognizes the need to continue to use perceptual compensation techniques in new and stressful situations, and he continues to use the upper extremity inhibition and control techniques learned in therapy. He has not been able to return to tennis, but he has practiced golf with fair results. He maintains an active social life, visiting with both family and friends, entertaining, and attending sports events. He performs some jobs at home, such as maintaining order in his office, balancing the checkbook, and paying bills. Despite a reduced work role, he does not wish to accept additional home care tasks, and continues to see them as the responsibility of others in the household. Although this occasionally causes friction between him and his wife, they are generally satisfied with their current duties.

Mr. Jackson has had to alter the way in which he performs previously routine tasks. The increased effort that is required to maintain attention while compensating for perceptual/motor deficits leads to more rapid fatigue. He becomes upset more easily, especially during periods of high activity or stress. He has therefore tried to reduce his exposure to large groups of people, busy or crowded store conditions, and highly demanding work projects. He has given up some favored sports activities and has not yet resumed driving. Overall, however, he has made a successful adjustment by substituting other interests for those that are too difficult, and by taking advantage of reduced work time in order to spend more time with family and friends. He has accepted these changes because they were necessary given his changed physical and cognitive status. Although he has not given up hope that his skills will return to their previous level, he acknowledges that by learning to adapt and perform his roles in new ways, he has achieved a measure of success. He feels thankful for the abilities that he has retained, and is proud of his efforts to overcome his limitations in order to contribute at home and at work. His supportive family, an accepting work environment, and his strong motivation to succeed have assisted him in adjusting to his limitations in order to achieve this positive outcome.

Part III

Evaluation and Treatment Guides

Chapter 10

Cognitive Evaluation Guide

This portion of the book is intended as a reference section and manual for identifying specific cognitive deficits that relate to function. Each section describes functional observations and tests for that deficit area. Functional observations should be done first whenever possible. A checklist can be used to note observations of cognitive and perceptual deficits during functional tasks (Exhibit 10-1). A simple three-point rating scale is suggested to provide a summary rating of the patient's status in each cognitive area. Tests can then be used to clarify and confirm observations if the therapist experiences difficulty in defining the underlying problem. Although several tests are listed for each deficit, the therapist should choose the test that will best fit his or her patient. Short, nonstandardized tests provide an opportunity to observe the patient's approach to a specific cognitive task. Standardized tests generally provide a higher degree of challenge and include norms that can help identify deficits in patients with subtle cognitive deficits. The standardized tests should be used if any type of patient research related to cognition and perception is contemplated. Many of the standardized tests can be purchased. The commercial source for these tests is provided.

AROUSAL

Functional Observations

Using the guidelines below, responses during activities of daily living (ADL) should be monitored to deter-

mine which types of stimulation produce optimal arousal. Frequently the patient with arousal deficits will be dependent on others for self-care or will be able to perform only a small part of a task, such as moving the washcloth during oral/facial hygiene. If the patient is dependent, the therapist can perform the task while noting the person's response to the various types of stimulation inherent in the activity.

Tactile. Note the patient's reactions to joint movement while dressing, water temperature during washing, changes in air temperature when removing blankets or moving between rooms, light touch versus deep pressure, and various textures (e.g., clothing, washcloth, lotion, etc.).

Vestibular. Observe changes in arousal during or following movement such as bending, rolling, bed mobility, transfers, traveling in the wheelchair, or reaching.

Auditory. Use various sounds such as voice, music, or bells and note the patient's response. Determine whether verbal commands, ambient sounds, familiar voices, or music have a positive effect on performance. Qualify the type of auditory stimulation that is most beneficial. Do loud sounds or soft sounds enhance arousal? Does background noise interfere with or improve responsiveness? Does fast or slow music lead to optimal arousal? Do unusual sounds such as a bell or buzzer stimulate increased responsiveness?

Visual. Define the amount, color, familiarity, and type of visual information that produces the highest

Exhibit 10-1 Record of Cognitive and Perceptual Component Skill Deficits during Self-Care Tasks

Skill Area	F D G	O F H	U E D	L E D	B A T H	T O I L	H M K	C O M	W R K	OTHER Describe _____
AROUSAL						X	X	X	X	
Describe length of time arousal maintained, environment (i.e., quiet, familiar, distracting), and type of stimulation (i.e., auditory, visual, tactile, vestibular, olfactory, gustatory).										
Skill Area	F D G	O F H	U E D	L E D	B A T H	T O I L	H M K	C O M	W R K	OTHER Describe _____
ATTENTION										
Describe type of attention, i.e., sustained, selective, alternating, and length of time.										
Skill Area	F D G	O F H	U E D	L E D	B A T H	T O I L	H M K	C O M	W R K	OTHER Describe _____
MEMORY										
Note whether STM (<1 hr) or LTM (>1 hr) were evaluated. Also describe sensory channels that are most effective: visual, auditory, tactile/kinesthetic.										
Skill Area	F D G	O F H	U E D	L E D	B A T H	T O I L	H M K	C O M	W R K	OTHER Describe _____
ORIENTATION										
Describe any difficulties with orientation to place, time, or people.										
Skill Area	F D G	O F H	U E D	L E D	B A T H	T O I L	H M K	C O M	W R K	OTHER Describe _____
PROBLEM SOLVING										
Describe where problem-solving difficulties occur: problem identification, generation of solutions, plan of action, implementation, safety, or self-monitoring.										
Skill Area	F D G	O F H	U E D	L E D	B A T H	T O I L	H M K	C O M	W R K	OTHER Describe _____
UNILATERAL VISUAL AWARENESS										
VISUAL SPATIAL AWARENESS (position of object, parts to whole)										
VISUAL ANALYSIS, SYNTHESIS (object identification, figure-ground, visual closure)										
VISUAL CONSTRUCTION (putting parts together)										
MIDLINE ORIENTATION										
UNILATERAL TACTILE AWARENESS										
TACTILE DISCRIMINATION (detection of shape, texture)										
Note specific deficits in tactile accommodation, body parts awareness, right-left discrimination, or bilateral integration.										
Skill Area	F D G	O F H	U E D	L E D	B A T H	T O I L	H M K	C O M	W R K	OTHER Describe _____
MOTOR PLANNING										
Describe whether activities were familiar or unfamiliar; note perseveration, sequencing difficulties, or object use problems.										

Key: FDG = feeding; OFH = oral/facial hygiene; UED = upper extremity dressing; LED = lower extremity dressing; TOIL = toileting; HMK = homemaking; COM = community; WRK = work; STM = short-term memory; LTM = long-term memory.

Rating: Choose ratings based on the descriptions in the functional observation section of the cognitive and perceptual workbook. N, no apparent deficit; P, partial deficit; S, severe deficit.
Below the rating note any information that will help qualify ratings.

level of arousal. For instance, Does the patient respond best to bright colors on a plain background? Does he or she become more alert when presented pictures of familiar people or objects? Does he or she respond best in a stark environment when asked to attend visually to one or two items?

Olfactory. Stimulate olfaction through use of lotions, colognes, extracts, and foods if appropriate. Present the stimuli for no longer than 10 seconds to avoid accommodation.

Gustatory. Note whether the tastes of certain foods seem to stimulate increased arousal. Do not test this sense until it has been determined that the patient is swallowing safely, since decreased arousal may make the patient more prone to choking. Small amounts of various tastes such as flavored ice, candy wrapped in gauze, or a flavored liquid can be applied with a swab to the appropriate receptors of the tongue. Note response to sweet, salty, bitter, and sour flavors (Table 10-1).

General

During selected activities such as oral/facial hygiene or feeding, note the amount of time before arousal is elicited and the length of time it is sustained. Choose several types of sensory stimulation that elicit the best patient response. Document the amount of elapsed time before a response occurs and the length of time that it is sustained. Allow approximately one to two minutes between stimuli in order to determine the latency of responses (Bermann and Bush 1988).

Clinical Observations

Interpretation

Note the types of stimulation that enhance arousal as well as the amount of stimulation required and the length of time that arousal is maintained. The following ratings can provide an overall rating for arousal.

No Apparent Deficit. The patient maintains wakefulness without prompting in all functional tasks.

Table 10-1 Location of Taste Receptors (Crouch and McClintic 1971)

Taste	Area of the Tongue
Sweet	Tip
Sour	Lateral edges, midway between the tip and back
Salty	Lateral edges, proximal and distal to the "sour" sensors
Bitter	Back portion

Partial Deficit. A partial deficit is any deficit that is between no apparent deficit and severe deficit. Specify the types of stimulation that are most effective.

Severe Deficit. The patient requires vigorous or highly specialized auditory, vestibular, visual, or other stimulation to maintain wakefulness for longer than 5 minutes. The patient may require noxious stimulation to elicit arousal. Specify the types of stimulation that are most effective.

ATTENTION

Functional Observations

Sustained Attention. Observe how well a patient attends to relevant information during task performance. The patient not only must appear to be intent on the task but must respond to important aspects of the task. For example, if a shirt becomes twisted when putting it on, the patient should indicate that he or she is aware of the mistake. When no difficulty is shown during simple routine tasks in a quiet environment, challenges should be increased by requiring performance of tasks that are more difficult and/or by increasing the stimulation in the environment.

Selective Attention

Observe the patient's ability to remain focused on functional activities such as eating, reading, exercising, following a map, playing a game, balancing a checkbook, or performing work simulation tasks while in a visually or auditorily stimulating environment. The ability to screen out or filter distractions implies that the person will respond to relevant distractors while ignoring those that decrease efficiency. The patient can be expected to respond to significant others or events in the environment, then return to the primary task.

Alternating Attention

To assess rapid alternating attention, observe the patient performing several tasks at once that require attention (e.g., writing a list while listening for a buzzer; setting the table while watching to ensure that cooking food does not burn; or conversing while exercising, cooking, or dressing). This type of attention can be expected only when at least one of the two tasks draws on automatic skills. For example, one could rapidly alternate attention between driving and conversing, or exercising and counting the number of repetitions. However, when one or both tasks require a high degree of concentration for accurate performance, this type of attention should not be expected.

Interpretation

Note the types of attention that are most problematic for the patient. Describe environmental or task features that limit attention. The following ratings can be used to provide a general description of attentional skills.

No Apparent Deficit. In a stimulating environment and during multistep tasks, the patient is able to determine relevant information, attend to critical factors for safe and accurate task performance, and, if distracted by pertinent events in the environment, can redirect self back to the task.

Partial Deficit. A partial deficit is any deficit that is between no apparent deficit and severe deficit. Specify the particular attentional problems.

Severe Deficit. In a *structured/quiet* environment, during one-step tasks, frequent cues are required to direct the patient to attend to relevant information and/or to redirect the patient when he or she is distracted. Frequent changes in activity (about every three minutes) are required. Specify the environmental and task features that enhance performance.

Tests: Sustained Attention

Name: Cancellation Task

Description

The patient is asked to scan several rows of letters and cross out those designated by the examiner.

Pros. This test is portable, is challenging, can be used to evaluate both unilateral neglect as well as visual attention, and seems to be more acceptable to some patients than the visual vigilance test described below. Some norms for performance are available.

Cons. Because recognition of letters is required, this test is not appropriate for aphasics.

Instructions

In a quiet, nondistracting room, administer the letter cancellation test described in the unilateral visual inattention section of Chapter 11.

Interpretation

If errors are scattered on both halves of the page and/or if errors tend to increase toward the end of the task, difficulties in visual vigilance may be suspected.

Name: Visual Vigilance Test (Abreu 1987)

Description

A series of cards is presented. The patient is required to watch for a predetermined shape or shapes (see Figure 4-5).

Pros. This test isolates visual attention from auditory attention, is easily transported, and is quickly administered.

Cons. Basic visual perceptual skills are required; therefore, the test cannot be used with patients who have severe visual perceptual deficits. The task is not standardized and may not be motivating to some patients.

Instructions

Source: Adapted from *Rehabilitation of Perceptual-Cognitive Dysfunction* by B. Abreu with permission of B. Abreu, © 1987.

In a quiet environment, the therapist says, "I am going to quickly show you different shapes like these [quickly flash cards]. Whenever you see this circle [show], respond like this [Knock once on the table, or say "circle," or nod head, etc. Choose the type of response that is easiest for the patient]. Ready? Let's begin." Sixty shape cards are quickly turned over by the examiner, one per second. Each card is placed on top of the previous one so that only one card is visible at a time. Cards are presented at the patient's midline or in their intact visual field. The therapist can inconspicuously make a hatch mark to denote each error. To document specific types of errors, the therapist can write *O* for an omission error, *C* for a commission error, and *P* for a perseveration error.

Interpretation

Clinical observations should include the number of errors and whether they became more numerous toward the end of the task. The errors can be described further by using Strub and Black's system (1985) as follows: (1) omission error—failure to respond when the correct stimulus has been presented; (2) commission error—response made when an incorrect stimulus has been presented; (3) perseveration error—continued response to subsequent incorrect stimuli.

Name: Random Letter Test (Strub and Black 1985)

Description

The patient is asked to listen to a series of letters and indicate when the specified letter is heard.

Pros. This test isolates auditory attention and is administered quickly. Preliminary norms are available.

Cons. The task may not be motivating to some patients and cannot be used with individuals who demonstrate receptive aphasia.

Instructions

Source: Adapted from *The Mental Status Examination in Neurology* (p. 43) by R.L. Strub and F.W. Black with permission of the F.A. Davis Co., © 1985.

In a quiet, nondistracting room, say to the patient: "I am going to read you a long series of letters; whenever you hear the letter *A*, respond like this." [Knock once on the table, or say "A," or say "yes," or nod your head, etc. Choose the type of response that is easiest for the patient.] Read the following list of letters in a normal tone at a rate of one letter per second:

    L T P E A O A I C T D A L A A
    A N I A B F S A M R Z E O A D
    P A K L A U C J T O E A B A A
    Z Y F M U S A H E V A A R A T

Interpretation

Preliminary norms show that average control subjects complete this test without error, whereas brain-damaged patients make an average of 10 errors (Strub and Black 1985). If errors are made, describe the types of errors seen: (1) omission error—failure to indicate when the correct letter has been presented; (2) commission error—patient responds to an incorrect letter; (3) perseveration error—patient continues to respond when subsequent incorrect letters are presented (Strub and Black 1985).

Tests: Selective Attention

Description

Any of the tests listed under "Sustained Attention" may be used in a distracting environment to test selective attention.

Pros. See "Sustained Attention."

Cons. See "Sustained Attention."

Instructions

Administer any of the tests listed under "Sustained Attention" in a distracting environment such as a noisy clinic, cafeteria, or lobby. This should be done only after the ability to sustain attention in a quiet environment is demonstrated.

Tests: Alternating Attention

Name: Trail Making Test

Originally part of the Army Individual Test Battery (1944) and now in the public domain, test forms and an administration manual can be obtained from Reitan Neuropsychology Laboratory, 1338 East Edison Street, Tucson, AZ 85719.

Description

This test has two parts, part A and part B, both of which consist of 25 circles containing numbers (part A) or numbers and letters (part B). Part A requires connecting a series of numbers in order. Part B requires alternating attention as the patient draws a line from a number to a letter in sequence. For example, the patient would draw a line from "1" to "A," then from "2" to "B," then from "3" to "C," etc. (See Figures 4-7 and 4-8).

Pros. This test is helpful for screening higher-level attentional deficits. It is easily transported, and norms exist for the standardized test.

Cons. Because the ability to recognize and put letters and numbers in order is required, it is not appropriate for aphasics.

Instructions

Begin with the part A sample sheet.

Part A: Sample

Provide the following instructions: "Begin at number one [point] and draw a line from one to two [point], two to three [point], three to four [point], and so on, in order, until you reach the end [point]. Draw the lines as fast as you can. Do not lift the pencil from the paper. Ready! Begin!"

The sample is used for teaching; therefore, the therapist should point out mistakes and explain them. For example, the therapist can instruct the patient to keep the pencil on the paper, re-explain the sequence of numbers, etc. After a mistake has been explained, the therapist should instruct the patient to "Go on from here." If performance is still inaccurate, guide the patient's hand through the sequence, using the eraser end of the pencil. Then say,

> Now you try it. Put your pencil point down. Remember, begin at number one [point] and draw a line from one to two [point], two to three [point], three to four [point], and so on,

in order, until you reach the circle marked "end" [point]. Do not skip around but go from one number to the next in the proper order. If you make a mistake, mark it out. Remember, work as fast as you can. Ready! Begin!

If mistakes continue to be made, repeat the teaching procedure until understanding is demonstrated or it is clear that this test is too difficult. If the patient performs correctly say, "Good! Let's try the next one," and proceed with part A.

Part A: Test

On this page are numbers from one to twenty-five. Do this the same way. Begin at number one [point] and draw a line from one to two [point], two to three [point], three to four [point], and so on, in order, until you reach the end [point]. Remember, work as fast as you can. Ready! Begin!

Start timing. Point out errors immediately, and have the patient continue from the place that the mistake occurred. Do not stop timing. Record the total number of seconds for test completion. Errors are recorded only as increased time for test performance. If part A is completed without error, continue with the sample part B. Say, "That's fine. Now we'll try another one."

Part B: Sample

Place the sample sheet for part B on the table and point to the sheet, saying,

On this page are some numbers and letters. Begin at number one [point] and draw a line from one to A [point to A], A to two [point], two to B [point to B], three to C [point to C], and so on, in order until you reach the end [point]. Remember, first you have a number [point to 1], then a letter [point to A], then a number [point to 2], then a letter [point to B], and so on. Draw the lines as fast as you can. Ready! Begin!

Again, use the sample for teaching. If a mistake was made, the examiner marks out the error and asks the patient to start from the last correct circle, saying, "Go on from here [point]. Use the guiding technique described in part A if errors continue, then say,

Now you try it. Remember you begin at number one [point] and draw a line from one to A [point to A], A to two [point], two to B [point

to B], B to three [point], three to C [point to C], and so on, in order, until you reach the circle marked "end" [point]. Ready! Begin!

If mistakes continue to be made, repeat the teaching procedure until understanding is demonstrated or it is clear that this test is too difficult. If the patient performs correctly say, "Good! Let's try the next one," and proceed with part B.

Part B: Test

Say:

On this page are both numbers and letters. Do this the same way. Begin at number one [point] and draw a line from one to A [point to A], A to two [point], two to B [point to B], B to three [point], three to C [point to C], and so on, in order, until you reach the end [point]. Remember, first you have a number [point to 1], then a letter [point to A], then a number [point to 2], then a letter [point to B], and so on. Do not skip around, but go from one circle to the next in the proper order. Draw the lines as fast as you can. Ready! Begin!

Start timing. Point out errors immediately, and have the patient continue from the place where the mistake occurred. Do not stop timing. Record the total number of seconds for test completion. Errors are recorded only as increased time for test performance.

Interpretation

This test requires the integration of various skills; therefore, careful observation of patient performance can help the therapist identify a range of difficulties. Visual perceptual skills are required to scan the unstructured array of figures efficiently and locate the numbers and letters; language skills are needed to identify the symbols; mental tracking skills are necessary to keep the numerical and alphabetical sequence simultaneously in mind; and alternating attention is required to attend to the relevant figures while switching between a number and a letter sequence. If the patient shows a wide discrepancy between performance on part A and part B, the problems may be attributed to difficulty with alternating attention and mental tracking. If the patient has problems with both parts of the test, primary attentional deficits, visual perceptual problems, or impaired language skills may be the cause (Reitan 1958). Since this test is timed, it is vulnerable to the effects of aging. Table 10-2 indicates scores in seconds for control subjects.

Name: Symbol Digit Modalities Test (Smith 1982)

This test is available from Western Psychological Services, 12031 Wilshire Boulevard, Los Angeles, CA 90025.

Description

The patient is asked to pair symbols with their corresponding numbers according to a code. The patient is given 90 seconds to work on this task (see Figure 4-9).

Pros. This is a standardized test with well-established reliability and validity data that can be administered quickly and is easily transported. It can be given as a written or an oral test.

Cons. The standardized directions are very long and require a high level of verbal comprehension.

Instructions

Source: Adapted from the *Symbol Digit Modalities Test Manual* by A. Smith with permission of Western Psychological Services, © 1982.

This test can be given in a written or verbal form. When using the written form, the examiner should omit the words in italics when giving instructions. When giving the verbal form, the examiner should omit the words in brackets and should write the numbers in the boxes for the patient. The verbal form should be used when the patient lacks the visual motor control to fill in the boxes quickly.

While sitting on the patient's nonaffected side, say:

Please look at these boxes at the top of the page. You can see that each box in the upper row has a little mark in it. Now look at the boxes in the row just underneath the marks. Each of the boxes under the marks has a number. Each of the marks in the top row is different, and under each mark in the bottom row is a different number. Now look at the next line of boxes [point] just under the top two rows. Notice that the boxes on the top have marks but the boxes underneath are empty. You are to fill in each empty box with the number that should go there according to the way they are paired in the key at the top of the page. *And tell me what the number is.* For example, if you look at the first mark, and then look at the key, you will see that the number 1 goes in the first box. *So you call out the number one for the first box.* Now what number should you put in the second box? *Just call it out to me* (five). That's right. *So you would say five to me* [so write the number five in the second box]. What number goes in the third box (two)? Two, right. That is the idea. You are to fill each of the empty boxes with the numbers that should go in them according to the key. *And call out the numbers to me.* Now for practice, *tell me the numbers that* fill in the rest of the boxes until you come to the double line. When you come to the double line, Stop!

Now when I say "go," *call out* [write in] the numbers just like you have been doing as fast as you can until I say stop. *I will write the numbers down for you.* When you come to

---

Table 10-2 Trail Making Test Scores for Control Subjects

Percentile	Age Group									
	20–39 (n = 180)		40–49 (n = 90)		50–59 (n = 90)		60–69 (n = 90)		70–79 (n = 90)	
	Part A	Part B	Part A	Part B	Part A	Part B	Part A	Part B	Part A	Part B
90th	21	45	22	49	25	55	29	64	38	79
75th	26	55	28	57	29	75	35	89	54	132
50th	32	69	34	78	38	98	48	119	80	196
25th	42	94	45	100	49	135	67	172	105	292
10th	50	129	59	151	67	177	104	282	168	450

Source: Adapted with permission from *Journal of Clinical Psychology* (1968;24:97), Copyright © 1968, Clinical Psychology Publishing Co., Inc.

the end of the first line, go quickly to the next line without stopping, and so on. *If you make a mistake, tell me what you think the correct answer is.* [If you make a mistake, do not erase, just write the correct answer over your mistake. I repeat, do not erase as you will waste time. Just write the correct answer over your mistake.] Do not skip any boxes and work as quickly as you can. Ready? Go! [Start stop watch and after 90 seconds say . . . Stop!]

Interpretation

To interpret the test fully, use norms and observations as described in the test booklet. This test requires visual perceptual skills, visual scanning, visual attention, shifting attention between two types of stimuli, intellect, and motor speed for the written form of the test. The correct responses are counted, beginning with the double line. Mean scores are shown in Table 10-3.

ORIENTATION

Functional Observations

Observe whether the patient's responses to questions and behavior during treatment indicate an awareness of his or her surroundings, an understanding of who you and other caretakers are, and an appreciation of time.

Tests

Name: Orientation Interview

Description

An interview is used to determine the patient's orientation to person, place, and time.

Pros. The questions elicit information about orientation and past roles in a brief format.

Cons. A high degree of verbal fluency is required, and the task may be repetitious if other disciplines routinely ask similar questions.

Instructions

Source: Adapted from *Rehabilitation of Perceptual-Cognitive Dysfunction* by B. Abreu with permission of B. Abreu, © 1987.

The sample interview questions below are intended as a guide. Items with an asterisk represent the questions that are considered essential to determining a person's orientation to critical factors about self, significant others, place, and time. Do not rate patients who have severe language deficits. Rather than reading the list, choose several questions from each category, attempting to use them in a conversation that flows naturally. Asking a long list of questions can be annoying to the patient.

Self

- What is your name*
- When were you born?
- Where do you live?
- Who do you live with?
- Do you have a family?
- What are their names?
- What type of work do you do?
- Using pictures or with family members present, ask "Who is this?" If family members or friends are not available, ask "Do you remember who I am?" ("Therapist" is a sufficient answer.)*
- What do you like to do in your spare time?

Place

- Where are you now?*
- Do you know what we do here?

Table 10-3 Symbol Digit Modalities Test Scores (N = 1,307)

	Years of Education: 12 or Less				Years of Education: 13 or More			
Age	Mean Score: Written	(STD)	Mean Score: Oral	(STD)	Mean Score: Written	(STD)	Mean Score: Oral	(STD)
18–24	54.40	(8.31)	61.31	(11.39)	61.93	(10.15)	69.91	(12.64)
25–34	53.30	(7.98)	60.57	(9.14)	57.72	(9.08)	65.71	(11.64)
35–44	51.50	(8.03)	59.87	(10.49)	54.20	(11.17)	60.95	(11.32)
45–54	47.26	(9.56)	53.91	(10.40)	52.27	(8.48)	58.31	(8.67)
55–64	42.80	(8.08)	49.03	(9.03)	47.60	(8.31)	54.47	(8.93)
65–78	33.31	(9.02)	42.05	(11.26)	43.55	(11.27)	52.89	(13.54)

Source: Adapted from the *Symbol Digit Modalities Test Manual*, by A. Smith with permission of Western Psychological Services, © 1982.

- How far is your home from here?
- What state/city are we in?
- Where is your room? (floor, room number)

Time

It is important to test both the patient's awareness of the specific time and date as well as awareness of the passage of time, since these are discrete skills.

- What is today's date? (the year, the month, and the day of the month) (Control subjects may err by one or two days, according to Benton 1983d.)*
- How long has it been since your accident/stroke?
- How long have we been talking? Or, How long has it been since your last meal? (Less than one half the actual time is considered an error.)*
- What time is it now? (Responds with the approximate time of day. Normal subjects may err by more than 30 minutes, according to Benton 1983d.)
- What day of the week is it? (Normal subjects very rarely are incorrect, per Benton 1983d.)
- What season is this?
- What is the next holiday?
- What holiday just passed?
- Name three holidays in winter.
- Who is the president?

Name: Estimation of Time (Benton 1964)

Description

The patient is asked to estimate the passage of one minute.

Pros. Information about the patient's awareness of time is provided. These deficits may not be apparent during functional observations because of the amount of structure that is inherent in a hospital setting.

Cons. Because of the language skills required, this test cannot be used with aphasic patients.

Instructions

Ask the patient to estimate the passage of one minute: "I would like you to try to tell me when 1 minute has passed. I will start the timer. You tell me when you think 1 minute has passed. Begin now." The examiner uses a watch or stopwatch to time the patient. Timing is stopped after 1 minute 38 seconds if no response has been given.

Interpretation

Errors of 21 to 22 seconds are average, errors of 33 seconds are moderately inaccurate, and errors of 38 seconds are extremely inaccurate (Benton [1964] as described by Lezak [1983]).

TOPOGRAPHICAL ORIENTATION

Functional Observations

Ask the patient to find the way from his or her room to other known areas such as the bathroom, the nurses' station, or a treatment area on another floor of the facility.

Have the patient describe the floor plan of the inpatient floor of the hospital (e.g., the cafeteria is on the second floor, occupational therapy is on the 10th floor, physical therapy is next to occupational therapy, etc.).

Once familiarized with the area outside the hospital, ask the patient to find his or her way to a given location, with or without a map.

Ask the patient to describe the floor plan of his or her house or a route from the house to a store or gas station. (Note: This is dependent on the family for verification.)

Interpretation

Just as with other areas of orientation, topographical awareness depends on a variety of cognitive and spatial skills. Memory deficits or visual spatial deficits may interfere with the patient's ability to remember where he or she has been or to visualize the relationship of one place to another. When drawing a floor plan, constructional apraxia must be ruled out.

No Apparent Deficit. Once familiarized with the territory, the patient can find his or her way within or outside the hospital. A map can be used when indicated to find new locations.

Partial Deficit. A partial deficit is any deficit that falls between no apparent deficit and severe deficit.

Severe Deficit. After several days, the patient continues to require direct supervision or assistance to locate his or her room or other areas that should be familiar.

MEMORY

Functional Observations

Short-Term Memory

Auditory. Note the patient's ability to recall relevant *new* information for approximately one minute. For example, ask the patient to remember the therapist's name or any instruction that was given.

Visual. Ask the patient to point to or describe a person, object, or location that was encountered.

Tactile/Kinesthetic. Ask the patient to repeat an action that was just demonstrated.

General. Note whether the patient retains information best when it is presented visually, verbally, or in a tactile/kinesthetic manner.

Long-Term Memory

Use tasks similar to those listed above; however, lengthen the time that memory is required. Note the patient's ability to retain specific instructions provided during the treatment hour. Prior to a shopping trip, for example, review with the patient two items to purchase. Note the patient's ability to retain this information once he or she has arrived at the store.

Once the patient is familiarized with a setting such as the kitchen or a treatment room, note his or her ability to remember the location of objects successfully (e.g., where utensils are kept in the kitchen, or where the exercise equipment is stored in the treatment room).

At the end of the treatment hour ask the patient to demonstrate or describe a few of the activities that he or she was involved in during the therapy session.

Interpretation

The therapist should determine which type(s) of memory are strongest in order to suggest corresponding methods for training the patient to perform activities in new ways. The following ratings can be used separately for each of the modes of memory (visual, auditory, and tactile/kinesthetic) as well as for recent and remote memory if performance varies. For example, the patient may show no apparent deficit for recent visual memory and a partial deficit for remote verbal memory. Overall the rating for memory would be partial deficit. The therapist would then qualify the rating.

No Apparent Deficit. The patient adequately recalls relevant visual, auditory, and tactile/kinesthetic information within a one-hour period retains important instructions for periods of time longer than one hour.

Partial Deficit. A partial deficit is any deficit that falls between no apparent deficit and severe deficit. Specify the type of memory deficits noted.

Severe Deficit. The patient is unable to recall visual, auditory, and tactile/kinesthetic information after one minute.

Tests: Sensory Memory

Name: Digit Repetition (Strub and Black 1985)

Description

The patient is asked to repeat a series of numbers immediately after the therapist.

Pros. This test is quickly administered and helps identify problems with immediate recall. It can also be used as a test of attention.

Cons. Because language skills are required, the test is not appropriate for aphasic patients.

Instructions

Source: Adapted from *The Mental Status Examination in Neurology* by R.L. Strub and F.W. Black with permission of the F.A. Davis Co., © 1985.

The therapist sits directly in front of the patient and verbally presents a series of digits at the rate of one number per second. The therapist states, "I am going to say some simple numbers. Listen carefully, and when I am finished, say the numbers after me." Begin with the first trial of two digits and continue until the patient fails:

3 - 7	9 - 2
7 - 4 - 9	1 - 7 - 4
8 - 5 - 2 - 7	5 - 2 - 9 - 7
2 - 9 - 6 - 8 - 8 - 3	6 - 3 - 8 - 5 - 1
5 - 7 - 2 - 9 - 4 - 6	2 - 9 - 4 - 7 - 3 - 8
8 - 1 - 5 - 9 - 3 - 6 - 2	4 - 1 - 9 - 2 - 7 - 5 - 1
3 - 9 - 8 - 2 - 5 - 1 - 4 - 7	8 - 5 - 3 - 9 - 1 - 6 - 2 - 7
7 - 2 - 8 - 5 - 4 - 6 - 7 - 3 - 9	2 - 1 - 9 - 7 - 3 - 5 - 8 - 4 - 6

Interpretation

Failure to perform adequately on this test may indicate a poor attention span as well as immediate recall problems. A patient should recall five to seven numbers for acceptable performance.

Tests: Short-Term Memory

Name: Visual Memory Test

Description

The patient is given nine photographs of functional objects to memorize (see Figure 4-10).

Pros. The test isolates visual memory.

Cons. The test is not standardized and cannot be used with patients showing severe visual perceptual deficits.

Instructions

The patient is told, "Look at these pictures and try to remember as many as you can." One minute is given to memorize the pictures. The pictures are removed, and the patient is then asked to recall as many objects as possible. If he or she is unable to answer because of language deficits or difficulty with recall, response sheets may be presented. The patient is then asked to point to the pictures that he or she remembers (see Figures 4-11A and B).

Interpretation

The patient should be able to remember five items, plus or minus two, for normal performance. If the response sheet is used, the task is made easier, since the patient is using recognition rather than free recall to retrieve the information. Differences between the patient's performance on the visual and auditory memory tests can indicate modality-specific memory deficits, whereas poor performance on both indicates more generalized problems possibly related to poor attention or poor ability to organize information.

PROBLEM SOLVING

Functional Observations

Begin observations with routine tasks or basic self-care. If the patient has shown good problem-solving abilities with these activities, gradually increase the level of challenge and the risk involved. Make the patient responsible for all decisions, and intervene only if harm is likely. For example, ask the patient to plan and carry out community trips; identify, plan, and participate in work simulation tasks; or plan a menu, purchase ingredients, and cook a meal. Suggestions for observing each of the components of problem-solving behavior follow.

Problem Identification

Does the patient recognize the difficulties imposed by current functional limitations? Does he or she recognize problems in the environment or in an activity when they occur?

Solution Generation

Can the patient identify solutions that have been effective in the past or try a new method to accomplish a task (e.g., open toothpaste or a container one-handed,

stabilize an object for cutting, or dress self). Observe the ability to apply judgment and weigh the consequences of various solutions before attempting the action (i.e., covert problem solving versus trial and error). Is safety consciousness and efficiency reflected in the chosen solutions? Is realistic awareness of current abilities demonstrated in the solutions to problems?

Planning

Does the patient plan the activity prior to beginning? Is he or she efficient in terms of energy conservation and work simplification principles? Do the steps of the plan follow logically?

Implementation

Does the patient implement the plan, or wait for direction to do so? Does he or she use the solutions and plans that were generated previously? If the patient moves directly to implementation without evidence of advanced planning or considering various solutions, are the resulting behaviors logical and effective? Is impulsivity noted? For example, does the patient remember to lock the wheelchair brakes; wait for assistance to stand when motor control is poor; or maintain awareness of obstacles, traffic, and other people when in the community? Note the effect of the environment on safety judgment. (Does a quiet structured environment improve problem solving? Is poor safety awareness seen only in certain environments, such as the kitchen or the community?)

Self-Monitoring

Is the patient aware of changes in the activity or the environment that necessitate a change in the plan? When the established plan is not effective, is he or she able to make spontaneous changes, or does he or she stick rigidly with the original approach? Is ongoing decision making evident?

Outcome

Was the final result safe and effective? Was the goal of the activity met? Was the activity completed in a timely manner?

Interpretation

The following scale, based on Allen's cognitive levels (1985), can be used to summarize observations of problem-solving behavior. For treatment planning purposes, however, the therapist should attempt to define which steps of the problem-solving process are faulty and what underlying cognitive and/or perceptual deficits are causing these problems. (Did difficulty arise with problem identification, planning, or self-monitoring? Are perceptual deficits, memory problems, or poor attentional skills interfering with problem solving?)

No Apparent Deficit. During basic and complex clinical tasks or ADL activities appropriate to his or her life style, the patient thinks through problems and considers alternatives before carrying out a plan. The patient effectively finds safe solutions to problems encountered without the therapist's intervention (Allen's level 6) or the patient uses a trial-and-error approach to problem solving and may not generally reflect on alternative courses of action or consequences of action. After experiencing the outcome of an action, results can be generalized to other situations (Allen's level 5).

Partial Deficit. The patient is able to solve a problem only if the usual solution is apparent. Thus the patient can solve familiar problems using routine patterns, but is unable to find new solutions to new problems (Allen's level 4).

Severe Deficit. The patient does not recognize the cause of problems and is unable to generate alternative strategies to allow successful performance (Allen's levels 1 to 3). Frequent intervention or monitoring (during more than 50 percent of the task) is required for safe, effective performance.

Not Examined. If the patient has been participating in structured activities and has not had the opportunity to make independent judgments, do not rate.

Tests

Name: Problem-Solving Simulations

Description

The patient is asked to solve verbally several functional problems.

Pros. Some insight into the patient's strategies for dealing with an emergency situation can be gained and the questions can be used early in the patient's admission if he or she has not yet had the opportunity to exhibit safety judgment in higher-level activities.

Cons. Verbal descriptions cannot substitute for observation of actual performance, since often verbal plans are not carried out when a problem occurs. Since this task relies heavily on language skills it is not appropriate for aphasic patients.

Instructions

Use these simulations only when the patient has good language skills. Follow up with functional obser-

vations, since a patient may be able to verbalize a response but not follow through. Present the following situations:

1. You need to use the bathroom at night. Your balance is not good enough for you to walk alone. You have called for the nurse, but no one has come. What should you do?
2. You locked yourself out of your house. What should you do?
3. You are at home alone and you fall. What should you do?

Interpretation

Analyze the patient's responses for evidence of insight into his or her disability, awareness of safety procedures, and ability to generate alternative strategies. Although verbal answers will indicate the patient's thoughts about the situation, the stress and demands imposed by a real emergency may cause performance to vary considerably. The patient must never be labeled "safe" on the basis of verbal responses alone.

Name: Three-Dimensional Block Design and Rey Figure

Description

The patient is asked to copy a complex two- or three-dimensional figure.

Pros. The therapist can observe both constructional and problem-solving skills in one test.

Cons. Because the test requires several different skills, it may be difficult to separate the visual perceptual, motor-planning, and problem-solving components. The problem-solving skills required for these tests are not as sophisticated as those required in complex daily living tasks.

Instructions

Present the tests as described in the visual construction section of the protocol (Chapter 11).

Interpretation

Note the patient's ability to organize the task, monitor the effectiveness of his or her choices, use mental manipulations versus a trial-and-error approach, and arrive at a successful conclusion. Determine which components of the task caused the most difficulty.

Name: Block Arrangement Problem

Description

The patient is asked to position a block on a small bulletin board by using the following materials: A small cardboard box (paper clip box), a thumbtack, a paper clip, a safety pin, a rubber band, a plastic cup, and a wooden block (see Figures 4-13 and 4-14).

Pros. This easy-to-administer test requires abstract thought, creative thinking, and physical manipulation rather than purely verbal problem solving. It can be done with one hand.

Cons. This is not a standardized test and is slightly bulky to transport. The problem-solving skills required are not as sophisticated as those needed to solve problems encountered in daily living tasks.

Instructions

The board is held vertically by the therapist, and the materials are presented to the patient with the following instructions: "I would like you to place this block on the bulletin board in any way you can, using these materials." The patient may ask for physical assistance if needed; however, the task can be completed with one hand.

Interpretation

Note the patient's ability to generate creative alternative solutions, test these solutions through covert versus overt methods, formulate a plan, monitor its effectiveness, modify the plan if needed, and arrive at a satisfactory solution. Solutions include tacking the box or cup to the board and placing the block on it; wrapping a rubber band around the block and attaching it to the board; or creating two struts with the pin and paper clip, and placing the block on them. As with other types of problem solving, the therapist should attempt to define the underlying cause(s) of difficulty, such as poor vis-

ual perceptual processing, poor solution generation, or poor self-monitoring. Results should not be generalized to functional performance, but problem areas noted during the simulation should be watched for during functional tasks.

Name: Financial Problems

Description

The patient is asked to solve two simple, functional, calculation problems.

Pros. This test is easy to administer and provides useful functional information for patients who will be involved in community or money-management tasks.

Cons. This test does not provide information about the broader problem-solving skills necessary for complex activities.

Instructions

Ask the patient to solve these problems: Lunch cost you $4.65. You want to leave a 15 percent tip. How much should you leave? [$.69 to $.70] Petunias cost $1.20 per pot. You have $5.00. How many can you buy? [4]"

Interpretation

These questions require mathematical problem solving related to specific functional tasks. The ability to perform these calculations should be narrowly interpreted as indicative of mathematical problem-solving skills only. The ability to perform the calculations mentally shows the capacity to keep track of several pieces of information simultaneously. If paper is required, difficulty with mental tracking may be suspected. Memory related to mathematical concepts is required. In addition, visual spatial skills are needed to arrange the numbers on paper or to visualize them in one's mind.

Chapter 11

Perceptual Evaluation Guide

This portion of the book provides guidelines for functional observations and formal tests to help the therapist detect various perceptual deficits. For each problem area, suggestions for making functional observations are provided. The therapist is urged to use these observations to identify problem areas affecting function. Paper-and-pencil tests, criterion-referenced tests, and standardized tests (when applicable) are also listed. Since all tests have benefits and limitations that influence how and when they are best used, some of the pros and cons are listed for each evaluation. The formal tests are to be used primarily to clarify problem areas and to validate observations as necessary. In some cases, they are also helpful to provide concrete examples of deficits to the patient and the family, to help demonstrate what the problems are and how they relate to function. Standardized tests are helpful with high-level patients, especially when independent living, return to work or school, or driving is contemplated. In addition, formal tests are useful when data are being collected for research or outcome studies. In all cases, the therapist should choose formal evaluations selectively based on his or her observations of the patient during functional activities. Resource information is provided for commercially available tests.

VISUAL PERCEPTION

• **Unilateral Visual Inattention**

Functional Observations

Note the patient's tendencies to neglect items in the right or left visual field during activities such as oral/ facial hygiene, dressing, setting time on a watch, copying an address, reading a menu, describing food on a plate, or propelling a wheelchair.

- Note whether the head and eyes move to both the right and left without requiring cues.

- Note whether the patient spontaneously positions a task in the right or left visual field to facilitate performance (i.e., a left-side hemiplegic may tend to write on the right half of a page or position tasks away from the involved side.

- When minimal deficits are seen in basic self-care, observe performance during higher-level cognitive, perceptual, and activities of daily living (ADL) tasks such as cooking, community activities, work tasks, or advanced leisure activities. As cognitive and perceptual demands increase, the therapist often observes more subtle forms of neglect.

Interpretation

No Apparent Deficit. In basic and more complex functional tasks, the patient shows no neglect of objects or details in the right or left visual field. Eyes and head move freely, and moving objects are detected quickly in both visual fields.

Partial Deficit: A partial deficit is any deficit that falls between no apparent deficit and severe deficit.

Severe Deficit. The patient consistently neglects objects and details in the right or left visual field. Items in the central as well as peripheral locations may be neglected. Difficulty maintaining the head and eyes in midline may be noted. Severely affected patients may orient their head away from the hemiplegic side.

Tests: Unilateral Visual Inattention

Name: Line Bisection (Schenkenberg et al. 1980)

This test can be obtained from Thomas Schenkenberg, Psychology Service (116B), Veterans Administration Medical Center, Salt Lake City, UT 84148.

Description

The patient is asked to mark the center of a series of horizontal lines on a page (see Figure 4-17).

Pros. Instructions and the concept of the test are simple; therefore, it can be used with confused patients. The test is fast to administer and is a useful screening test for spatial neglect (Friedman 1990). Impaired line bisection correlates with lower ADL scores.

Cons. Percentage deviation scores are time-consuming to calculate; therefore, an alternate method based on the charts found in the article by Schenkenburg et al. (1980) and the findings of Van Deusen (1983) is suggested. The test cannot be used as an independent predictor of ADL function (Friedman 1990).

Instructions

Source: Adapted with permission from *Neurology* (1980;30:509), Copyright © 1980, AdvanStar Communications.

The paper is positioned horizontally in the patient's midline. The subject is not allowed to move the paper. Tape may be used as necessary. Read the following instructions:

1. Use your right (or left) hand; keep your other hand off the table.
2. Cut each line in half by placing a small pencil mark through each line as close to its center as possible. [The examiner demonstrates the procedure using the top line.]
3. Do not make more than one mark on any line.
4. Mark each of the lines without skipping any.

If a patient skips a line, allow him or her to continue. After completing the sheet, point out the missed lines, note the location of those missed, and ask the patient to bisect them.

Interpretation

Two scores are obtained. First, record the number of lines missed. Skipping two or more lines on *one* half of the page indicates neglect. Lines missed on *both* the right and left portion of page may indicate a general reduction in attention rather than unilateral neglect. Marks that deviate significantly from true center also indicate unilateral neglect. Deviation may be calculated formally by measuring the left lines and the center lines, then determining the difference between true center and the patient's mark. The mathematical formula is found in the article by Shenkenburg et al. (1980). Standard deviations can also be calculated. See the article by Van Deusen (1983) for details specific to the elderly population. For simplicity, when exact scientific scores are not required, transparent overlays can be used to show the true center for each line as well as deviations in 5-percent increments. Generally, normal subjects varied approximately 5 percent from true center, with approximately a 5 percent standard deviation. Deviations of more than 10 percent thus can be considered to indicate neglect.

Name: Drawing and Copying Tasks

Description

Based on anticipated level of skill, the patient is asked to draw from memory a clock and a person, or to copy a house and/or the Rey figure.

Pros. These tests are easy to administer and can be adapted to various levels of function. Copying the house is the most basic task, and copying the Rey figure is the most complex. Drawing from memory tests the patient's ability to form a visual image, organize it, and reproduce it on paper. These tests are often sensitive to unilateral inattention as well as visual spatial and visual construction deficits. The complex Rey figure is able to detect difficulties with visual attention and spatial orientation, as well as with absorbing and organizing detailed visual information.

Cons. Because these tests require integration of various skills, it may be hard to determine which problem areas are causing the most difficulty. For example, free drawing of a person requires visual memory of the human form, visual attention, motor planning, visual spatial abilities, and organizational skills. These tests are not standardized.

Instructions

See the visual construction section in this chapter.

Interpretation

Note any tendency to neglect features or details in the right or left portion of the drawing. Note whether neglect occurs only when details are positioned at the far right or far left or whether neglect is also noted in more central positions. Note whether the patient centers the drawing on the page or tends to place the drawing to the right or left of center. Note the patient's head and eye positions. Are spontaneous head and eye movements seen to both the right and the left, or is cuing required? Marked deviations of the position of the drawing on the page or neglect of details in one half of the drawing indicate neglect. See the visual construction section for additional observations and interpretations.

Name: Albert's Test (Fullerton et al. 1986)

Description

The patient is asked to cross out 41 randomly oriented lines arranged in roughly six rows on the page (see Figure 4-18).

Pros. The test is easy to administer and has supporting norms. Because the lines are scattered on the page, it is challenging to the patient's organizational skills and may be more sensitive to inefficient scanning patterns than tests in which information is arranged in neat rows or columns. Literature supports a high correlation between test performance and functional skills as well as mortality six months after the stroke (Fullerton et al. 1986). The test does not rely on sophisticated language skills and can be used with aphasics if unilateral visual inattention is suspected.

Cons. There are no serious drawbacks to this test. Because it requires visual organization, it can be too difficult for some patients who may benefit from a more structured task.

Instructions

Source: Adapted with permission from *Lancet* (1986:430), Copyright © 1986, Lancet Ltd.

Present the test sheet to the patient. Point out some lines, including those to the extreme right and left. Tell the patient to cross out all the lines. The therapist should demonstrate, using the line in the center of the page. When the patient indicates that he or she is finished, ask, "Have you crossed all the lines?" If the patient has language deficits, use nonverbal cues to encourage him or her to check the work.

Interpretation

Record the number of lines missed. Albert (1973) states that 37 percent of right-brain-damaged subjects and 30 percent of left-brain-damaged subjects failed to cross out one or more lines, while none of the control subjects failed to cross out a line. The mean number of errors was approximately five for right brain damage and one for left brain damage. Fullerton and associates (1986) classified performance of stroke patients as shown in Table 11-1. Note the patient's organization of the task. Are lines crossed in a right to left pattern, or is another system used (i.e., up and down, or in concentric circles)? If the patient uses a random approach to crossing the lines, without any pattern or technique, poor organization of the visual scanning process is suspected and oculomotor control should be tested further. Patients showing this type of difficulty may benefit from visual scanning training.

Name: Letter Cancellation Task (Diller et al. 1974)

Description

The patient is asked to look at a page with six rows of 52 typed letters and to put a mark through all the letters *C* and *E* (see Figure 4-19).

Pros. The test is related to visual scanning used in reading. It may be more challenging than cancellation of shapes or colors, since it relies on higher-level language skills. The letters are arranged in structured rows and thus require less organizational skill than when the forms are scattered on the page in a random array. This allows the therapist to look more closely at attention without the confounding factor of visual organization. There are limited norms for performance.

Cons. The test requires language skills sufficient to identify letters; thus it may not be appropriate for aphasics. The letters may be too small for patients with low vision.

Table 11-1 Relationship of Albert's Test Performance to Presence of Neglect

Classification	Number of Lines Missed	Percent of Lines Uncrossed
No neglect	1 or 2	4.3%
Neglect uncertain	3–23	4.3%–56.8%
Definite neglect	>23	>56.8%

Source: Adapted with permission from *Lancet* (1986:430), Copyright © 1986, Lancet Ltd.

Instructions

The therapist places the test sheet at the patient's midline and points to the trial line, asking the patient to mark the *C*s and *E*s. If the patient is unable to perform the trial, further instruction may be given. If correct, the therapist will then proceed to give instructions as follows: "Look at the letters on this page. Put one line through each *C* and *E*. Ready, begin here." The therapist points to the first letter in the first row and begins timing the patient.

Interpretation

Note the time and total number of errors. According to Diller et al. (1974) 13 control subjects had a median error of one with a performance time of 100 seconds. Compare errors on the right with those on the left side of the page. Randomly scattered errors indicate poor sustained attention. Errors concentrated on one half of the page indicate unilateral neglect. Observe the patient's general approach to the task (i.e., does the patient work from left to right or move randomly over the page; is the response time slowed; does the patient selectively choose the correct response, or frequently mark nontarget letters?).

Name: Reaction Time Measure of Visual Field (Gianutsos and Klitzner 1981)

Available from Life Science Associates, One Fenimore Road, Bayport, NY 11705; telephone (506) 472-2111.

Description

This is a computerized test that measures the patient's speed of response to stimuli present in either visual field.

Pros. The test can be administered quickly and introduces speed, a factor that is important in dynamic tasks—especially in the community. Norms are available.

Cons. The computer may be threatening to some patients. Since a computer is required, the test is not easily portable.

Instructions

Instructions are available from Life Science Associates.

Interpretation

Use interpretive information supplied with the test. Difficulties may reflect problems that will interfere with community-level activities and driving.

• **Visual Spatial Awareness**

Functional Observations

Observe the patient's ability to orient his or her shirt correctly for dressing, to put parts of an electric razor or mixer together, to put a lid on a container, to distribute items correctly when setting a table, to arrange items on a shelf, or to organize the contents of a drawer neatly. *Note:* All functional tasks have a motor component and therefore are not pure tests of visual spatial awareness.

Clinical Observations

Note misplacements, deviations, or poor relationships of a part to the whole during craft projects, puzzle construction, or design copying. Constructional apraxia must be ruled out in order to interpret these errors as spatial relations deficits.

Interpretation

Inability to position objects correctly in relation to oneself or to other objects indicates spatial relationship problems; however, motor-planning problems, decreased attention, or general confusion must be ruled out.

No Apparent Deficit. The patient correctly positions objects during activities.

Partial Deficit. A partial deficit is any deficit that falls between no apparent deficit and severe deficit.

Severe Deficit. The patient frequently orients objects incorrectly and requires assistance to correct errors, i.e., twists shirt and pants, orients comb or brush improperly, misaligns utensils when setting a table, is unable to put parts of an electric razor together. (Apraxia must be ruled out.)

Visual Spatial Tests

Name: The Cross Test (Kim et al. 1984)

Description

This test, based on the format used by Kim et al. (1984), consists of 10 stimulus cards (15 cm high and 20 cm wide) and 10 corresponding response cards. Each stimulus card has one small black cross (0.5 cm by 0.5 cm) printed on it. Five response cards have an identical cross located in exactly the same position. Five of the response cards have a cross that varies slightly from the stimulus (i.e., not more than 1 cm away from the stimulus location). The two cards are presented together, one above the other. The patient uses a yes/no response to indicate whether the stimulus cross and the response cross are in the same location (see Figure 4-20).

Pros. The Cross Test is easy to administer and does not require a motor response; thus it is a pure spatial test. Limited scoring criteria exist.

Cons. It is not a true standardized test as it doesn't have extensive reliability data.

Instructions

Source: Adapted with permission from *Neuropsychologia* (1984;22(2):180), Copyright © 1984, Pergamon Press.

Present the stimulus card to the patient at midline. Present the response card directly below the stimulus card. Ask the patient, "Are the two crosses in the same location?" The patient can respond yes or no orally or by gesturing.

Interpretation

Based on a study of 20 patients with right hemisphere lesions, 20 patients with left hemisphere lesions, and 10 normal control subjects, Kim et al. (1984) found mean error rates as shown in Table 11-2. Two or more errors can be considered defective performance, suggesting visual spatial deficits or poor awareness of subtle differences between two items.

Name: Judgment of Line Orientation (Benton 1983b)

Available from Science and Medical Marketing Manager, Oxford University Press, 200 Madison Avenue, New York, NY 10046.

Description

The patient is asked to view two lines and determine their angles on the page by comparing them with a numbered array. The patient may respond verbally or by pointing to the answer (see Figure 4-21).

Pros. This is a pure test of spatial relations. It includes well-documented norms and interpretive information and is challenging for higher-level patients.

Cons. The test can become monotonous for the patient and the therapist and requires approximately 10 to 15 minutes to administer.

Instructions

Source: Adapted from *Contributions to Neuropsychological Assessment: A Clinical Manual* (pp 46–47) by A Benton with permission of Oxford University Press, © 1983.

Beginning with the practice item, point to the upper stimulus page and say: "See these two lines? Which two lines down here [point to the response card] are in exactly the same position and point in the same direction as the two lines up here? Tell me the number of the lines." If the patient is aphasic say, "Show me these lines down here. Point to them." If the patient is correct, say, "That's right" and proceed with the next practice item. If the patient does not understand the task, say, "Let us just look at this line. [Cover the line in position 6 with your hand.] Which line down here [point] points in the same direction as this one [point] and is also in the same position. That is, it's on the same side of the page as this line up here." The patient can be corrected on each of the trial items by using the extended instructions above. If the patient is unable to identify both lines correctly on at least two practice items, do not administer the test. After completing the trial items, open the booklet to the page labeled "Test Items" and say, "Now we are going to do more of these, except now the lines which you see up here [point] will be shorter, because part of the line has been erased. Tell me [or show me] which two lines down here are pointing in the same direction as the lines up here?" Encourage the patient to make his or her best guess if there is no response within 30 seconds.

Interpretation

The extensive information available in the test manual must be read for a thorough understanding of scoring and interpretation. A summary of scores is found in Table 11-3.

VISUAL ANALYSIS AND SYNTHESIS

Functional Observations: Visual Analysis

Ask the patient to discriminate between various colors, sizes, and shapes of common objects as he or she is able. Is the patient able to analyze the relevant features and recognize the object? Note whether the patient can

Table 11-2 Performance on the Cross Test

Subjects	Mean Error Rates
Control	1
Right hemisphere lesion	3.5
Left hemisphere lesion	2.5

Source: Adapted with permission from *Neuropsychologia* (1984;22(2):180), Copyright © 1984. Pergamon Press.

Table 11-3 Judgment of Line Orientation

Age (yr)	Mean Corrected Scores*	
	Men	Women
16–49	25.6	25.3
50–64	25.3	25.2
65–74	25.7	25.8

*Score corrections: 50–64 years, add 1 point to obtained score; 65–74 years, add 3 points to obtained score; women, add 2 points to obtained score. Scores can be further classified as follows: 19–20, borderline; 17–18, moderative defective; <17, severely defective (Benton 1983b).

Source: Adapted from *Contributions to Neuropsychological Assessment: A Clinical Manual* (p 49) by A Benton with permission of Oxford University Press, © 1983.

---

locate items in a drawer, find a washcloth on a white sheet, or pick out an object in the clinic.

Functional Observations: Visual Synthesis

When only part of an object is exposed, can the patient recognize the whole? For instance, if just the handle of his or her toothbrush is visible, can the patient identify it?

Interpretation

No Apparent Deficit. The patient is able to discriminate and locate items in a cluttered environment such as a drawer, a cabinet, or the clinic and can identify objects when only part of the item is showing.

Partial Deficit. A partial deficit is any deficit that falls between no apparent deficit and severe deficit.

Severe Deficit. Frequently (more than half the time) the patient is unable to correctly locate items in a cluttered environment or identify objects that are partially obscured. The patient may or may not correctly identify the color, shape, and size of objects.

Visual Analysis Tests

Name: Visual Discrimination of Abstract Shapes

Description

The patient is required to analyze subtle distinctions between various abstract designs (see Figure 4-22).

Pros. This is an easy-to-administer screening tool.

Cons. It is nonstandardized and does not clearly distinguish complex analysis problems from more basic unilateral visual inattention.

Instructions

Present the visual discrimination work sheets vertically within the patient's visual field. If necessary, the therapist can cover all of the designs except the one the patient is working on, to avoid confusion. Point to the picture at the top. Say, "Can you point to the design below that matches the one on top?"

Interpretation

Incorrect responses may relate to difficulty attending to and discriminating fine differences in visual information. Rule out unilateral neglect and poor spatial relations by testing those areas separately. Since disorganized visual scanning may result in poor integration of information, use Albert's Test to check the patient's approach to a visual scanning problem.

Name: Visual Form Discrimination (Benton 1983f)

Available from Science and Medical Marketing Manager, Oxford University Press, 200 Madison Avenue, New York, NY 10046.

Description

This multiple-choice test requires analysis of the subtle features of a design. The patient responds by pointing to or verbally matching the stimulus design to one of four choices (see Figure 4-23).

Pros. For more advanced patients, this is a high-level test with well-developed norms.

Cons. Since the test is standardized, it requires more time to administer than do screening tests.

Instructions

Source: Adapted from *Contributions to Neuropsychological Assessment: A Clinical Manual* (p. 57) by A. Benton with permission of Oxford University Press, © 1983.

Complete instructions are available in the test manual published by Oxford University Press. It is critical to read the complete instructions to administer and score the test correctly. Begin with the first trial item and say, "See this design? Find it among these four designs [point]. Which one is it? Show me." Confirm correct responses and proceed. If errors are made, show the patient the correct answer and point out differences between it and the incorrect items on the response card. Continue with the test items, encouraging the patient to make a selection after 30 seconds by saying, "Which one do you think is the same? What is your best guess?"

Interpretation

Use norms and information that accompanies the test to analyze performance fully. Correct responses are awarded two points; peripheral errors are given one point; and major rotations, major distortions, and failure to respond receive zero points. A summary of scores in the manual is found in Table 11-4.

Name: Figure-Ground Screening Test

Description

This is a nonstandardized screening test that evaluates a patient's ability to analyze visual information and attend to relevant material while suppressing irrelevant information. This skill is required to discriminate foreground from background information (see Figure 4-25).

Pros. This test is easy and fast to administer and can be used with most aphasic patients, since limited verbal comprehension is required.

Cons. The test is not standardized. Because visual analysis is by nature a skill requiring visual perceptual and cognitive integration, poor test performance may relate to a variety of underlying causes, including poor vision, poor visual scanning, unilateral neglect, decreased selective attention, or difficulty in understanding the abstract nature of the test. It is important for the therapist to attempt to define the underlying difficulty through further observation and/or evaluation in order to direct treatment appropriately.

Table 11-4 Visual Form Discrimination: Means, Medians, and Ranges of Scores in Control Patients

Age (yr)	Men	Women
16–54	Mean = 30.8 Median = 31.0 Range = 28–32 (*n* = 28)	Mean = 29.9 Median = 30.0 Range = 24–32 (*n* = 30)
55–75	Mean = 29.3 Median = 30.0 Range = 23–32 (*n* = 15)	Mean = 31.3 Median = 31.0 Range = 27–32 (*n* = 12)

Source: Adapted from *Contributions to Neuropsychological Assessment: A Clinical Manual* (p 58) by A Benton with permission of Oxford University Press, © 1983.

Instructions

Present the test sheets within the patient's visual field. While pointing to the stimulus design, say to the patient: "Look at this design. Now look at these designs below [point]. Find this design [point to stimulus design] in one of these designs [point to forms below]. Look very carefully."

Interpretation

Try to distinguish the nature of the disability. Rule out poor visual acuity, poor scanning strategies, and unilateral neglect through other tests. If the patient is able to complete other visual tests and is able to comprehend other simple abstract concepts yet has trouble with figure-ground, analyze the problem further. Possibly the patient has difficulty discriminating relevant from irrelevant visual information or inhibiting the unimportant visual lines in order to attend to those that define the target shape. Perhaps visual search strategies are inefficient when given an unstructured task.

Name: Ayres Figure-Ground Test (Ayres 1966)

Description

This is a multiple-choice test requiring the patient to identify three shapes in each embedded figure design. Because the limited norms were developed in 1973, the 1966 version of the test (rather than the updated version) must be used (see Figure 4-26).

Pros. Norms for adults are available, although they are based on a relatively small sample. Test items range from simple to difficult. The test is portable and offers information about the patient's ability to process relatively complex visual information.

Cons. Norms are not well established. In addition, the test is somewhat abstract and may not be motivating to some patients.

Instructions

Source: Adapted from *Southern California Figure-Ground Visual Perception Test* (pp. 10–11) by J. Ayres with permission of Western Psychological Services, © 1966.

Using the Ayres test booklet presented within the patient's visual field, begin with the trial items and say: "Three of these pictures [point to response plate] are up here [point to stimulus plate]. Which three are they?" After the patient identifies the correct items, point out the three pictures not in the stimulus plate and say: "These three are not up here." Then say: "That is the way it will be each time I turn the page. You are to find the three pictures down here which also are up here. Look carefully, because it can be tricky." If the patient is incorrect, use the trial item to clarify the procedure. Turn to the test plates and begin timing the patient. Discontinue each item after one minute. Discontinue the test if the patient's responses to the trial items are incorrect. When the geometrical figures are reached, re-explain the directions as follows:

> Now you will look at designs instead of pictures of things. Three of these designs [point] are part of this one [point]. They are hidden in this upper design, just as some of these pictures [point to *8B*] were part of this upper figure [point to *8A*]. This design is a cross, but it is not like the crossed lines up here, so it is not part of the upper design. This one [point to item *b*] is part of the design up here. Can you see it? [trace design] Can you see this one up here? [point] Which one of these [point to *d*, *e*, *f*] is hidden in this design? [point] The rest of the designs will be something like this one. Find the three designs up here [point to multiple-choice plate] that are up here [point].

Interpretation

Attempt to define the underlying cause of difficulty. Rule out poor visual acuity, unilateral neglect, and poor comprehension of the instructions. Note difficulty with abstraction, poor organization of the task, and lack of systematic visual scanning processes. Use the information below to interpret scores. The mean score for the patient's age plus or minus one standard deviation will indicate normal ranges of performance. Performance below one standard deviation from the mean can be considered a partial deficit, whereas three standard deviations below mean can be considered severely impaired. Data for scoring were collected through a pilot normative study conducted at Boston University (Mahoney and Siev 1973) (Table 11-5).

Visual Synthesis Tests

Name: Hooper Visual Organization Test (Hooper 1983)

This test is available from Western Psychological Services, 12031 Wilshire Boulevard, Los Angeles, CA 90025.

Description

The patient is asked to identify an object by looking at a series of pictures that have been cut and shifted on the page. This is a test of the patient's ability to look at parts of an object and synthesize, or integrate, the parts to form a whole.

Pros. The test is portable, and its norms are well established. It is challenging for high-level patients, since it requires mental manipulation of visual information to construct a whole from its parts.

Cons. The test is too abstract for some patients. It requires the integration of visual skills and cognitive abilities such as analysis of component parts, mental rotation of pieces, and mental organization of these parts into a coherent whole. Language skills are also required to label the items. When a patient has difficulty with this test, it may be difficult to define which specific skill deficit(s) underlie the problem. Performance on this test is also related to age, intelligence, and educational level.

Instructions

Source: Adapted from *The Hooper Visual Organization Test Manual* (p. 4) by H.E. Hooper with permission of Western Psychological Services, © 1983.

Present the booklet in midline or within the patient's visual field. Do not allow the patient to rotate the book. Begin by saying: "This is a test of your ability to recognize pictures of objects when the pictures have been cut up and rearranged. Look at each picture and decide what it might be if it were put together. [Present item 1.]

Table 11-5 Ayres Figure-Ground Test: Preliminary Norms

Age (yr)	Standard Deviation	Number of Subjects	Mean Score
20–29	9.7	22	31.9
30–39	8.9	12	32.6
40–49	7.8	10	22.8
50–59	5.7	12	23.9

Source: Adapted from *Perceptual and Cognitive Dysfunction in the Adult Stroke Patient* (p 158) by Sieve, Frieshtat, and Zoltan with permission of Slack Publishers, © 1986.

For example, look at the first picture. What would it be if it were put together?" If the respondent says "fish," say: "That's right. It's a fish. Now do the other pictures in the same way. Toward the end they become rather hard. Try to give an answer even if you are not sure of it."

If the patient cannot decide what the object is in item 1, or answers incorrectly, give the following help: "The correct answer is 'fish.' You see, here is the head, the fins, and the tail. If it were put together correctly, it would be a fish. Now do the other pictures in the same way. Toward the end they become rather hard. Try to give an answer even if you are not sure of it."

Turn the pages for the patient after each item is presented. If the subject delays more than one minute on any of the items, encourage him or her to make a guess.

Interpretation

Use the extensive materials available in the test manual. According to the 1983 version of the manual, research results are somewhat controversial regarding the use of this test for screening generalized neurological deficits versus using it to specify problems with visual organization. Thus it is recommended that interpretations are based on observations of a variety of test or functional situations. A summary of quantitative scores is found in Table 11-6.

VISUAL CONSTRUCTION

Functional Observations

Observe performance in everyday tasks that incorporate visual spatial skills; visual discrimination; visual synthesis; and motor activity such as putting on clothing, wrapping a package, arranging flowers, setting a table, constructing a puzzle, making a sandwich, or making a craft project.

Table 11-6 Scores for the Hooper Visual Organization Test

Raw Score	Probability of Impairment*
24–30	Very Low
21–23	Low
19–20	Moderate
16–18	High
<16	Very High

*Additional scoring information is found in the test manual which provides adjustments for age and educational level.

Source: Adapted from *The Hooper Visual Organization Test Manual*, (p 7) by HE Hooper with permission of Western Psychological Services, 1983.

Interpretation

Attempt to define the problem area that interferes with performance: Does the patient neglect a body side or visual space (unilateral neglect)? Does difficulty seem to be due to improper spatial orientation of the activity or incorrect relationship of the part to the whole (poor awareness of spatial relationships)? Does organization of the task seem to be lacking (cognitive deficits)? Does the patient fail to attend to relevant details (decreased attention)? Does performance seem apraxic, perseverative, or improperly sequenced, or are objects used inappropriately (motor-planning problems)? Answers to these questions may indicate particular deficits and lead the therapist to test suspected problem areas further.

No Apparent Deficit. The patient is able to perform activities requiring high-level visual motor integration without difficulty. These include activities such as putting together parts of a razor, mixer, blender, or flashlight; wrapping a package; setting a table; making a craft project; or doing other construction tasks familiar to the patient.

Partial Deficit. A partial deficit is any deficit that falls between no apparent deficit and severe deficit.

Severe Deficit. The patient has difficulty with simple constructional tasks such as putting a lid on a container, making a three-piece sandwich, or putting a letter in an envelope, such that the desired outcome is not attained.

Visual Construction Tests

Name: Copying a Picture: Simple Figure Test

Description

The patient is asked to copy a house.

Pros. This test is easy to administer, is more concrete than the freehand drawing task, and allows the therapist to detect a wide range of potential problem areas in one simple task.

Cons. The test is not standardized, and the therapist may have difficulty distinguishing the underlying deficit. Accuracy may be impaired if the patient is drawing with the nondominant hand.

Instructions

Place a work sheet showing a picture of a house in the patient's midline. Ask the patient to copy the picture.

Interpretation

Note unilateral neglect of the right or left portion of the picture. Total omission of half of the picture implies a more severe deficit than omission of details on one half of the page. Note the proportion and relationships of parts. Inaccuracies indicate spatial organizational difficulties; embellishment of one aspect of the picture while poorly executing others may indicate adequate attention to detail without the ability to visualize the whole. Note perseveration such as repeatedly copying a portion of the picture, which points to motor-planning problems. Observe the patient's ability to proceed in an organized manner.

Name: Freehand Drawing of a Clock and a Person

Description

The patient is asked to draw a clock and a person from memory.

Pros. This test correlates highly with functional skills, is easy to administer, and does not require sophisticated verbal skills. The therapist can detect a variety of underlying problem areas through careful observation of performance. Compared with the simple design copying task, this task requires more organizational skills and the ability to form a mental image of an object.

Cons. The test is not standardized and it may be difficult to define the underlying problem(s), since many skills are used together to produce a faithful picture. Patients with receptive language difficulties may not understand the directions. Accuracy may be impaired if the patient is drawing with the nondominant hand, and poor artistry must be ruled out in the drawing of a person.

Instructions

Present the patient with a blank sheet of paper and a pen/pencil placed at midline. Ask the patient to draw a person. If difficulty is noted with freehand drawing, introduce copying tasks. If the patient is able to comply with the request to draw a person, present a clean sheet of paper and ask him or her to "draw a clock and set the time at 11:25."

Interpretation

Note unilateral neglect of the right or left portion of the picture. Total omission of half of the picture indicates a more severe deficit that does omission of details on one half of the page. Note the proportion and relationships of parts. Difficulties indicate poor perception of spatial relationships. Note perseveration, which may indicate motor-planning problems. Unrelated drawing activities, such as adding unnecessary details or extra lines, may relate to poor attention to the whole or poor task organization. Note whether the task is approached in a systematic manner (see Figures 4-29 through 4-34).

Name: Copying a Picture: Complex Figure Test (Rey 1941; Osterrieth 1944)

Description

The patient is asked to copy the Rey figure (see Figure 4-28).

Pros. In addition to the positive aspects of the simple copying tasks, this test is helpful in detecting deficits in high-level patients who are not challenged by the simple tests. A high degree of visual organization is required, as well as the ability to detect subtle features and recognize the spatial relationships of one part to another. Some scoring guidelines are available.

Cons. The test is not standardized. Accuracy may be impaired if the patient is drawing with the nondominant hand.

Instructions

Source: Adapted from *Psychological Appraisal of Children with Cerebral Defects* (pp. 397–398) by E.M. Taylor with permission of Harvard University Press, © 1959.

Present the Rey figure work sheet in the patient's midline. Give the patient one of five colored pencils and say, "Copy this picture as accurately as you can." Time the patient. As the patient completes each section of the drawing, a colored pencil of a different color can be presented. This allows the therapist to study the organizational approach used by the patient. The patient can be asked to draw the picture from memory immediately after completion of the copied picture (Lezak 1983).

Interpretation

The activity should be analyzed qualitatively with the intention of identifying underlying deficit(s). Note unilateral neglect of the right or left portion of the picture as well as its position on the page. Total omission of half of the picture indicates a more severe deficit than omission of details on one half of the page. Note proportions and relationships of parts to each other and to the whole. Note perseveration, such as repeatedly copying a portion of the picture. Note organization of the task. Right-side hemiplegics often proceed in a piecemeal fashion, joining little sections together to create the whole. Left-side hemiplegics often show a disorganized approach.

A formal scoring system may be used if more precise measurements are needed. Using the reference diagram (Figure 11-1), consider each of the 18 units separately. Appraise the accuracy of each unit and its relative position within the design. For each unit, score as shown in Table 11-7.

Name: Block Design Construction

Description

The patient is asked to copy a three-, five-, and ten-block design (see Figure 4-35).

Table 11-7 Scoring System for the Rey Complex Figure Test

Performance Measurement	Score
Correct shape placed properly	2 points
Correct shape placed poorly	1 point
Distorted or incomplete component placed properly	1 point
Distorted or incomplete component placed poorly	1/2 point
Absent or unrecognizable component	0 points
Maximal total	36 points
Average adult copy score	32 points, with no normal score <29
Average adult memory score	22 points

Source: Adapted from *Psychological Appraisal of Children with Cerebral Defects* (p 399) by EM Taylor with permission of Harvard University Press, © 1959.

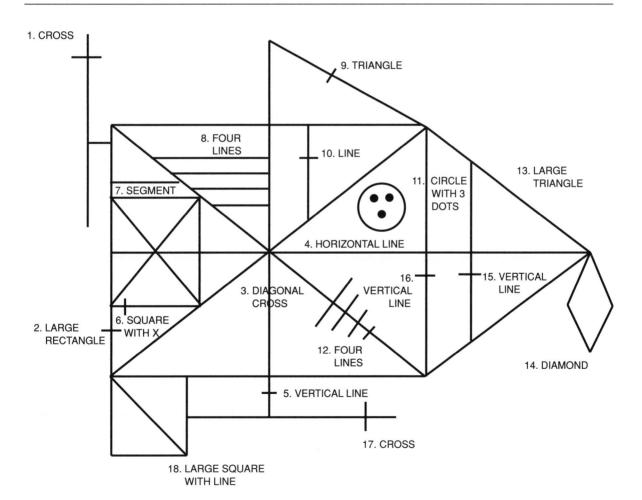

Figure 11-1 Copying a figure: Complex Figure Test. *Source:* Adapted from *Psychological Appraisal of Children with Cerebral Defects* (pp 398–399) by EM Taylor with permission of Harvard University Press, © 1959.

Pros. The test is an easily and quickly administered screening test that evaluates three-dimensional spatial awareness and planning skills.

Cons. It is a nonstandardized test that is too simple to detect subtle problems in higher-level patients. It may be considered childish by some patients.

Instructions

Beginning with the three-block design, make a model. Do not let the patient see you construct the model. For convenience, you may glue the model together so that it does not need to be rebuilt during each testing session. Use one-inch cubes of the same color. Present the model in the patient's midline and say, "Copy this design [point] using these blocks" [point to a set of ten blocks that match the model in color, shape, and size]. Proceed with the five- and ten-block design in the same way, referring to the diagram for design construction details. If the patient incorrectly completes the design, ask, "Are the two models the same, or different?" If the patient says that they are different, ask, "What is the difference between my model and yours?" The therapist can then move the blocks to the position the patient describes and ask, "Now are they the same?"

Interpretation

Note omissions, additions, and displacements (i.e., separations, misplacements, and angular deviations greater than 45 degrees). To distinguish between spatial relationship problems and constructional problems, analyze the patient's ability to correct the model verbally. If he or she can describe the correct relationships of the blocks and the differences between the stimulus model and his or her design but has difficulty arranging them manually, the problems may be constructional. If the patient can neither describe nor position the blocks correctly, difficulties with spatial organization or analysis are likely. Patients who have trouble with the block design test but not the Hooper Visual Organization Test may have a constructional deficit (Lezak 1983).

Name: Three-Dimensional Block Construction (Benton 1983e)

The test is available from Science and Medical Marketing Manager, Oxford University Press, 200 Madison Avenue, New York, NY 10046.

Description

The patient is asked to copy a 6-, an 8-, and a 15-block design using either a picture or a model as a guide.

Pros. This test is challenging to a higher-level patient and helps elicit subtle visual perceptual or constructional problems. The norms are well referenced, and validity information is available.

Cons. This test is bulky to transport and is more time-consuming to administer than the screening test. It is too difficult for low- or moderate-functioning patients.

Instructions

Source: Adapted from *Contributions to Neuropsychiatric Assessment: A Clinical Manual* (pp. 110–112) by A. Benton with permission of Oxford University Press, © 1983.

Seat the patient with the model (or picture) and the tray of blocks within his or her visual field. It is easiest to glue the models together; however, this makes the test even more difficult to carry. Tell the patient:

> Use these blocks and put some of them together so that they look like this model. Make the model as it looks as you face it, as you see it, not as I see it. You will not need all the blocks here, and you will have to pick out the ones you need to make a copy of the model. Make your model as carefully as you can. This is more important than how long you take. Place the blocks in the same position and with the same angles as they are in the model. Tell me when you are finished.

Use the score sheet to record observations.

Interpretation

Read the information that is found in the test manual for details of scoring and interpreting performance. Table 11-8 shows norms for test performance.

BODY AWARENESS

Functional Observations

Tactile Sensory Loss

Note responsiveness to touch, and the ability to use the extremity without visually monitoring the activity.

Table 11-8 Three-Dimensional Block Construction

Norms	Block Model Presentation (N=30)		Photographic Presentation (N=30)	
	Form A	Form B	Form A	Form B
Mean	25.4	24.5	20.7	20.2
Standard deviation	7.4	8.5	8.8	8.0

Source: Adapted from *Contributions to Neuropsychiatric Assessment: A Clinical Manual* (pp 110–112) by A Benton with permission of Oxford University Press, © 1983.

Unilateral Tactile Inattention

Note any tendency to neglect one body side, especially when the patient is engaged in a task.

Tactile Accommodation

Does the patient drop, lose control, or forget about an item in the affected hand after a few seconds have elapsed, despite adequate sensation and motor control?

Tactile Extinction

Does the patient forget about an item in the affected hand when attempting to do two things at once (i.e., carry an object and walk)? This indicates that the patient is unable to maintain awareness of multiple forms of sensory input and tends to extinguish sensations that are less prominent.

Bilateral Integration

Note the patient's ability to use both body sides together in a smooth, coordinated manner. Does the patient use available motor function in the affected side appropriately to stabilize an item, propel a wheelchair, or place the upper extremity or lower extremity into clothing? Does the patient avoid crossing midline?

Body Parts Identification

Does the patient attend appropriately to various body parts during dressing, grooming, bathing, and other functional tasks? Aphasic patients should not be required to point to or name body parts, because it is a test of language skills. Rather, their ability to locate and monitor their body during functional tasks should be observed.

Right-Left Identification

Observe the patient's ability to follow instructions regarding right and left during mobility or other functional tasks. Since this skill is heavily reliant on language, it is not appropriate for aphasic patients.

Midline Orientation

Observe the patient's awareness of body position during static and dynamic tasks. Distinguish motor loss from poor body awareness by assisting the patient's movement and asking the patient to tell you when he or she feels upright and symmetrical.

BODY AWARENESS TESTS

Unilateral Tactile Inattention Tests

Name: Bilateral Simultaneous Stimulation

Description

The patient is touched by examiner on the right and left sides of the body simultaneously to determine whether tactile information is extinguished (see Figure 4-37A, B).

Pros. This test is short and easy to administer.

Cons. No scoring information is available.

Instructions

The examiner first tests to ensure that the patient is able to feel light touch on both the hands and the cheeks. The following sequence is used, touching the patient as indicated each time, asking, "Did I touch you? Where did I touch you?"

1. Right and left hand simultaneously
2. Both cheeks
3. Right hand and left cheek
4. Left hand and right cheek
5. Left hand and right hand

Interpretation

Failure to identify two stimuli indicates extinction and may affect the patient's ability to use the hand while concentrating on another aspect of the task. Although both deficits indicate problems with tactile attention, difficulty identifying bilateral hand stimuli is not as serious as difficulty identifying hand and cheek stimuli.

Name: Face-Hand Test (Goldman 1966)

Description

The patient is touched by the examiner on the right and left sides of the body to determine whether tactile information is extinguished.

Pros. The test provides valuable information about tactile inattention for patients with both obvious and more subtle deficits.

Cons. The test is more lengthy than the screening protocol above.

Instructions

Source: Adapted with permission from *Neurology* (1952;2:48), Copyright © 1952, AdvanStar Communications.

The therapist sits facing the patient and says: "I am going to touch you. Point to where I touch you." The subject is told, "Please close your eyes," and is then touched with one or two brisk strokes on the cheek and dorsum of the hand simultaneously, according to the list below. If the patient does not identify one of the two stimuli during the first four trials, he or she is asked, "Anywhere else?"

1. Right cheek—left hand
2. Left cheek—right hand
3. Right cheek—right hand
4. Left cheek—left hand
5. Right cheek—left cheek
6. Right hand—left hand
7. Right cheek—left hand
8. Left cheek—right hand
9. Right cheek—right hand
10. Left cheek—left hand

If the subject makes repeated errors with the eyes closed, the procedure can be repeated with the eyes open, giving the following instructions: "Now I am going to touch you again. But this time I want you to keep your eyes open and watch carefully where I touch you."

Interpretation

The most common error is extinction, or the failure to feel two stimuli presented simultaneously on opposite body sides. When two stimuli are presented on the same side of the body, they should be perceived correctly if the patient is following the directions correctly. Displacement is seen when the patient is touched in one place but indicates that he or she felt it in another (Shapiro et al. 1952). According to the literature, 80 to 90 percent of the people who make continual errors with their eyes closed will continue to do so with their eyes open (Pollack et al. 1958).

More than six errors with the eyes closed can be considered a positive sign of brain injury. Problems with extinction will affect the patient's use of the hand, especially when he or she is also attending to another activity.

Name: Bilateral Integration: Double Circles (Roach and Kephart 1966)

Description

The patient is asked to make two large circles in the air with his or her hands (see Figure 4-40).

Pros. This test is easy to perform.

Cons. Normal or nearly normal movement and sensation in the affected extremity are required for this nonstandardized test.

Instructions

Evaluate only when normal or nearly normal movement and sensation are present. Ask the patient, "Make two large circles in the air using your right arm and your left arm at the same time."

Interpretation

Note the patient's ability to move both arms together in a coordinated manner. If the patient is able to move each arm separately in a coordinated way, but performance declines with bilateral movement, bilateral integration problems may exist. If both arms move in the same direction, clockwise, for example, confusion regarding laterality and directionality may exist (Roach and Kephart 1966). Unilateral neglect or sensory impairment may interfere with the patient's spontaneously incorporating the affected extremity in functional tasks.

Tactile Discrimination Tests

Name: Finger Localization (Benton 1983a)

Test materials, complete instructions, and interpretive information are available from Science and Medical Marketing Manager, Oxford University Press, 200 Madison Avenue, New York, NY 10046.

Description

This standardized test requires the patient to distinguish which fingers were touched.

Pros. It is a well-established test with norms for sensory discrimination. It is useful when subtle deficits in tactile processing are suspected of causing difficulty with high-level skills.

Cons. Patients may not understand the purpose of the test; therefore, the therapist must have a strong rationale and explain the purpose clearly to the patient.

Instructions

Source: Adapted from *Contributions to Neuropsychiatric Assessment: A Clinical Manual* (p. 85) by A. Benton with permission of Oxford University Press, © 1983.

If the patient is able to maintain a relaxed hand position with the palms up, use this standardized position. If not, place the patient's hands palm down on the table (nonstandardized hand position). Apply the stimulus for two seconds to the finger tip (palm up) or to the finger between the distal interphalangeal joint and nail (palm down), using firm pressure with the sharp end of a pencil. If mild sensory or attention deficits are present, the stimulus can be provided for three to four seconds. Position yourself across from the patient. Say to the patient: "I am going to touch different fingers on your hand; you tell me which finger I touch. You can name the fingers, if you wish, or you can point to them on this card." Proceed to touch the fingers in the order shown on the test sheet. The patient is allowed to see his or her hand during this portion of the test. After

completing part A, say: "Now put your [right, left] hand under this platform. You won't see me touching your fingers, but you will feel it." Guide the patient's hand under the box and continue with the test. After completion of this portion of the test, say: "Now I am going to touch two of your fingers at the same time. Tell me which fingers I touch. Again, either name the fingers or point to them on the card or call their numbers on the card."

Interpretation

Use information available in the test manual. Normative scores and classifications are found in Tables 11-9 and 11-10. If the nonstandard test position is used, the norms are not valid.

Name: Tactile Form Perception Test (Benton 1983c)

Complete instructions, materials, and interpretive information are available from Science and Medical Marketing Manager, Oxford University Press, 200 Madison Avenue, New York, NY 10046.

Description

This is a standardized test that requires the patient to feel a sandpaper shape while his or her vision is occluded. The patient then responds by pointing to the correct shape on a multiple-choice card (see Figures 4-41 and 4-42).

Pros. Tactile exploration is used to interpret spatial information in this standardized test. This can be useful to determine whether manual exploration might substitute for vision when analyzing spatial information. Reliability, validity, and norms are well established.

Cons. The test is time-consuming and may seem too abstract to the patient.

Table 11-9 Finger Localization Scores Based on 104 Subjects

Score	Classification
54–60	Normal
51–54	Borderline
48–50	Moderately defective
0–47	Severely defective

Source: Adapted from *Contributions to Neuropsychiatric Assessment: A Clinical Manual* (p 110–112) by A Benton with permission of Oxford University Press, © 1983.

Table 11-10 Performance Patterns Based on Finger Localization Norms

Classification	Score	Right-Left Difference
Normal bilaterally	Total score: 51–60; single hand scores: 25–30	0–3 points
Borderline bilaterally	Total score: 49–51; one single hand score: 23–24; and one single hand score: 26–27	0–3 points
Bilateral symmetrical defect	Single hand scores: <26	0–3 points
Bilateral asymmetrical defect (specify R or L)	One hand with score <26	4 or more points lower
Unilateral defect (specify R or L)	One hand with score of 26 or greater	4 or more points lower
Normal (specify R or L)	Single hand score: 26–30	Other hand not tested
Borderline (specify R or L)	Single hand score: 25	Other hand not tested
Defective (specify R or L)	Single hand score: <25	Other hand not tested

Source: Adapted from *Contributions to Neuropsychiatric Assessment: A Clinical Manual* (p 110–112) by A Benton with permission of Oxford University Press, © 1983.

Instructions

Source: Adapted from *Contributions to Neuropsychiatric Assessment: A Clinical Manual* (p. 71–73) by A. Benton with permission of Oxford University Press, © 1983.

The examiner is seated across from the patient. Ten cards with sandpaper shapes are arranged in order under the wooden platform and the response card is placed on top. Say to the patient: "Now I want to see how good you are at finding out what I put in this box by feeling it with your fingers. I will put some sandpaper figures on cards in the box. The figures look like the ones on this card here." Place the practice card in the box and say: "Feel around and touch all parts of this card so that you won't miss anything." As the subject feels the card, say: "Now, can you show me which figure it was? Point to the figure on this card, which is the same as the one in the box." Repeat this step while pointing to the correct figure if the patient was incorrect. Then continue the test by saying: "Place your hand in the box and feel the next figure there. Make sure that you have touched all the parts before you make your choice. After you have felt the whole card I want you to point to the figure on this board, which is the same shape as the figure you just felt. If you don't know for sure, make a guess." Begin the stopwatch. Allow the patient 30 seconds to feel the card, then tell him or her to make a choice. If the patient does not give an answer within the next 15 seconds, encourage him or her to guess. If the patient does not respond, present the next item. Present each figure by saying: "Here is another figure for you to feel. Once again, feel the whole card." If motor control is sufficient, present the second set of cards to test the other hand.

Interpretation

Norms and interpretations are described in the test manual. Table 11-11 describes some typical performance patterns.

Table 11-11 Tactile Form Perception: Performance Patterns

Classification	Score	Right-Left Difference
Normal	16–20	0–2
Borderline	15	0–2
Bilateral symmetrical defect	0–14 total score; single hand scores: 0–7	0–2
Bilateral right or left asymmetrical defect	3–11 total score; single hand scores: 0–7	3 points lower
Unilateral right- or left-hand defect	8–17 total; single hand score: 8–10	3 or more points lower
Normal right or left hand	8–10	Other hand not tested
Borderline right or left hand	7	Other hand not tested
Right- or left-hand defect	0–6	Other hand not tested

Source: Adapted from *Contributions to Neuropsychiatric Assessment: A Clinical Manual* (p 77) by A Benton with permission of Oxford University Press, © 1983.

Name: Graphesthesia, Rey's Skin Writing Procedure (Adapted from Rey 1964)

Description

Numbers are traced with the therapist's finger tip on the patient's palm.

Pros. This test is easy to administer and is an established test in neurological literature. It tests the patient's ability to discriminate moving spatial information through the sense of touch.

Cons. The test may be abstract to the patient. It cannot be given to patients with aphasia or primary sensory deficits.

Instructions

Source: Adapted from Rey 1964.

Using your finger tip, trace the following numbers on the dominant palm: 5, 1, 8, 2, 4, 3; and the numbers 3, 4, 2, 8, 1, 5 on the nondominant palm. After tracing each number, ask the patient, "Tell me the number I wrote on your hand."

Interpretation

Use the scale shown in Table 11-12. Patients having more errors than shown under the cutting score column can be considered to have impairment. Errors on the right or the left only indicate a contralateral lesion. Bilateral errors indicate difficulty with tactile processing.

Right-Left Discrimination Tests

Name: Left-Right Awareness (Adapted from Chapparo and Ranka 1980)

Description

The patient is asked to identify right and left on self, in space, and on others.

Pros. The test is administered quickly and may be helpful when patients will be required to follow right-left directions in the community or for driving training.

Cons. The test is not standardized, and, because it is heavily language-dependent, it may not relate to functional activities other than following verbal directions. It should not be given to aphasic patients. Often clinical observations will provide the same information.

Instructions

The therapist should sit in front of the patient and begin asking the following questions:

1. "Show me your right hand."
2. "Show me your left hand."
3. [Give the patient a pen or a pencil.] "Put the pen in my right hand."
4. "Is this pen on your right side or your left side?"[Place pen on the patient's left side.]
5. "Show me your right leg."
6. "Show me your left leg."
7. "Is this pen on your right side or your left side?" [Place pen on patient's right side.]
8. [Give the patient a pen.] "Put the pen in my left hand."

Interpretation

Record incorrect responses and describe differences in identifying right and left on self versus on others or in space. Rule out poor attention and difficulty following directions. Language plays a strong role in this task; therefore, it would not be appropriate for aphasic patients.

Midline Orientation Tests

Name: Estimation of Midline

Description

The patient's awareness of midline is observed during unsupported sitting with or without assistance, de-

---

Table 11-12 Graphesthesia Scores

Classification	Mean Deviation from Norm	Cutting Score Right	Cutting Score Left
Manual/unskilled (*n* = 51)	0	2	2
Technical/clerical (*n* = 25)	0	2	1
Baccalaureate (*n* = 55)	0	1	1
Elderly (ages 68–83) (*n* = 14)	0	3	3

Source: Adapted from *L'examen Clinique in Psychology* by A Rey, Presses Universitaires de France, 1964.

pending on motor control. This test may be performed in standing or other upright developmental positions if sufficient motor skill is present.

Pros. The test provides structured observations to determine a patient's awareness of an upright position.

Cons. This is a nonstandardized test that requires the ability to follow simple instructions as well as the ability to perceive midline. Clinically, it appears more accurate when the patient has adequate motor control to sit unsupported.

Instructions: Assuming Midline

Place the patient in a sitting position on a mat or a bench (use a higher-level developmental position when appropriate). Displace the patient's trunk approximately 45 degrees toward the affected side. Ask the patient: "Please sit [stand, kneel, etc.] up straight and centered."

Visual Cues. If the patient is unable to assume midline, place a mirror in front of him or her. Again ask the patient: "Please sit [stand, kneel, etc.] up straight and centered."

Physical Assistance. If the patient remains unable to assume midline, provide physical assistance. Begin to move the patient slowly toward midline. Ask the patient to "Tell me when you feel centered." If the patient has language difficulties, place the patient in various positions, some upright and some off center. Say after each position change, "Now are you straight?" Ask the patient to use a verbal or nonverbal yes/no response.

Interpretation

Describe the patient's ability to assume midline (i.e., can assume the position independently, requires visual feedback from the mirror, requires assistance from the therapist) and his or her perception of midline (i.e., patient errs by approximately 0 degrees, 15 degrees, or 30 degrees in perception of the upright position). In addition, note how long the position can be maintained without cues. Rapid decline in posture could be due to motor-control problems or due to a poor ability to attend to one's position in space. After a stroke, remaining at midline often becomes a cognitive task, requiring conscious control, rather than an automatic response. When the patient is required to maintain posture and attend to an activity, cognitive control of midline may be lost as the patient shifts attention to the task. Posture may therefore deteriorate.

MOTOR PLANNING

Functional Observations: Familiar Tasks

Sequencing. Observe the patient's ability to sequence routine and habitual tasks such as feeding, oral/facial hygiene, toileting, and dressing. Observe his or her ability to perform all steps of an activity independently. For example, to brush his or her teeth, the patient would *obtain the toothbrush and toothpaste, open the toothpaste, apply the toothpaste to the brush,* turn on the water, wet the brush, turn off the water, *clean the teeth,* spit out the toothpaste, obtain a cup, turn on the water, fill the cup, rinse the mouth, rinse the brush, turn off the water, and put away the toothpaste and toothbrush. Failure to follow this particular sequence does not necessarily indicate problems, because each person will have a slightly different procedure. However, omission of the key steps (in italics), use of correct steps at an improper point in the sequence, use of incorrect steps, or excessive hesitancy about how to proceed to the next part of the task suggest difficulty with sequencing. More complex tasks may also be analyzed; however, as tasks become less automatic, cognitive factors become more important. Therefore it becomes more difficult to decide whether the difficulty is due to disruption of habitual motor patterns and sequences or due to higher-level cognitive problems.

Perseveration. Observe the performance of simple functional tasks. Does the patient continue to shave the same area excessively; comb one portion of the hair for a prolonged period; or wash the face, put down the cloth as if finished, only to pick it up again and resume face washing?

Object Use. Note the patient's ability to use appropriately and effectively objects that were handled frequently prior to the stroke. Observe the patient's use of objects such as eating utensils, a comb, a toothbrush, a washcloth, a razor, toilet paper, kitchen utensils, and/or familiar tools such as a hammer. It is helpful to observe the use of objects during very habitual tasks such as eating as well as during familiar, but less habitual, activities such as crafts or cooking. If inappropriate tool use occurs, classify the problem. Does the patient fail to use objects (i.e., uses hands to eat stew or pudding, or attempts to "drink" a bowl of cereal by lifting it to the mouth rather than using a spoon)? Does he or she use objects for the wrong purpose (i.e., combs hair with a toothbrush, or chooses the improper eating utensil)? Does the patient orient the object incorrectly (i.e., turns spoon upside down when attempting to eat cereal, or fails to adjust its position as it is brought toward the mouth)?

Gestures. Can the patient wave, shake hands, make the "OK" sign, and use gestures to make needs known (i.e., hunger, need to use the bathroom, desire to go to his or her room)?

Facial Motions. Can the person blow out a match, wink, or blow on hot liquid to cool it?

Motor Patterns. Does the patient use ineffective movements (i.e., uses ineffective patting motions to wash body or face, or light up-and-down movements to cut food)? Does he or she resist movement (i.e., when attempting to roll or transfer, the patient moves in a counterproductive manner)? Does he or she have difficulty initiating familiar movement patterns such as moving supine to sitting (i.e., pushes backward with the nonaffected side)? This must be distinguished from fear of or resistance to movement.

Interpretation

Difficulties in any of the above areas can indicate motor-planning problems. Incorrect object use implies ideational apraxia, and incorrect movement patterns and perseveration suggest ideomotor apraxia. Incoordination due to a purely motor or sensory loss or due to use of the nondominant hand must be distinguished from apraxia. One must remember that even when the chosen activities are familiar to the patient, the loss of motor function caused by hemiplegia makes it necessary for the patient to learn to do them in a new way.

No Apparent Deficit. The patient uses objects and tools appropriately, and accurately sequences the steps for performance of familiar tasks.

Partial Deficit. A partial deficit is any deficit that falls between no apparent deficit and severe deficit.

Severe Deficit. The patient frequently uses objects inappropriately and may require physical assistance to perform a task correctly. Frequent demonstration, hand-over-hand assistance, or cuing is required to sequence the steps of a task. Perseveration during performance may be noted frequently.

Functional Observations: Unfamiliar Tasks

Sequencing. Observe the patient performing tasks that were not performed prior to the stroke (for instance, pushing a wheelchair by using arms and legs together). Can the patient sequence and time actions so that the movement is effective? Does he or she tend to be able to move only one limb at a time, rather than moving the arm and leg together, thus interfering with maximal efficiency?

Perseveration. When learning a new task such as an exercise sequence, does the patient tend to repeat one pattern, and have difficulty switching to the next exercise? What types of cues are most helpful in moving to the next step (i.e., demonstration, verbal cues, or hand-over-hand guidance)?

Object Use. After initial training, is the patient able to comprehend the purpose and correct use of unfamiliar equipment such as a rocker knife, a dressing stick, a suction denture brush, the bed controls, or wheelchair parts? Can the patient benefit from cues, demonstration, and assistance, or does he or she continue to show difficulty while using new equipment?

Motor Patterns. Can the patient follow demonstration or cuing to produce unfamiliar motor patterns with the unaffected arm, such as shrugging shoulders, using the leg to propel a wheelchair, "pinching" the shoulders back (scapular adduction), or grasping the affected thumb or fingers correctly for self-range of motion exercises? When the patient attempts to learn these movements, is physical assistance necessary? Do movement attempts seem uncoordinated and ineffective?

Interpretation

Difficulties in any of the above areas may indicate motor-planning problems with unfamiliar activities. Incorrect object use implies ideational apraxia, while incorrect movement patterns and perseveration suggest ideomotor apraxia. Incoordination due to a purely motor or sensory loss must be distinguished from apraxia.

No Apparent Deficit. The patient uses objects and tools appropriately, and accurately sequences the steps for performance of unfamiliar tasks.

Partial Deficit. A partial deficit is any deficit that falls between no apparent deficit and severe deficit.

Severe Deficit. After repeated instruction, the patient frequently continues to use unfamiliar objects inappropriately. Demonstration, hand-over-hand assistance, or cuing is often required to use unfamiliar objects or to sequence the steps of an unfamiliar task. Perseveration during performance may be noted frequently.

Motor-Planning Tests: Unfamiliar Tasks

Name: Imitation of Postures

Source: Adapted from *Patterns of Sensory Integrative Dysfunction in Adult Hemiplegia*, Project Report R-112 and Test Manual, Rehabilitation Institute of Chicago, 1980.

Description

The patient is asked to imitate a series of unfamiliar postures.

Pros. This test provides a method of looking specifically at the patient's ability to copy fine versus gross movements.

Cons. This nonstandardized test requires visual analysis skills and the ability to understand abstract concepts; therefore, it is not appropriate for some patients.

Instructions

The therapist and the patient sit facing each other. If the patient is a right-side hemiplegic, the therapist uses his or her right arm to demonstrate the test items, and vice versa. The patient is asked to mirror the examiner with the nonaffected arm. The therapist says: "You make your arms and hands do the same thing that mine do. See how fast you can do it." Quickly assume the trial position, using your right arm if the patient is a right-side hemiplegic. Assume each position quickly so that the patient cannot see you motor plan the task. Hold each position for three seconds, counting to yourself. If the patient is correct on the trial item, state, "That's right, it's as though you were looking in a mirror." If the patient is *incorrect*, assist him or her to assume the correct position, and say, "Now your arm looks like mine. It is as if you were looking in a mirror." Proceed with the test items, saying, "Now do this one; do it quickly." The therapist should assume the following positions for the patient to imitate:

- Put your fist on your chin (trial).
- Put your hand under your elbow.
- Pinch one thumb with the opposite thumb and middle finger.
- Clasp your hands and bring them to your hip.
- Clench your fist. Place your hand on your chest. Make a *V* with your index finger and middle finger.

Imitation of Postures with Verbal Cues

If the patient has difficulty performing the tasks, provide verbal cues along with the demonstration. Say:

- "Put your fist on your chin."
- "Put your hand under your elbow."
- "Pinch your thumb with your middle finger and thumb."

- "Clasp your hands and bring them to your hip."
- "Clench your fist. Place your hand on your chest. Make a *V* with your index finger and middle finger."

Interpretation

Note difficulties with fine versus gross motor patterns. If verbal cuing improves performance, it may indicate that the patient's internal language system is unable to code the information. These patients may be helped by providing external language cues or by asking the patient to verbalize the steps of an activity. If the patient talks himself or herself through the test, he or she may be using language skills to compensate for difficulties in perceiving or planning the task.

Name: Sequencing an Unfamiliar Task

Description

The patient is asked to imitate a three-step action.

Pros. This test helps the therapist focus on the patient's ability to sequence an unfamiliar movement pattern.

Cons. This nonstandardized test often is unnecessary and should be used only when routine clinical activities have not provided an opportunity to observe sequencing of an unfamiliar action.

Instructions

The therapist and the patient sit facing each other. The patient is asked to mirror the examiner. The therapist says: "You make your arms and hands do the same thing that mine do. See how fast you can do it." Perform the following action: clasp your hands, touch the right shoulder, touch the left knee. Repeat this sequence touching the left shoulder and the right knee. If the patient has difficulty following the demonstration, use language to assist performance. Say: "Clasp your hands. Touch your right [or left] shoulder. Touch your left [or right] knee."

Interpretation

Note the patient's difficulty in performing the proper sequence of activities and any tendency to perseverate. Visual spatial deficits that impair the patient's ability to detect the correct spatial configuration should be ruled out.

Chapter 12

Goal Writing and Treatment Ideas

This chapter provides suggestions for writing goals and gives guidelines for treatment. Based on evaluation results and the patient's interests, the occupational therapist (OT) should define primary problem areas that are limiting functional achievement. Each problem area is followed by several goals ranging from the most basic to the most complex. The therapist should choose the goal level that best fits the patient. Each goal contains modifiers placed within parentheses that allow the therapist to customize each goal further. Following many of the core goals are additional qualifiers that may be used as appropriate. Blank spaces in the sample goals are to be filled in with relevant activities, times, etc. For example, the goal "Patient will attend to (oral/facial hygiene, basic self-care, feeding, work-related task, leisure activity, financial management task) (for _____ minutes, until completed) in a quiet environment *with (min., mod., max.) cues*" can be customized by choosing the descriptions in parentheses that are most appropriate for the patient. The customized goal might state: "Patient will attend to feeding for 10 minutes in a quiet environment with min. cues." Following the goals for each area are brief descriptions of treatment ideas that can help in remediation or compensation for deficit. For further explanation of these activities, consult Chapters 6 and 7.

COGNITIVE GOALS AND TREATMENT

Arousal

Description of Problem

Patient has difficulty maintaining adequate level of arousal for participation in treatment.

Goals

1. Patient will demonstrate (arousal, attention) for _____ (minutes, seconds) following (olfactory, gustatory, tactile, vestibular, proprioceptive, auditory, visual, etc.) stimulation
2. Caregiver will (perform, describe) sensory stimulation techniques
   with (min., mod., max.) cues
   with written instructions
3. Patient will remain alert for _____ minutes to complete (oral/facial hygiene, self-feeding, etc.)
   with (min., mod., max.) cues
   following (tactile, vestibular, olfactory, verbal) stimulation

Treatment Suggestions

1. Provide sensory stimulation in conjunction with purposeful activity.
2. Use movement to increase arousal.
3. Schedule treatment to correspond to the patient's optimal period of arousal.
4. Teach the family methods of providing structured sensory input.

Attention: Sustained

Description of Problem

Patient has difficulty maintaining attention to a repetitive task in a quiet environment.

Goals

1. Patient will attend to (oral/facial hygiene, basic self-care, feeding, work-related task, leisure ac-

tivity, financial management task) (for _____ minutes, until completed) in a quiet environment *with (min., mod., max.) cues*

2. Caregiver will (use, describe) methods to structure the environment to minimize distraction during functional activities

Treatment Suggestions

1. Use activities relevant to the patient.
2. Grade the amount of time required for attention to the task.
3. Balance the motoric and cognitive demands of a task to provide optimal challenge.
4. Structure the environment to decrease amount of irrelevant stimuli.

Attention: Selective

Description of Problem

Patient has difficulty screening distractions when working in a multistimulus environment.

Goal

1. Patient will attend to (basic self-care task, leisure activity, home management activity, financial management task, work-related task, etc.) (for _____ minutes, until completed) in a (distracting, community, clinic, work) environment *with (min., mod., max.) cues*

Treatment Suggestions

1. See treatment suggestions for sustained attention.
2. Grade the types and amounts of competing stimuli.

Attention: Alternating

Description of Problem

Patient has difficulty alternating attention between visual and verbal information or when doing two tasks at once (for instance, talking while chopping vegetables).

Goal

1. Patient will attend to several facets of (meal preparation, community, work, leisure) activity simultaneously
   in a (distracting, quiet) environment
   with (min., mod., max.) cues

Treatment Suggestions

1. See treatment suggestions for sustained and selective attention.
2. Involve the patient in activity requiring attention to several tasks simultaneously (e.g., meal preparation, carrying on a conversation while performing an automatic activity).
3. Choose activities that require alternating between different sensory systems (e.g., auditory and visual, motor and auditory, etc.).
4. Grade the cognitive complexity of the two or more tasks chosen to provide optimal challenge.

Memory: Short-Term

Description of Problem

Patient is unable to retain information for one minute. This may be caused by ineffective encoding of information. If so, the underlying cause(s), such as poor attention or impaired perception should be addressed. The problem may also be caused by inability to store the information in a meaningful way or inability to retrieve the information when needed.

Goal

1. Patient will retain and use (visual, verbal, tactile kinesthetic, orientation) (information, instructions) related to current (basic self-care, community, leisure, meal preparation, etc.) task for _____ seconds
   using a (list, memory book)
   with (min., mod., max.) cues

Treatment Suggestions

1. Maintain a consistent routine and environment from day to day.
2. Use information relevant to the patient.
3. Organize information into small, logical groups.
4. Repeat information periodically during the treatment session.
5. Use the patient's strongest sensory system(s) to improve retention.
6. Grade the amount of structure and types of adaptations provided as the patient improves.
7. Allow the patient to experience the consequences of memory loss to improve motivation to address this area.
8. Introduce the concepts of compensation strategies and their value in managing memory problems when the patient is aware of the deficit.

9. Once the patient is aware of the memory deficit and appears motivated to improve, assist him or her in utilizing compensatory techniques or strategies for memory retrieval. Use visual cues (pictures, lists, timetables, memory book, visualization of the object or a feature) or auditory cues (alarm clock; verbal or silent repetition of information, stating its relevance; asking questions to jar memory, mnemonic devices such as rhymes; or using the letters of a word to recall a list).

Memory: Long-Term

Description of Problem

Patient has difficulty retaining information for longer than a minute. Carry-over of new learning is impaired.

Goal

1. Patient will retain (verbal, visual, tactile kinesthetic, personal, historical, orientation (information, instructions) related to (basic self-care, previous roles, community, leisure, work, etc.) for _____ (minutes, hours, days)
    using (visual, verbal) compensatory aids
    with (min., mod., max.) cues

Treatment Suggestions

1. See treatment suggestions for short-term memory.

Orientation

Description of Problem

Patient is unable to recall information, such as place, date, familiar others, and time related to who and where he or she is in the environment.

Goals

1. Patient will be oriented to (date, time, passage of time, place, daily schedule, familiar others, personal historical information)
    using (compensatory techniques, memory book, calendar, clock)
    with (min., mod., max.) cues
2. Caretaker will (use, describe) techniques to facilitate orientation
    to (person, place, time)
    with written instructions

Treatment Suggestions

1. Use techniques described under "Short-Term Memory."
2. Provide opportunities to estimate the passage of time and to monitor schedule.

Problem Solving: Problem Identification

Description of Problem

Patient has difficulty recognizing an actual or potential problem. Patient may be impulsive because of inability to process a wide range of information, resulting in stimulus-response behavior.

Goal

1. Patient will (identify, anticipate) at least (one, two, three) problems interfering with performance of _____ activities of daily living (ADL) task
    with (min., mod., max.) cues
    through trial and error

Treatment Suggestions

1. Allow the patient to experience trouble with tasks at various levels of difficulty to facilitate awareness of problem areas.
2. Provide opportunities for trial-and-error problem identification if the patient is unable to anticipate problems.
3. Initially emphasize problem solving in routine, familiar, ADL, or leisure tasks, progressing to higher-level or unfamiliar home management work and community-level activities.
4. Provide graded problem-solving activities such as performing familiar tasks with one hand, planning and organizing a meal, planning a trip, doing financial management tasks, using a menu, following a train schedule, using a phone book.
5. Use cuing to help the patient anticipate problems.
6. Encourage the patient to slow down through cues or self-monitoring techniques (e.g., counting to five, describing two possible problems before acting, etc.) to promote improved awareness of possible problem situations.

Problem Solving: Solution Generation

Description of Problem

Patient has difficulty generating effective solution(s) to an identified problem. Patient may persist in using an ineffective approach to a problem and may be unaware of subtle details of the problem.

Goal

1. Patient will identify (one, two, or more) logical solutions to problems encountered in _____ (self-care, work, etc.) task
    with (min., mod., max.) cues

Treatment Suggestions

1. See treatment suggestions for problem identification.

Problem Solving: Planning

Description of Problem

Patient shows difficulty organizing activities that are not habitual. Patient may have difficulty anticipating the materials, time, and sequence needed to complete a task.

Goals

1. Patient will identify (materials, time, sequence) needed for performing _____ (basic, complex) ADL task
    with (min., mod., max.) cues
2. Patient will successfully plan and carry out _____ (basic, complex) ADL task
    within given time limits
    using work simplification principles
    with (min., mod., max.) cues
3. Patient will effectively (plan, follow) (daily, weekly) schedule of work, self-care, leisure, and rest
    using work simplification principles
    with (min., mod., max.) cues

Treatment Suggestions

1. See treatment suggestions for problem identification and planning.
2. Provide planning practice by asking the patient to plan for a hypothetical situation, but follow up by planning a real activity.
3. Grade the amount of materials and the number of steps needed to complete a task.
4. Grade time requirements by having the patient plan a half-hour treatment session before planning a weekly schedule; place time constraints on activity after basic planning skills are demonstrated.
5. Gradually decrease the amount of cuing and structure, eventually allowing the patient to plan the activity without the OT's intervention.

6. Incorporate work simplification training, gradually requesting that the patient apply energy-conservation techniques in new situations.

Problem Solving: Implementation of Solution

Description of Problem

Patient has difficulty following through with identified solutions to problems. He or she may persist in using an approach to a problem without assessing its effectiveness.

Goal

1. Patient will (implement, assess effectiveness of) identified solutions to problems encountered in _____ (self-care, work, etc.) task
    with (min., mod., max.) cues

Treatment Suggestions

1. See treatment suggestions for problem identification, planning, and generating solutions.

Problem Solving: Self-Monitoring

Description of Problem

Patient has difficulty monitoring the effectiveness of various actions. Patient may show decreased awareness of the subtle features of a problem and respond only to the most obvious factors, neglecting psychosocial, cultural, or other details that would lead to an optimal decision.

Goal

1. Patient will demonstrate judgment adequate for making (rapid, successful) decisions related to _____ (complex ADL skills, work, leisure, community participation, finances, time management)
    with (min., mod., max.) cues

Treatment Suggestions

1. See treatment suggestions for problem identification, planning, generating solutions, and implementing solutions.
2. Begin with routine tasks and progress to higher-level activities that demand quick, effective analysis of more subtle features for successful completion.
3. Use financial problem-solving work sheets, a daily or weekly schedule, community activities, computer games, high-level games of strategy.

Problem Solving: Safety

Description of Problem

Patient has difficulty responding to task demands in a safe manner. Difficulties may be due to poor attention to the environment, limited ability to process all of the information relevant to the situation, impulsivity, difficulty anticipating the consequences of a particular action, or poor awareness of limitations. These deficits may result in breakdown of any part of the problem-solving sequence listed above.

Goals

1. Therapist may choose a goal listed above, depending on which aspect of problem solving is affected or may write a specific safety goal as suggested below.

2. Patient will safely complete _____ (basic self-care, complex ADL skill)
    in a (structured, unstructured, quiet, distracting) environment
    with (min., mod., max.) cues

3. Caretaker will identify (cognitive, perceptual, motor) deficits that interfere with safe performance of (basic, complex) ADL tasks
    and describe at least _____ interventions to promote safety
    with (min., mod., max.) cues

Treatment Suggestions

1. See treatment suggestions for the aspect of problem solving that limits safety.

2. Structure the environment to minimize distraction and/or risks.

3. Grade structure and cuing to allow the patient to exercise safety judgment.

4. Discuss possible consequences prior to a task, and review performance immediately after the activity to reinforce safe practices and identify those that could be improved.

PERCEPTUAL GOALS AND TREATMENT

Visual Perceptual: Unilateral Visual Inattention

Description of Problem

Patient unconsciously neglects visual information in one half of space.

Goals

1. Patient will visually (attend to, locate) (a) (stationary, slowly moving, rapidly moving) (self-care object, familiar face, complex visual information)
    (in, through (midline, midrange, extreme ranges) of (right, left, both) visual field(s) during (basic self-care, complex ADL skills, community activities, work activities) with (min., mod., max.) (verbal, tactile, visual) (cues, physical assist)

2. Patient/caregiver will describe the impact of unilateral visual inattention on function and (describe, demonstrate) at least (one, two, three) compensation techniques
    with (min., mod., max.) cues

Treatment Suggestions

1. Begin by using visual stimuli that elicit the most consistent response.

2. Alter the environment to increase or decrease stimuli as needed.

3. Use movement to enhance response to visual activities.

4. Use multisensory tasks to enhance visual registration.

5. Grade distance required for visual attention and scanning (i.e., begin with items positioned at midline, gradually increasing horizontal scope).

6. Grade speed and level of complexity of information presented.

7. Teach compensation techniques, such as consciously turning the head to scan the environment, use of colored margin markers when reading, positioning items to maximize visual field, scanning to find where the border of a page meets the table, using the finger as a guide.

Visual Perceptual: Visual Analysis and Synthesis

Description of Problem

Patient has difficulty interpreting complex visual information. Problems may be seen in analyzing parts (such as in figure-ground), discriminating forms, or combining parts to create a whole (such as in visual closure or construction). The problems may be due to underlying deficits in visual scanning, visual spatial skills, problem solving, or visual attention.

Goals

1. When the underlying deficit is known, therapist will structure goals to address that area.

2. Patient will demonstrate visual perceptual skills sufficient for safe performance of _____ (functional task)
    with (min., mod., max.) cues

3. Patient will (identify white shirt on white sheet; find item in drawer; find item in refrigerator; find item on store shelf; identify color, shape, or size of functional objects; identify relevant visual information; identify cross-walk sign; identify uneven surfaces)

   during _____ (structured, unstructured, table top, functional activity)

   when (stationary, moving slowly, moving quickly, presented at a rate of _____)

   using _____ compensation techniques

   with (min., mod., max.) cues

4. Patient will compensate for visual perceptual deficits in _____ (structured, unstructured) (functional task) by (supplementing visual information with tactile information, slowing pace and double-checking work, organizing work area to minimize visual clutter, verbally analyzing visual information to determine part-to-whole relationships and subtle characteristics, minimizing other distractions, using systematic visual scanning pattern)

   with (min., mod., max.) cues

5. Patient/caregiver will describe impact of (figure-ground, form discrimination) deficits on safety and quality of functional performance and (describe, demonstrate) compensation techniques for use during _____ (functional task)

   with (min., mod., max.) cues

Treatment Suggestions

1. Use movement to enhance response to visual perceptual activities. For example, combine color, shape, and size discrimination with rolling or sitting balance activity. Vary the developmental position used when working on higher-level visual perceptual tasks. Balance the perceptual and motor demands of the task to optimize performance.

2. Use the tactile system to enhance visual perceptual processing. Encourage the patient to feel the shapes of objects, use a finger to trace designs in powder if unable to use a pen.

3. Use language by asking the patient to describe visual information, such as how one part relates to the whole, or verbally describe his or her visual search strategy when solving a visual perceptual problem.

4. Grade from familiar, concrete tasks to unfamiliar, abstract activities.

5. Grade the visual complexity of the activity. For example, three-dimensional, complex figure-ground discrimination will be more difficult than two-dimensional, familiar embedded figures. Including more elements or requiring attention to subtle details will increase the task difficulty. Speed of presentation will change task demands. As visual processing improves, increase the speed that is required to attend to the information. Computer programs and community activities may be used to add time demands.

6. Teach compensation techniques, such as visually checking work, allowing more time to complete an activity, organizing work area, or minimizing external distractions when increased attention to visual information is required.

7. Describe to the patient and the caregiver how visual perceptual deficits affect ADL tasks and how clinical activities relate to functional performance.

8. Provide opportunities for the caregiver and the patient to practice suggested treatment activities and compensation methods in a variety of functional tasks.

Visual Perceptual: Visual Construction and Visual Spatial Awareness

Description of Problem

Patient has difficulty analyzing the spatial relationships of objects and putting parts together in two or three dimensions to form a whole.

Goals

1. Patient will show (visual spatial, visual construction) skills sufficient to perform _____ (functional task)

   with (min., mod., max.) (cues, assistance)

2. Patient will correctly orient (shirt, pants, items when setting the table, parts of a craft activity)

   with (min., mod., max.) (cues, assistance)

3. Patient will correctly combine parts to (wrap a gift, make a model, make a craft project, copy a drawing, make a sandwich, set the table, dress self, perform _____ work activity, perform _____ self-care activity)

   from (memory, verbal instructions, written directions, diagrams)

   with (min., mod., max.) (cues, assistance)

4. Patient/caregiver will identify impact of visual construction and visual spatial deficits on safety and quality of functional performance

   and will (demonstrate, describe) (at least one, two, three) strategies to compensate for deficits

   with (min., mod., max.) (cues)

5. Patient will compensate for visual (spatial, construction) deficits in _____ (structured, unstructured) (functional task) by (describing the plan and sequence of steps prior to and during performance, supplementing information with tactile information, slowing pace and double-checking work, organizing work area to minimize visual clutter, verbally analyzing visual information, minimizing other distractions, using systematic visual scanning pattern)
with (min., mod., max.) cues

Treatment Suggestions

1. See suggestions under visual analysis and synthesis.
2. For difficulties organizing the motor component of a task, ask the patient to describe the plan and task steps verbally before and during an activity. Provide written or verbal cues to enhance performance. Hand-over-hand guidance or tactile cues may be needed if motor-planning problems are more severe.

Body Awareness: Tactile Sensory Loss

Description of Problem

Primary tactile sensory loss interferes with patient's normal protective and discriminative responses.

Goals

1. Patient/caregiver will describe sensory deficits and their impact on safe and efficient performance of _____ (functional activity)
and will (describe, demonstrate) at least (one, two, three) compensation techniques to enhance performance
with (min., mod., max.) (cues, assistance)
2. Patient will compensate for sensory loss by
properly positioning (right, left) upper extremity (in bed, in wheelchair, during _____ functional task)
visually monitoring (right, left) (upper, lower) extremity during (wheelchair propulsion, oral/facial hygiene, bathing, meal preparation, ironing, _____ functional task)
protecting (right, left) (upper, lower) extremity from (sharp, hot, cold) objects/conditions
with (min., mod., max.) (cues, assistance)
3. Therapist can use tactile discrimination goals if sensory deficits are mild.

Treatment Suggestions

1. Describe and demonstrate area of sensory loss to caregiver.
2. Describe and demonstrate effects of these deficits on tasks such as shaving, bathing, cooking, wheelchair mobility, use of sharp objects, or ironing, and effects of hot or cold outdoor temperatures.
3. Provide suggestions for positioning, handling, and compensation.
4. Provide opportunities for caregiver/patient to practice these techniques in functional settings.
5. Provide graded single sensory input (e.g., rubbing lotion, using texture such as that of a washcloth, soap, shaver) on body during daily ADL activities.
6. Use movement to enhance response to sensory input.
7. If sensory deficits are subtle, see tactile discrimination treatment suggestions.

Body Awareness: Unilateral Tactile Inattention, Bilateral Integration

Description of Problem

Unilateral tactile inattention is characterized by neglect of body parts and/or tactile information on one side of the body. Sensation may be intact, diminished, or absent. Patient is unable to compensate for sensory loss or use sensation that is present, especially when attending to another aspect of a task. Bilateral integration refers to the ability to use both sides of the body together in the absence of sensory and motor deficits.

Goals

1. Patient will (locate, position, attend to) (right, left) upper extremity during (bed mobility, wheelchair mobility, therapeutic activities, _____ functional activities, bilateral simultaneous stimulation)
with (min., mod., max.) (cues, assistance)
2. Patient will show tactile attention sufficient to (carry an object while walking, grasp clothing during dressing, stabilize an object, perform _____ functional task)
with (min., mod., max.) (cues, assistance)
3. Patient will show bilateral integration sufficient for using two hands together to (fold clothes, wring a cloth, use a rolling pin, shuffle cards, push wheelchair, type, etc.)
with (min., mod., max.) (cues, assistance)

4. Patient/caregiver will identify the effects of unilateral tactile inattention on the efficiency and safety of _____ functional task
    and (describe, demonstrate) at least (one, two, three) compensation strategies
    with (min., mod., max.) (cues, assistance)

Treatment Suggestions

1. Improve awareness of body through movement and tactile stimulation.
2. Provide activities with a variety of tactile qualities, such as weight, shape, and texture. Begin with materials having gross differences in these qualities, eventually asking the patient to attend to more subtle differences.
3. Provide unilateral, then bilateral stimulation activities, encouraging the patient to attend to the tactile qualities of the task.
4. Begin in a nondistracting environment, gradually increasing the amount of stimulation during tasks requiring tactile attention.

Body Awareness: Tactile Discrimination

Description of Problem

Patient has difficulty discriminating subtle characteristics of an object through the sense of touch.

Goal

1. Patient will tactilely discriminate (subtle, gross) differences in (size, shape, texture) of _____ functional objects during ADL tasks
    with (min., mod., max.) cues

Treatment Suggestions

1. Use methods described under tactile sensory loss for patients with severe tactile discrimination deficits.
2. Use methods described under unilateral tactile inattention.
3. Provide graded tactile activities requiring improved selectivity of response.

Body Awareness: Body Parts Identification, Right-Left Identification

Description of Problem

Patient has difficulty identifying body parts and right and left. Performance requires language, attention, visual spatial, and sensory processing.

Goals

1. Patient will correctly (identify, follow directions related to) (right-left, body parts) during (_____ self-care tasks, work tasks, functional mobility, community activities, therapeutic activities)
    with (min., mod., max.) (cues, assistance)

Treatment Suggestions

1. Improve awareness of body through movement and tactile stimulation.
2. Provide activities that enhance awareness of self before emphasizing body scheme or right-left discrimination on others.
3. Use names of body parts and right-left directions during ADL tasks and therapeutic activities.

Body Awareness: Midline Orientation

Description of Problem

Patient has difficulty identifying and maintaining a symmetrical upright posture. This interferes with establishing the correct postural set on which to base movements outside of midline.

Goals

1. Patient will (identify, maintain, assume) proper midline orientation during (static sitting, _____ functional, _____ therapeutic) activity
    for _____ minutes
    with (min., mod., max.) (tactile, verbal, visual) (cues, assistance)
2. Patient/caregiver will describe impact of poor midline orientation on safety and efficiency of _____ functional task
    and will (describe, demonstrate) use of (compensation techniques, positioning equipment)
    with (min., mod., max.) (cues, assistance)

Treatment Suggestions

1. Teach the patient or caregiver compensatory techniques such as the use of a mirror, vertical object, positioning equipment, tactile cues, and verbal cues to enhance midline orientation.
2. Help the patient to feel correct body orientation during tasks by positioning or guiding movement, describing the qualities of proper midline position, using multisensory input and movement to enhance awareness, and encouraging him or her to attend to the characteristics of midline orientation.

3. Begin with static midline positions, gradually requiring more dynamic movements into and out of midline in various developmental positions.

4. Balance the cognitive and perceptual demands of the task to maximize performance.

Motor Planning: Familiar Tasks

Description of Problem

Despite adequate strength, coordination, and range of motion (ROM), patient experiences difficulty carrying out previously routine activities. Patient may have difficulty with conceptualizing a task; i.e., he or she is unable to identify or demonstrate the use of common objects, has difficulty mentally sequencing the steps of a task, or does not attend to critical points when changes in the routine or sequence are needed. The patient may also have difficulty with the execution of a task. For instance, movement may be clumsy or perseverative, or spatial orientation of objects may be incorrect; patient may be able to describe steps verbally, identify another person's correct and incorrect performance, or arrange pictures in sequence, but has difficulty carrying out an activity.

Goal

1. Patient will demonstrate motor planning sufficient to
   (perform, sequence) _____ familiar task use (toothbrush, comb, razor, toilet paper, spoon, hammer, pen, etc.) appropriately with (min., mod., max.) cues with (demonstration, hand-over-hand assistance, tactile prompts)

Treatment Suggestions

1. Assist the patient in identifying the name and use of objects.

2. Provide repetition, consistent approach, and opportunity to use objects in their usual context. For example, perform oral/facial hygiene as part of morning routine, or practice utensil use during a regular meal.

3. Grade the complexity of the tasks in terms of skill required to use objects or the number of steps that must be sequenced. For example, using a washcloth requires less skilled movement than applying makeup, and eating a bowl of ice cream requires less sequencing than preparing a toothbrush and brushing one's teeth.

4. Use activities that encourage an automatic response (for example, catching a ball, dressing, washing, shaking hands).

5. Minimize the need for the patient to learn a new technique for self-care until adequate performance of routine tasks is shown.

6. Ask the patient's family to observe self-care performance. Point out the effects of motor-planning deficits.

7. Provide an opportunity for the family to practice intervention strategies.

8. Use multisensory cues to enhance the patient's use of objects. For example, provide demonstration of object use, provide correct context to stimulate proper use, use hand-over-hand guidance when necessary, verbally identify objects and their use, and have the patient verbally identify objects and their use when able.

9. Involve the patient in gross and fine motor activities that require sequencing, including exercises, functional tasks, functional mobility, and gross motor games.

10. Use rhythm and music as appropriate during therapeutic activities.

11. Give cues to assist sequencing. For instance, offer verbal guidance; provide pictures, lists, or diagrams; structure the task by giving the patient only the materials he or she needs for that step. Have patient talk himself or herself through the procedure.

12. Provide opportunities to practice skills under various conditions and in various situations to improve generalization.

Motor Planning: Unfamiliar Tasks

Description of Problem

Patient has difficulty learning the motor sequence needed to perform new activities, despite adequate strength, coordination, and ROM. Conceptualization and execution difficulties may be seen as described under "Motor Planning: Familiar Tasks."

Goal

1. Patient will demonstrate motor planning sufficient to
   (perform, sequence) (wheelchair mobility, transfers, one-handed ADL techniques, upper extremity ROM, _____ unfamiliar task) use (sock donner, rocker knife, wheelchair, one-handed can opener, adapted cutting board, electric razor, etc.) with (min., mod., max.) cues with (demonstration, hand-over-hand assistance, tactile prompts)

Treatment Suggestions

1. Use treatment suggestions for motor planning familiar tasks.
2. Provide a consistent teaching approach and limit the number of unfamiliar activities taught.

GROUP GOALS

Depending on the size and nature of the groups offered in a department, almost any of the goal areas described in the cognitive and perceptual goal workbook can be modified to be addressed appropriately in a group setting. The therapist must be sure that the size of the group, the focus of the group, and the levels of other group members are conducive to focusing on that goal. In some cases (for instance, when the group is large or the members of the group have diverse skill levels) the goals will need to be less specific than those addressed in individual treatment.

Experience has shown that specifying goals in the group policy as well as on referral and feedback forms leads to more appropriate referrals and expectations. In addition, group treatment is then more goal-directed, with better-defined entrance and exit criteria. Samples of some of the perceptual and cognitive areas addressed by various groups in the occupational therapy department of the Rehabilitation Institute of Chicago (RIC) follow. Goals can be customized to correspond to the types of groups offered in various facilities. Although most of the groups also address motor and ADL function, those goals are not included unless they relate directly to cognition and perception. The goals listed below are short-term goals specific to various groups. The therapist can select the goals that are appropriate to the patient. The group leader then gives feedback regarding progress toward that goal. When the patient's goals have been reached, they can be upgraded, or the patient can graduate from the group. The patient's documentation should also include functional long-term goals relevant to each area. For example, the first short-term goal listed below reads: "Patient will work on a project at an acceptable rate (with cues, independently)." The long-term goal related to this area might be: "Patient will increase speed of task performance to allow completion of morning ADL routine in 45 minutes."

Sample Group Goals

This is an abbreviated list showing a small number of goals that are addressed in various department groups.

1. Patient will work on a project at an acceptable rate (with cues, independently).

2. Patient will demonstrate attention and problem solving sufficient to complete a project (with assistance, independently).
3. Patient will attend to tasks for 10 minutes (without, with minimal, with moderate) (cues, physical prompting).
4. Patient will follow a simple one-step command (without, with minimal, with moderate) cues.
5. Patient will interact appropriately with another group member (without, with minimal, with moderate) cues.
6. Patient will remember another group member's name (without, with minimal, with moderate) cues.
7. Patient will locate and position affected upper extremity safely (without, with verbal, with tactile) cues.
8. Patient will use affected upper extremity as (an active, a passive) assist in bilateral activities (with cues, independently).

GROUP TREATMENT

Groups of various types are available to stroke patients at The Rehabilitation Institute of Chicago (RIC). They have been developed as a cost-effective way to address defined skills. In addition, the benefits of socialization, peer support, and variety make groups popular and effective. All groups have formal policies and procedures for patient selection and operation as well as defined methods of monitoring their effectiveness. The groups that are commonly used to address cognitive and perceptual deficits are described briefly below.

Eat Group

Focus: To promote independence in eating.

Patient Selection Criteria

Patients who have dysphagia, perceptual, or cognitive deficits that interfere with independent eating are eligible. Patients must be capable of eating at least one-quarter of the meal without direct supervision.

Staffing

One speech pathologist, one occupational therapist, and one rehabilitation technician. The ratio never exceeds one patient to three staff members.

Structure

The group meets daily for breakfast and lunch on the patient floor. Efforts are made to minimize distractions.

Specific Activities

Each dysphagia patient has a distinctive wheelchair bag that contains specific instructions such as diet, feeding techniques, and cues required for safe eating. Equipment and techniques used by the OT to promote function can also be found in the bag. The staff members help the patients begin their meals and then spend time with individuals according to their needs. Thermal stimulation or review of specific swallowing techniques may precede the meal. Depending on their problems, patients may be encouraged to use adaptive equipment, may have their tray simplified to promote improved attention, or may be reminded to attend to the affected visual field.

GROW (Group Rehabilitation on Ward)

Focus: Patients are assisted to meet individual goals through interdisciplinary co-treatment.

Patient Selection Criteria

Patients who have Occupational Therapy (OT), Speech Therapy (ST), and Physical Therapy (PT) needs and can benefit from receiving interdisciplinary co-treatment are eligible.

Staffing

One occupational therapist, one physical therapist, and one speech therapist. The patient-to-staff ratio is one to one.

Structure

Three patients and therapists from OT, PT, and ST meet daily in a small treatment room on the nursing unit. Each patient is seen daily by each discipline during the three-hour morning treatment session. Rest breaks are provided for the patients as needed. Therapists set mutual goals each week and work together to meet those goals. When beneficial, two therapists can co-treat the patient to maximize performance. Occasionally all patients are treated for a portion of the period in a small group.

Specific Activities

Therapists use treatment activities appropriate to their disciplines to promote goal attainment. The OT may use neurodevelopmental techniques, sensorimotor activities, self-care tasks, cognitive and perceptual remediation activities, or other techniques appropriate to the patients. Co-treatment allows two sets of hands for mobility, incorporation of ambulation into functional tasks, and improved speech production through movement. Consistency in the way the patient is taught

is enhanced due to the therapist's close working relationship.

Avocational Group

Focus: Attention, memory, problem-solving, or perceptual skills are facilitated through participation in craft activities.

Patient Selection Criteria

The patient must be capable of working independently with minimal supervision for a 50-minute treatment session and must have an interest in avocational activities.

Staffing

One certified occupational therapy assistant (COTA) and one therapy aide. The ratio can be as high as five patients to one staff member.

Structure

The group meets daily. Each patient works independently on his or her chosen project with intermittent assistance available.

Specific Activities

The patients work toward completing woodwork, ceramics, tile work, leather work, macramé, decoupage, needle work, or other craft projects. The activity may be graded from a simple sanding and staining project to designing, drawing plans, and creating a wooden item. Assistance is available for selected steps in the project or to facilitate problem solving and sequencing of the activity.

Perceptual Motor Orientation Group

Focus: Patients with moderate to severe cognitive and perceptual deficits work to improve these areas through a variety of activities.

Patient Selection Criteria

Patients must be able to participate in a highly structured group setting without disrupting other members, must be able to follow simple directions with demonstration or cuing, and must show some carry-over from day to day with cues if necessary.

Staffing

One occupational therapist and one therapy aide. Patient-to-staff ratio must remain at or below three to one.

Structure

The group meets daily to review orientation information, engage in gross perceptual motor activities, and participate in a game or other task appropriate to the level of the group members.

Specific Activities

Orientation activities usually begin the session. They may include: use of an orientation board, introduction of each group member, writing out name tags, introducing another person in the group, reading a weather report, or discussing the hospital routine.

Gross motor activities are designed to increase the patient's level of arousal and integrate movement with cognition and perception. A large spandex loop of fabric can be held by all group members who can then follow a series of directions from the group leader, i.e., lift up, pull back, push in, or pass it to the right/left. A scarf can be tied to the band which is then moved to the right or left. When the scarf stops near a person, he or she can be asked a question, can ask another group member a question, can pick the next person to receive the scarf, or can choose an exercise for the group. Music can be incorporated to make the game similar to "hot potato."

Balloon games are generally popular and can be graded from simply tossing the balloon from one to another, to calling out a name before tossing it, to playing simulated volleyball with the group members keeping score. When a team loses the ball, they can be asked a simple question. If they answer it correctly, no points are lost.

Parachute activities are also used. For example, a balloon might be placed in the center of the parachute with the goal being to roll it off on the opponent's side. A more cooperative effort might be to keep the balloon on the parachute. Bean bags of various colors or small plastic items could be placed on the parachute and bounced. The leader can remove one and ask the group to identify the missing item. Objects could be placed on the floor in the middle of the circle. As the parachute is raised, the group can try to name the objects.

Simple cognitive and social skills may be addressed by giving a functional object to each group member. Each person can be asked to demonstrate or describe the use of his or her object. Simple range of motion and mobility exercises can be performed with a focus on identifying body parts and following instructions. Body awareness and spatial awareness can be enhanced through games that require throwing or sliding a particular colored bean bag at a target, horse shoes, ring toss, bowling, or basketball, using a floor-based hoop.

The group participates in a wide variety of cognitive and perceptual activities. For example, the group may make a collage or bake cookies; play color, shape, or number bingo; or play dominoes. A map or puzzle of the United States, state, or city can be used to identify and discuss facts and remembrances of various places. Colored pegs, pieces of a simple puzzle, or parquetry blocks can be passed to group members. All group members are encouraged to work together to construct a specific design or picture. A large loop of yarn can be placed on a table and group members can be asked to make various shapes by pulling the yarn into a square, triangle, or circle. Objects can be placed on the table for viewing for approximately 30 seconds. They are then hidden beneath a towel and group members are asked to remember what they saw. Alternately, group members can be asked to feel and name the object without seeing it. Cards with simple everyday problems written on them can be placed in a pile. Each group member chooses a card, reads it to the group, and discusses possible solutions with other group members. Games such as Concentration, Pictionary, Hangman, or Uno, may be appropriate for higher level groups. Based on the skills of the group and the creativity of the leader, many other activities may also be used to promote cognitive and perceptual skills in an enjoyable manner.

Stroke Group

Focus: To promote independence in self range of motion exercise and upper extremity management.

Patient Selection Criteria

Patients must be able to follow instructions, show carry over of learning from day to day with minimal cues, and participate in a group without disruption.

Staffing

One occupational therapist and one therapy aide. The ratio is one staff member for every four patients.

Structure

The group meets daily with a focus on upper extremity management and practicing a series of range of motion exercises. Cognitive and perceptual goals are secondary to upper extremity management; however, cognitive and perceptual functions are addressed through mobility activities, sequencing steps of an exercise, following instructions, remembering exercise techniques, and group interaction.

Specific Activities

Patients are asked to remove splints, wheelchair arm rests, or slings, and are to position their feet on the floor. Assistance is given when needed. A structured program of exercises is followed to promote body alignment and upper extremity mobility. When able, group members are encouraged to lead all or a portion of the exercises. Some of the group time each week is allotted to gross motor activities or to use of the affected arm. The gross motor activities are similar to those used by the perceptual motor orientation group described above. Functional activities to promote the use of the affected arm as a passive or active assist may be chosen by the group and the leader together.

Stroke Re-Entry Group

Focus: To promote independence in community skills or teach the caregiver methods of assisting the patient in the community.

Patient Selection Criteria

The patient must be able to tolerate two hours in the wheelchair, be able to cognitively and physically participate in community activities with assistance, or have a designated caregiver who is willing to learn the necessary skills.

Staffing

One occupational therapist, one physical therapist, and one recreational therapist as appropriate. The staff-to-patient ratio for trips is generally one to one. Aides, students, or caretakers may provide additional assistance when needed.

Structure

This group meets three times per week. One session is devoted to planning, one to a simple community activity, such as a box lunch picnic, a shopping trip to a nearby store, or following a map through the local streets. The third session is devoted to going to a more distant location such as a museum, restaurant, or shopping mall.

Specific Activities

The group is encouraged to choose activities that they might enjoy following discharge. They are involved in planning the steps required to carry out the trip. They may place phone calls to determine hours, accessibility, and directions for the chosen destination. They are directed to consider time constraints and to plan the scope of the activity accordingly. The importance of taking medications, planning ahead for use of the bathroom, and considering weather conditions and ozone levels is stressed. Discussion during and after the trip about problems encountered and how they were handled are facilitated by group leaders. Outdoor mobility, clothing management, money handling, identifying community resources, and issues of accessibility are addressed in a functional setting.

Functional Occupations Program

Focus: To improve prevocational work skills.

Patient Selection Criteria

The patient must show potential to improve a variety of preliminary work competencies such as awareness of deficits, goal directed behavior, and ability to remain focused on a task. The patient must have met with vocational rehabilitation specialists and defined a potential work role (i.e., secretarial, custodial, management, manufacturing, etc.). A four-hour evaluation then determines specific motor, mobility, lifting, work skills, ADL skills, and executive functions.

Staffing

A registered occupational therapist (OTR) performs the evaluation and plans treatment. Treatment is provided by one OTR or COTA to every four patients.

Structure

The group meets daily for two three-hour sessions. Each patient's schedule is determined based on his or her current level of endurance and anticipated work schedule. Patients perform work-related tasks to build organizational skills, attention, memory, ability to follow instructions, endurance, strength, and coordination. Tasks vary depending on the potential work role of the patient.

Specific Activities

Activities relate to potential jobs such as collating papers, filing, distributing mail, cleaning, or constructing equipment. Simulated job tasks using the Baltimore Therapeutic Equipment (BTE) or other devices are also performed as appropriate.

Guidelines for ADL Goals versus Component Skill Goals

ADL goals can be customized to address component skills that are limiting performance. For example, if the patient's goal is independence in feeding and the component skill most limiting performance is inappropriate utensil use, the goal can be stated: "Patient will demonstrate appropriate utensil use to promote independence in feeding." In this way, any component deficit can be attached to a functional goal to clarify the subskill and the self-care skill being addressed. Alternatively, if the components interfering with function are well defined in the occupational therapy documentation and self-care training will be the focus of treatment, ADL goals may be written without specifying the component areas. This type of goal might read: "Patient will perform upper extremity dressing with minimal assistance." When component goals are not written, attainment of ADL goals implies improvements in the component areas. The benefit of writing ADL goals without qualifiers is that they are functional and are readily understood by patients. In addition, the goals can be written more succinctly, and paper work can be streamlined by focusing only on the self-care goals.

For newer staff, or when detailed treatment plans are not written, component goals can serve as a nice guide for treatment. Specific component goals, such as those described earlier in this section, help ensure that treatment addresses the skills required for function and help reimbursers understand how treatment techniques apply to self-care improvements. Component goals are also helpful when one or more subskills affect performance in many areas of self-care. A goal for that particular area will be most practical. For example, a low-level patient might need to sustain attention for two minutes before any self-care area will improve. A short-term goal might be: "Patient will sustain attention to a basic ADL task for two minutes in a quiet environment with moderate cues." A high-level patient who hopes to return to work as a teacher may show no clearcut change on a seven-point ADL rating scale; however, improvement in planning may enhance his or her job potential. A goal might state: "Patient will successfully plan and carry out a 20-minute lesson."

Clearly, there are occasions when ADL goals alone are sufficient and appropriate as well as occasions when component goals clarify the treatment sequence. The occupational therapy department at RIC allows variation in the types of goals written based on individual preference, the experience level of the staff member, and the specific needs of the patient. Generally, when a staff member is newer and notes serve as an objective guide for therapy as well as a method of monitoring treatment focus, more specific component goals are encouraged. Component goals have been detailed previously. The ADL goals employ the RIC functional assessment scale (RIC-FAS), which is used throughout the hospital to record status and progress in basic skills. This scale is based on the functional independence measure system developed by the American Congress of Rehabilitation Medicine.

The following core skills are always evaluated, and goals are written when appropriate: feeding, upper extremity dressing; lower extremity dressing; oral/facial hygiene; bathing; toileting; and the mechanical aspects of communication, such as use of a pen, a telephone, or a typewriter. In addition, complex ADL skills are addressed according to the patient's functional level, previous roles, and expected discharge status. Each complex ADL is described by a main category, such as meal preparation, which is then divided into levels to allow more specific·ratings of a particular aspect of the skill. Rather than rating meal preparation in general, the therapist chooses the appropriate level, such as cold meal preparation, and rates the patient according to his or her ability to plan and perform all aspects of the task. The activity analysis used in the department to determine a rating includes physical factors such as strength, endurance, and mobility as well as cognitive factors such as organization, problem solving, safety, and time management. The complex ADL tasks addressed by OTs at RIC and the levels for each are listed below.

Meal Preparation

1. Self-serve meal (e.g., prepared sandwich or Meals on Wheels)
2. Cold meal
3. Hot beverage, soup, or prepared food (such as frozen pizza or frozen dinner)
4. Hot one-dish meal (e.g., casserole, hamburger)
5. Hot multidish meal (e.g., full dinner) (adapted from Moss Rehabilitation Hospital occupational therapy department Kitchen Evaluation Form, 1980, pp. 82–83)

Clothing Care

1. Handwashing
2. Machine washing/drying
3. Ironing
4. Mending

Cleaning

1. Routine light (e.g., cleaning spills, dishes, dusting, and making bed)
2. Routine heavy (e.g., cleaning tubs, washing floors, emptying garbage, changing sheets)
3. Seasonal/occasional (e.g., cleaning windows, closets, and drapes)

Household Maintenance

1. Indoor (e.g., unlocking and opening doors and windows, changing light bulbs or fuses, making minor repairs)
2. Outdoor (e.g., shoveling snow, working in garden, trimming bushes, caring for lawn)

Emergency Procedures and Household Safety

1. Emergency communication (i.e., able to use emergency telephone number or emergency call system)

2. Recognition and prevention (i.e., able to identify hazards in home, make changes to promote safety, plan emergency evacuation, and handle medical emergency)

Money Management

Use levels one and two when shopping is the *only* community skill that will be addressed.
   1. Shopping and making purchases: structured/routine (i.e., able to order items over the telephone or make purchase in a familiar store at a quiet time)
   2. Shopping and making purchases: unstructured/ unfamiliar (i.e., able to make purchase in an un- familiar store at a busy time)
   3. Household money management (i.e., able to pay bills, plan budget, balance checkbook)

Community Skills

Use when a *variety* of community activities will be addressed. Goals may be written for the composite skill (e.g., "Patient will independently plan and carry out a trip to the movies") or goals may address a subskill (e.g., "Patient will require minimal assistance for com- munity safety during trip to unfamiliar bank").
   • Structured routine (i.e., familiar task in familiar environment, performed during quiet times with no time constraints and low possibility of un- planned problems occurring)
      1. Planning
      2. Money management
      3. Pathfinding (topographical orientation)
      4. Community safety
      5. Transportation/mobility
      6. Time management
      7. Social interaction
   • Unstructured/unfamiliar (i.e., unfamiliar task in unfamiliar environment, performed during busy times with time constraints and with the possibil- ity of problems arising)
      1. Planning
      2. Money management
      3. Pathfinding (topographical orientation)
      4. Community safety
      5. Transportation/mobility
      6. Time management
      7. Social interaction

Care of Others

Use when the *patient* must take care of another per- son.

   • Child care
      1. Playing/nurturing (i.e., able to select appropri- ate toys and use age-appropriate interaction; is aware of strategies for behavior management and facilitation of emotional growth)
      2. Physical daily care (i.e., able to perform the following safely, using appropriate equipment and techniques: feeding, oral/facial hygiene, diapering/toileting, dressing, bathing)
      3. First aid/community resourcing (i.e., able to perform first aid for cuts, choking, etc.; can take temperature, babyproof a home, give medications, and handle other emergencies; has access to child care supplies/physician; can use stroller and car seat and can instruct baby sitter)
   • Adult care
      1. Visiting/nurturing (i.e., can provide age-appro- priate activities; is able to attend to emotional and social needs)
      2. Physical daily care (i.e., able to perform the following safely, using appropriate equipment and techniques: feeding, oral/facial hygiene, diapering/toileting, dressing, bathing)
      3. Household management (can obtain and moni- tor assistants who provide direct care and ser- vices, such as cleaning, or can assist with chores such as cleaning, shopping, and meals)

Leisure

   1. Solitary indoor activities (i.e., games, crafts that can be performed alone within the home)
   2. Social indoor activities (i.e., games, parties that require interaction with others but can be per- formed within the home)
   3. Social/community activities (may use subskills listed under "Community Skills" to delineate this area further)

Work

   1. Prerequisite work behaviors/component skills (i.e., skills such as strength, coordination, atten- tion, problem solving, time awareness, etc., which are necessary even if a particular job has not been identified)
   2. Work-related task performance (i.e., ability to engage in one or more portions of a job; for in- stance, sorting mail, taking telephone messages, sweeping the floor)
   3. New work role (i.e., significant modification in work role is needed for patient to resume em- ployment)

4. Previous work role (i.e., patient can resume previous job once particular aspects of the job are modified or certain component skills improve)

Rating System

All ADL skills are rated using the seven-point RIC-FAS. Activity analysis guidelines are provided to assist the therapist in determining the RIC-FAS score. If the patient requires assistance with more than three fourths of the task as defined through department protocols and activity analysis, a score of *dependent* would be given. The rating levels and descriptions follow:

7. Independent. Patient performs activity safely with no physical or verbal assistance, without specialized equipment or adaptation, and within a reasonable amount of time. No caretaker intervention is required.

6. Independent with Equipment/Modified Environment. Patient performs activity safely without physical or verbal assistance, but requires any one or more of the following: specialized equipment, excessive time to complete the task, or adapted environment. No caretaker intervention is required.

5. Independent with Setup/Distant Supervision. Patient requires caretaker presence to initiate and/or complete the task, or for setup and cleanup, or only during unpredictable occurrences, but independently completes the interim components. Caretaker must be present to set up and clean up the activity and may need to be within calling distance in case of unpredictable occurrences.

4. Minimal Assistance/Intermittent Supervision. Patient performs more than three fourths of the task. Because of physical or cognitive impairment, caretaker must be present to supervise and/or provide physical or verbal assistance at various points throughout the activity.

3. Moderate Assistance/Continuous Supervision. Patient performs one half to three fourths of the task without physical assistance, and/or continuous verbal cuing/supervision may be necessary. Caretaker must be present throughout the entire activity to provide physical or verbal assistance.

2. Maximal Assistance. Patient performs between one fourth to one half of task or may be physically unable to perform any part of the activity, but can accurately direct the caregiver. Caretaker must be present throughout the entire activity to provide physical or verbal assistance.

1. Dependent. Patient performs less than one fourth of task and is unable to direct the caretaker. Caretaker must be present throughout the entire activity and performs most of the task.

Abreu, B. 1987. *Rehabilitation of perceptual-cognitive dysfunction.* New York: Joseph P. Calnan.

Abreu, B.G. 1990. *The quadraphonic approach: Management of cognitive and postural dysfunction.* Handouts from a workshop presentation, 98–99.

Abreu, B.G., and J.P. Toglia. 1987. Cognitive rehabilitation: A model for occupational therapy. *American Journal of Occupational Therapy* 41:439–448.

Affolter, F. 1987. *Perception, interaction and language, interaction of daily living as the root of development.* Heidelberg, West Germany: Springer-Verlag, Berlin.

Albert, M. 1973. A simple test of visual neglect. *Neurology* 23:658–664.

Alexander, M.P. 1988. Clinical determination of mental competence. *Archives of Neurology* 45:23–26.

Allen, C., et al. 1989. A medical review approach to Medicare outpatient documentation. *American Journal of Occupational Therapy* 43:743–800.

Allen, C.K. 1985. Measurement and management of cognitive disabilities. *Occupational therapy for psychiatric diseases.* Boston: Little, Brown & Co.

American Automobile Association. Night Sight Meter—Model No. 3538. Instructions for use. Falls Church, Va.

American Occupational Therapy Association (AOTA). 1989. *Uniform terminology for occupational therapy.* 2nd ed. Rockville, Md.

Anderson, E.K., and E. Choy. 1970. Parietal lobe syndromes in hemiplegia. *American Journal of Occupational Therapy* 24:13–18.

Anderson, T.P., et al. 1974. Predictive factors in stroke rehabilitation. *Archives of Physical Medicine and Rehabilitation* 55:545–553.

Andrews, K., et al. 1980. The prognostic value of picture drawings by stroke patients. *Rheumatology and Rehabilitation* 19(3):180–188.

Arnadottir, G. 1990. *The brain and behavior: Assessing cortical dysfunction through activities of daily living.* St. Louis: C.V. Mosby Co.

Ayres, A.J. 1966. Southern California Figure-Ground Visual Perception Test. Los Angeles: Western Psychological Services.

Bach-y-Rita, P. 1980. Brain plasticity as a basis for therapeutic procedures. In *Recovery of function: Theoretical considerations for brain injury rehabilitation,* ed. P. Bach-y-Rita. Bern, Switzerland: Hans Huber Publishers.

Bach-y-Rita, P. 1981. Brain plasticity as a basis of the development of rehabilitation procedures for hemiplegia. *Scandinavian Journal of Rehabilitation Medicine* 13:73–83.

Balla, J.I., et al. 1990. The application of basic science concepts to clinical problem-solving. *Medical Education* 24:137–147.

Barney, K. 1991. From Ellis Island to assisted living: meeting the needs of older adults from diverse cultures. *The American Journal of Occupational Therapy* 45(7):586–593.

Baum, C.M. 1991. Addressing the needs of the cognitively impaired elderly from a family policy perspective. *The American Journal of Occupational Therapy* 45(7):594–606.

Baum, B., and K.M. Hall. 1981. Relationship between constructional praxis and dressing in the head-injured adult. *The American Journal of Occupational Therapy* 35(7):438–442.

Benton, A. 1985. Visuoperceptual, visuospatial, and visuoconstructive disorders. In *Clinical neuropsychology*, eds. K.M. Heilman and K.E. Valenstein, 151–185. New York: Oxford University Press.

Benton, A. 1983a. Finger localization. In *Contributions to neuropsychological assessment: A clinical manual*, 84–97. New York: Oxford University Press.

Benton, A. 1983b. Judgment of line orientation. In *Contributions to neuropsychological assessment: A clinical manual*, 44–53. New York: Oxford University Press.

Benton, A. 1983c. Tactile form perception. In *Contributions to neuropsychological assessment: A clinical manual*, 70–83. New York: Oxford University Press.

Benton, A. 1983d. Temporal orientation. In *Contributions to neuropsychological assessment: A clinical manual*, 3–8. New York: Oxford University Press.

Benton, A. 1983e. Three-dimensional block construction. In *Contributions to neuropsychological assessment: A clinical manual*. New York: Oxford University Press.

Benton, A. 1983f. Visual form discrimination. In *Contributions to neuropsychological assessment: A clinical manual*. New York: Oxford University Press.

Benton, A.L., et al. 1983. *Contributions to neuropsychological assessment: A clinical manual*. New York: Oxford University Press.

Benton, A.L., et al. 1979. Visuospatial judgement: A clinical test. *Archives of Neurology* 35:364–367.

Benton, A.L., et al. 1964. Temporal orientation in cerebral disease. *Journal of Nervous and Mental Disease* 139:110–119.

Bermann, D., and T. Bush. 1988. Treatment of sensory-perceptual and cognitive deficits. In *Head injury: A guide to functional outcomes in occupational therapy*, eds. K. Kovich, and D. Bermann. Gaithersburg, Md.: Aspen Publishers, Inc.

Bernspang, B., et al. 1989. Impairments of perceptual and motor functions: Their influence on self-care ability 4 to 6 years after a stroke. *Occupational Therapy Journal of Research* 9:27–37.

Bolger, J.P. 1982. Cognitive retraining: A developmental approach. *Clinical Neuropsychology* 4:66–70.

Boll, T.J., et al. 1981a. A quantitative and qualitative approach to neuropsychological evaluation. In *Neuropsychological evaluation*, 67–80. New York: Academic Press, Inc.

Bosse, J.C., and P.J. Lederer. 1988. Visual acuity: Are you getting the whole picture? Testing contrast sensitivity can sharpen your diagnostic and management skills. *Review of Optometry* June:59–67.

Bouska, M.J., et al. 1985. Disorders of the visual perceptual system. In *Neurological rehabilitation*, ed. D.A. Umphred, 552–585. St. Louis: C.V. Mosby Co.

Bouska, M.J. 1981. Visual function in adults with brain-damage. *Newsletter of the American Occupational Therapy Association* 4(2):1–2.

Bowman, O.J. 1990. Balancing art and science and private and public knowledge: A matrix for successful practice. *American Journal of Occupational Therapy* 44:583–587.

Boys, M., et al. 1988. The OSOT perceptual evaluation: A research perspective. *American Journal of Occupational Therapy* 42:92–98.

Brooks, N., and N.B. Lincoln. 1984. Assessment for rehabilitation. In *Management of memory problems*, eds. B.A. Wilson and N. Moffat, 28–45. Gaithersburg, Md.: Aspen Publishers, Inc.

Burns, M.S., et al. 1985. *Clinical management of right hemisphere dysfunction*. Gaithersburg, Md.: Aspen Publishers, Inc.

Butler, S.R. 1971. Organization of cerebral cortex for perception. *British Medical Journal* 4:544–547.

Butters, N., et al. 1983. The effect of verbal mediators on the pictorial memory of brain-damaged patients. *Neuropsychologia* 21:307–323.

Cambridge Automated Perimeter, Bio-Rad Ophthalmic Division. 1990. Use of automated perimetry to evaluate brain injured drivers. Cambridge, Mass.

Campbell, D., and J. Oxbury. 1976. Recovery from unilateral visuo-spatial neglect. *Cortex* 12:303–312.

Carr, J., and R. Shepherd. 1989. *Motor Relearning following Stroke*. From a course presented at the Rehabilitation Institute of Chicago, June 23–24.

Carr, J.H., and R.B. Shepherd. 1987. *A motor relearning programme for stroke*, 2nd ed. Gaithersburg, Md.: Aspen Publishers.

Carter, T.L., et al. 1983. Effectiveness of cognitive skill remediation in acute stroke patients. *American Journal of Occupational Therapy* 37:320–326.

Cassin, B., et al., eds. 1990. *Dictionary of eye terminology*. Gainesville, Fla.: Triad Publishing Co.

Chapparo, C. and J. Ranka. 1980. Patterns of sensory integrative dysfunction in adult hemiplegia. Project report R-112, and test manual. Chicago: Rehabilitation Institute of Chicago.

Chedru, F. 1976. Space representation in unilateral spatial neglect. *Journal of Neurology, Neurosurgery and Psychiatry* 39:1057–1061.

Christenson, M.A. 1990a. Adaptations of the physical environment to compensate for sensory changes. *Physical and Occupational Therapy in Geriatrics* 8(3/4):3–30.

Christenson, M.A. 1990b. Enhancing independence in the home setting. *Physical and Occupational Therapy in Geriatrics* 8(3/4):49–63.

Chusid, J.G. 1973. *Correlative neuroanatomy and functional neurology*. Los Altos, Calif.: Lange Medical Publications.

Cohen, A.H., and R. Soden. 1981. An optometric approach to the rehabilitation of the stroke patient. *Journal of the American Optometric Association* 52:795–800.

Colarusso, R.P., and D.D. Hammill. 1972. *Motor-free visual perception test manual*. Novato, Calif.: Academic Therapy Publications.

Committee on Medical Aspects of Automotive Safety. 1969. Visual factors in automobile driving and provisional standards. *Archives of Ophthalmology* 81:865–871.

Crouch, J.E., and J.R. McClintic. 1971. *Human anatomy and physiology*. New York: John Wiley and Sons, Inc.

Csikszentmihalyi, M. 1975. *Beyond boredom and anxiety*. San Francisco: Jossey-Bass, Inc.

Damasio, A., et al. 1980. Neglect following damage to the frontal lobe or basal ganglia. *Neuropsychologia* 18:123–132.

Dannenbaum, R.M. 1990. Evaluating sustained touch-pressure in severe sensory deficits: Meeting an unanswered need. *Archives of Physical Medicine and Rehabilitation* 71:455–459.

David, S.K., and W.T. Riley. 1990. The relationship of the Allen cognitive level test to cognitive psychopathology. *American Journal of Occupational Therapy* 44:493–497.

Davies, A. 1968. The influence of age on trail making test performance. *Journal of Clinical Psychology* 24:96–98.

Davis, J. 1989. Bobath techniques for the occupational therapist in the treatment of adult hemiplegia. Workshop presented by International Clinical Educators at Community Hospital of Los Gatos-Saratoga, Calif., Jan. 30–Feb. 4.

Denes, G., et al. 1982. Unilateral spatial neglect and recovery from hemiplegia. *Brain* 105:543–552.

Diller, L., et al. 1974. *Studies in cognition and rehabilitation in hemiplegia* (Rehabilitation monograph no. 50). New York: New York University Medical Center Institute of Rehabilitation Medicine.

Diller, L., and W.A. Gordon. 1981. Interventions for cognitive deficits in brain-injured adults. *Journal of Consulting and Clinical Psychology* 49:822–834.

Dombovy, M.L., et al. 1987. Disability and use of rehabilitation services following stroke in Rochester, Minnesota, 1975–1979. *Stroke* 18:830–836.

Dougherty, P.M., and M.V. Radomski. 1993. *The cognitive rehabilitation workbook: A dynamic assessment approach for adults with brain injury*. 2nd ed. Gaithersburg, Md.: Aspen Publishers, Inc.

Dunn, W., and L. McGourty. 1989. Application of uniform terminology to practice. *American Journal of Occupational Therapy* 43:817.

Easton, J.D. 1981. *TIA, progressing stroke, and stroke: Recognition and response* (Telecourse #374). New York: Network for Continuing Medical Education.

Erickson, R.C., and M.L. Scott. 1977. Clinical memory testing: A review. *Psychological Bulletin* 84:1130–1149.

Farber, S.D., and J. C. Moore. 1990. Regional neuroanatomy of the nervous system. In *AOTA self study series: Neuroscience foundations of human performance*, ed. C.B. Royeen. Rockville, Md.: The American Occupational Therapy Association.

Farber, S.D. and B. Zoltan. 1989. Visual-vestibular systems interaction: Therapeutic implications. *Journal of Head Trauma Rehabilitation* 4:9–16.

Farver, P.F., and T.B. Farver. 1982. Performance of normal older adults on tests designed to measure parietal lobe functions. *American Journal of Occupational Therapy* 36:444–449.

Feigenson, J.S., et al. 1977. Factors influencing outcome and length of stay in a stroke rehabilitation unit. *Stroke* 8:651–656.

Filskov, S., and T. Boll. 1981. *Handbook of clinical neuropsychology*. New York: John Wiley and Sons, Inc.

Fine, S.B. 1991. Resilience and human adaptability: Who rises above adversity. *The American Journal of Occupational Therapy* 45(6):493–503.

Fisher, A.G., et al. 1992. Cross-cultural assessment of process skills. *The American Journal of Occupational Therapy* 46(10):876–885.

Fleming, M.H. 1991. Clinical reasoning in medicine compared with clinical reasoning in occupational therapy. *The American Journal of Occupational Therapy* 45(11):988–996.

Fleming, M.H. 1991. The therapist with the three track mind. *The American Journal of Occupational Therapy* 45(11):1007–1014.

Fox, J.V.D. 1963. Effect of cutaneous stimulation on performance of hemiplegic adults on selected tests of perception. Thesis, University of Southern California.

Fraser, C.M. and A. Turton. 1986. The development of the Cambridge apraxia battery. *A paper published by the OT department, Addenbrooke's Hospital, Cambridge, England.*

Friedman, P.J. 1990. Spatial neglect in acute stroke: The line bisection test. *Scandinavian Journal of Rehabilitation Medicine* 22:101–106.

Fullerton, K., et al. 1986. Albert's test: A neglected test of perceptual neglect. *Lancet* (February): 430–432.

Galski, T., et al. 1990. An assessment of measures to predict the outcome of driving evaluations in patients with cerebral damage. *American Journal of Occupational Therapy*:709–713.

Gianutsos, R., and C. Klitzner. 1981. Computer programs for cognitive rehabilitation: Personal computing for survivors of brain injury. *Proceedings of the Johns Hopkins first national search for applications of personal computing to aid the handicapped.* Baltimore: Johns Hopkins University.

Gianutsos, R., et al. 1988. Rehabilitative optometric services for survivors of acquired brain injury. *Archives of Physical Medicine and Rehabilitation* 69:573.

Gianutsos, R., et al. 1989. Rehabilitative optometric services for persons emerging from coma. *Journal of Head Trauma Rehabilitation* 4(2):17–25.

Glasgow, R.E., et al. 1977. Case studies on remediating memory deficits in brain-damaged individuals. *Journal of Clinical Psychology* 33:1049–1054.

Goldman, H. 1966. Improvement of double simultaneous stimulation perception in hemiplegic patients. *Archives of Physical Medicine and Rehabilitation* 47:687–691.

Golper, L.C., et al. 1980. Aphasic adults and their decisions on driving: An evaluation. *Archives of Physical Medicine and Rehabilitation* 61:34–40.

Gouvier, W.D., et al. 1989. Psychometric prediction of driving performance among the disabled. *Archives of Physical Medicine and Rehabilitation* 70:745–750.

Harlowe, D., and J. Van Deusen. 1984. Construct validation of the St. Marys CVA evaluation: Perceptual measures. *American Journal of Occupational Therapy* 38:184–186.

Hartman, N., and S. Hutchinson. 1989. Medical review of dysphagia claims for speech-language pathology, occupational therapy and physical therapy services.

Hasselkus, B.R. 1991. Ethical dilemmas in family caregiving for the elderly: Implications for occupational therapy. *American Journal of Occupational Therapy* 45(3):206–212.

Hawkins Watts, J., et al. 1986. The assessment of occupational functioning: A screening tool for use in long-term care. *American Journal of Occupational Therapy* 40:232–234.

Heaton, R.K., and M.G. Pendleton. 1981. Use of neuropsychological tests to predict adult patients' everyday functioning. *Journal of Consulting and Clinical Psychology* 49:807–821.

Heilman, K.M., and R.T. Watson. 1978. Changes in the symptoms of neglect induced by changing task strategy. *Archives of Neurology* 35:47–49.

Herman, E.W. 1992. Spatial neglect: New issues and their implications for occupational therapy practice. *American Journal of Occupational Therapy* 46(3):207–216.

Higbee, K.L. 1988. *Your memory: How it works and how to improve it.* New York: Prentice-Hall.

Hooper, H.E. 1983. The Hooper visual organization test. Los Angeles: Western Psychological Services.

Hopewell, C.A., and A.H. van Zomeren. Neuropsychological aspects of motor vehicle operation. Dallas Rehabilitation Institute. Dallas, TX: Neuropsychological Institute.

Hopewell, C.A., and R.J. Price. 1985. Driving after head injury. *Journal of Clinical Experimental Neuropsychology* 7:148.

Illinois Vehicle Code. 1990. As amended through Public Act 86-1028. Available from the secretary of state of the state of Illinois, Springfield, IL.

Jensen, A.R., and W.D. Rohwer, Jr. 1966. The Stroop color-word test: A review. *Acta Psychologia* 25:36–93.

Jones, R., et al. 1983. Assessment and training of brain-damaged drivers. *American Journal of Occupational Therapy* 37:754–760.

Jongbloed, L. 1986. Prediction of function after stroke: A critical review. *Stroke* 17:765–776.

Kaplan, J., and D.B. Hier. 1982. Visuospatial deficits after right hemisphere stroke. *American Journal of Occupational Therapy* 36:314–315.

Katz, N., et al. 1989. Loewenstein occupational therapy cognitive assessment battery for brain injured patients: Reliability and validity. *American Journal of Occupational Therapy* 43:184–191.

Kielhofner, G., ed. 1985. *A model of human occupation.* Baltimore: Williams & Wilkins Co.

Kielhofner, G., and J.P. Burke. 1985. Components and determinants of human occupation. In *A model of human occupation*, ed. G. Kielhofner. Baltimore: Williams & Wilkins Co.

Kim, Y., et al. 1984. Visuoperceptual and visuomotor abilities and locus of lesion. *Neuropsychologia* 22:177–185.

Kimble, G. 1985. Psychology of Learning. In *Psychology and learning: Master lecture series*, vol. 4, ed., B. Hammonds, 9–44. Washington, DC: American Psychological Association.

Kinsbourne, M. 1974. Cognitive deficit and the aging brain: A behavioral analysis. *International Journal of Aging and Human Development* 5(1):41–49.

Kotila, M., et al. 1986. Four year prognosis of stroke patients with visuo-spatial inattention. *Scandinavian Journal of Rehabilitation Medicine* 18:177–179.

Lackner, J.R. 1988. Some proprioceptive influences on the perceptual representation of body shape and orientation. *Brain* 111:281–297.

Legh-Smith, J., et al. 1986. Driving after stroke. *Journal of the Royal Society of Medicine* 0141-0768186.

Levine, R.E., and L.N. Gitlin. 1990. Home adaptations for persons with chronic disabilities: An educational model. *The American Journal of Occupational Therapy* 44(10):923–929.

Levine, D.N. 1990. Unawareness of visual and sensorimotor defects: A hypothesis. *Brain and Cognition* 13:233–281.

Lezak, J. 1983. *Neuropsychological assessment.* 2nd ed. New York: Oxford University Press.

Logan, G.D. 1980. Attention and automaticity in stoop and priming tasks: Theory and data. *Cognitive Psychology* 12:523–553.

Loverro, J., and M. Reding. 1988. Bed orientation and rehabilitation outcome for patients with stroke and hemianopsia or visual neglect. *Journal of Neurological Rehabilitation* 2:147–150.

Luria, A.R. 1970. The functional organization of the brain. *Scientific American* 222(3):66–70.

Luria, A.R. 1973. *The working brain: An introduction to neuropsychology.* New York: Basic Books, Inc.

Luria, A.R. 1980. *Higher cortical functions in man*, trans. B. Haigh. New York: Basic Books, Inc. (Original work published 1962.)

MacDonald, J.C. 1960. An investigation of body scheme in adults with cerebral vascular accidents. *American Journal of Occupational Therapy* 14:75–79.

Mahoney, J., and E. Siev. 1973. Provisional normative study of normal adults on the Southern California figure ground, position in space and kinesthesia test. Unpublished data in *Perceptual and cognitive dysfunction in the adult stroke patient: a manual for evaluation and treatment.* Thorofare, N.J.: Slack, Inc.

Maino, D.M. 1986. Out of office oculomotor and hand-eye therapy. *Cognitive Rehabilitation.* November/December:16–19.

Mark, V.W., and K.M. Heilman. 1990. Bodily neglect and orientational biases in unilateral neglect syndrome and normal subjects. *Neurology* 40:640–643.

Mayer, M.A. 1988. Analysis of information processing and cognitive disability theory. *American Journal of Occupational Therapy* 42:176–183.

Mesulam, J.M. 1981. A cortical network for directed attention and unilateral neglect. *Annals of Neurology* 10(4):309–325.

Milkie, G.M. 1974. *Vision: Its role in driver licensing.* Joint publication of the American Optometric Association and the American Association of Motor Vehicle Administrations. St. Louis: American Optometric Association.

Miller, G.J. 1989. Evaluating reaction time, threat recognition, and crash avoidance. Abstract for AOTA conference, scientific/technical session 107-B. 19–22.

Miller, V.T. 1983. Lacunar stroke: A reassessment. *Archives of Neurology* 40:129–134.

Moore, J., and Warren, M. 1990. Sensory Learning: Application of a Sensory Integration Treatment Approach to Adult Stroke and Head Injury. Presented at a course at the Rehabilitation Institute of Chicago, October 19–21.

Morse, A.R. 1986. Neuropsychological tools and techniques of cognitive assessment. In *Brain injury: Cognitive and prevocational approaches to rehabilitation*, ed. P.A. Morse, 51–88. New York: Tiresias Press, Inc.

Mosey, A.C. 1986. *Psychosocial components of occupational therapy*. New York: Raven Press.

Moss Rehabilitation Hospital. 1980. Occupational therapy department kitchen evaluation form. In *Sample forms for occupational therapy*, ed., the Division of Professional Development, American Occupational Therapy Association, 82–83. Rockville, Md.: AOTA Inc.

Neistadt, M.E. 1988. Occupational therapy for adults with perceptual deficits. *American Journal of Occupational Therapy* 42:434–439.

Neistadt, M.E. 1989. Normal adult performance on constructional praxis training tasks. *American Journal of Occupational Therapy* 43:448–455.

Neistadt, M.E. 1992. Occupational therapy treatments for constructional deficits. *The American Journal of Occupational Therapy* 46(2):141–148.

Nottingham Rehab Catalogue. 1989/1990. Chesington O.T. Neurological Assessment Battery, 170–171. West Bridgford, Nottingham NG26HD, England: Nottingham Rehab.

Osterrieth, P.A. 1944. Le test de copie d'une figure complexe. *Archives de Psychologie* 30:206–356.

Ottenbacher, K. 1982. Sensory integration therapy: affect or effect? *The American Journal of Occupational Therapy* 36(9):571–578.

Oxbury, J.M., et al. 1974. Unilateral spatial neglect and impairments of spatial analysis and visual perception. *Brain* 97:551–564.

Pedretti, L.W., and S. Pasquinelli-Estrada. 1985. A frame of reference for occupational therapy in physical dysfunction. In *Occupational therapy: practice skills for physical dysfunction*, 2nd ed., ed., Pedretti, L.W. St. Louis: CV Mosby Co.

Pfeiffer, E. 1975. A short portable mental status questionnaire for the assessment of organic brain deficit in elderly patients. *Journal of the American Geriatrics Society* 23:433–441.

Picariello, G. 1986. A guide for teaching elders. *Geriatric Nursing* 7:38–39.

Pizzamiglio, L., et al. 1990. Effect of optokinetic stimulation in patients with visual neglect. *Cortex* 26:535–540.

Pollack, M., et al. 1958. Factors related to individual differences in perception in institutionalized aged. *Journal of Gerontology* 13:192–197.

Price, A. 1980. The issue: Neurotherapy and specialization. *American Journal of Occupational Therapy* 34:809–815.

Quigley, F., and J.A. DeLisa. 1983. Assessing the driving potential of cerebral vascular accident patients. *American Journal of Occupational Therapy* 37:474–478.

Randt, C.T., et al. 1980. A memory test for longitudinal measurement of mild to moderate deficits. *Clinical Neuropsychology* 2:184–194.

Reitan, R. 1958. Validity of the Trail Making Test as an indicator of organic brain damage. *Perceptual and Motor Skills*. Southern University Press 8, 271–276.

Reitan, R., and D. Wolfson. 1985. *The Halstead-Reitan neuropsychological test battery: Theory and clinical interpretation*. Tucson, Az.: Neuropsychology Press.

Resnick, L. 1985. Cognition and Instruction. In *Psychology and learning: Master lecture series*, vol. 4, ed., B. Hammonds, 127–180. Washington, DC: American Psychological Association.

Rey, A. 1964. *L'examen clinique in psychology*. Paris: Presses Universitaires de France.

Rey, A. 1941. L'exmen psychologique dans les cas d'encephalopathie traumatique. *Archives de Psychologie* 28:44.

Riddoch, M., and G. Humphreys. 1983. The effect of cueing on unilateral neglect. *Neuropsychologia* 21(6):589–599.

Roach, E.G., and N.C. Kephart. 1966. *The Purdue perceptual-motor survey*. Columbus, OH: Charles E. Merril Publishing Company.

Robertson, I.H., et al. 1990. Microcomputer-based rehabilitation for unilateral left visual neglect: A randomized controlled trial. *Archives of Physical Medicine and Rehabilitation* 71:663–668.

Ross, F.L. 1992. The use of computers in occupational therapy for visual-scanning training. *The American Journal of Occupational Therapy* 46(4):314–322.

Roth, E.J. 1988. The elderly stroke patient: Principles and practices of rehabilitation management. *Topics in Geriatric Rehabilitation* 3(4):27–61.

Roy, E.A. 1983. Neuropsychological perspectives on apraxia and related action disorders. In *Advances in Psychology*, vol. 12, 293–320. Amsterdam, North-Holland: Memory and Control of Action.

Roy, E.A. 1982. Action and performance. In *Normality and pathology in cognitive function*, ed. A. Ellis, 265–298. London: Academic Press.

Roy, E.A., and P.A. Square. 1985. Common considerations in the study of limb, verbal and oral apraxia. In *Neuropsychological studies of apraxia and related disorders*, ed., E. A. Roy, 111–161. North Holland: Elsevier Science Publishers.

Saint-Cyr, J.A., et al. 1988. Procedural learning and neostriatal dysfunction in man. *Brain* 3:941–959.

Schenkenberg, K., et al. 1980. Line bisection and unilateral visual neglect in patients with neurological impairment. *Neurology* 30:509–517.

Schwartz, A.S., et al. 1977. A sensitive test for tactile extinction: Results in patients with parietal and frontal lobe disease. *Journal of Neurology, Neurosurgery and Psychiatry* 40:228–233.

Schwartz, R., et al. 1979. Verbal and nonverbal memory abilities of adult brain-damaged patients. *American Journal of Occupational Therapy* 33:79–83.

Shapiro, M.F., et al. 1952. Exosomethesia or displacement of cutaneous sensation into extrapesonal space. *Archives of Neurology and Psychiatry* 68:481–490.

Simms, B. *Drivers with brain damage.* (unpublished paper.)

Simpson, E.L. 1980. In *Adult development and approaches to learning*. U.S. Dept. of Health, Education, and Welfare. Washington, D.C.: U.S. Government Printing Office.

Sivak, M., et al. 1980. Perceptual/cognitive skills and driving: Effects of brain damage. Publication of the University of Michigan Highway Safety Research Institute, 1–54. Ann Arbor.

Soderbak, I., and L.A. Normell. 1986. Intellectual function training in adults with acquired brain damage. *Scandinavian Journal of Rehabilitation Medicine* 18:139–146.

Spreen, O., and E. Strauss. 1991. *A compendium of neuropsychological tests: Administration, norms, and commentary.* New York: Oxford University Press.

Stedman's medical dictionary. 25th ed. 1990. Baltimore: Williams & Wilkins Co.

Strano, C.M. 1989. Effects of visual deficits on ability to drive in traumatically brain injured population. *Journal of Head Trauma Rehabilitation* 4:35–43.

Strub, R.L., and F.W. Black. 1985. *The mental status examination in neurology.* 2nd ed. Philadelphia: F.A. Davis Co.

Tan, M., and R. Zemke. 1991. Performance on the Motor-Free Visual Perception Test by Persons 60–89 Years Old. American Occupational Therapy Association Conference, Cincinnati, OH, June 5.

Titus, M.N., et al. 1991. Correlation of perceptual performance and activities of daily living in stroke patients. *The American Journal of Occupational Therapy* 45(5):410–418.

Tobis, J.S., et al. 1990. Falling among the sensorially impaired elderly. *Archives of Physical Medicine and Rehabilitation* 71:144–147.

Toglia, J.P. 1991. Generalization of a treatment: a multicontext approach to cognitive perceptual impairment in adults with brain injury. *The American Journal of Occupational Therapy* 45(6):505–516.

Towle, D., et al. 1988. Use of computer presented games with memory-impaired stroke patients. *Clinical Rehabilitation* 2:303–307.

Umphred, D. 1983. Conceptual model of an approach to the sensorimotor treatment of the head-injured client. *Physical Therapy* 63:1983–1987.

Van Deusen, J. 1983. Normative data for ninety-three elderly persons on the schenkenburg line bisection test. *Physical and Occupational Therapy in Geriatrics* 3(2):49–53.

Van Deusen, J., and D. Harlowe. 1987. Continued construct validation of the St. Mary's CVA evaluation: bilateral awareness scale. *American Journal of Occupational Therapy* 41:242–245.

Van Deusen-Fox, J., and D. Harlowe. 1984. Construct validation of occupational therapy measures used in CVA evaluation: A beginning. *American Journal of Occupational Therapy* 38:101–106.

van Zomeren, A.H., et al. 1987. Acquired brain damage: A review. *Archives of Physical Medicine and Rehabilitation* 68:697–705.

Vizzetti, D. 1987. A model for grading tasks based on cognitive demand. Paper written for Rehabilitation Institute of Chicago project. Chicago.

Vizzetti, D. 1989. Understanding cognition to improve functional performance. Paper written for Rehabilitation Institute of Chicago presentation. Chicago.

Walker, K.F. 1989. Clinically relevant features of the visual system. *Journal of Head Trauma Rehabilitation* 4:1–8.

Warren, M. 1981. Relationship of constructional apraxia and body scheme disorders to dressing performance in adult CVA. *American Journal of Occupational Therapy* 35:431–437.

Warrington, E.K., et al. 1986. The WAIS as a lateralizing and localizing diagnostic instrument: A study of 656 patients with unilateral cerebral lesions. *Neuropsychologia* 24:223–239.

Webster, J.S., and R.R. Scott. 1983. The effects of self-instructional training on attentional deficits following head injury. *Clinical Neuropsychology* 5:69–74.

Weinberg, J., et al. 1979. Training sensory awareness and spatial organization in people with right brain damage. *Archives of Physical Medicine and Rehabilitation* 60:492–496.

Weinberg, J., et al. 1977. Visual scanning training: effect on reading-related tasks in acquired right brain damage. *Archives of Physical Medicine and Rehabilitation* 58:479–486.

Whiting, S., et al. 1985. Rivermead perceptual assessment battery. In *NFER-Nelson 1988 Catalogue*, Windsor, Berkshire: England, p. 88.

Williams, N. 1967. Correlation between copying ability and dressing activities in hemiplegia. *American Journal of Physical Medicine* 46(4):1332–1340.

Wilson, B., et al. 1987. Development of a behavioral test of visuospatial neglect. *Archives of Physical Medicine and Rehabilitation* 68:98–102.

Wilson, T., and T. Smith. 1983. Driving after stroke. *International Rehabilitation Medicine* 5:170–177.

Zarit, S., and R. Kahn. 1974. Impairment and adaptation in chronic disabilities: Spatial inattention. *Journal of Nervous and Mental Disease* 159:63–71.

Zoltan, B., et al. 1986. *The adult stroke patient: A manual for evaluation and treatment of perceptual and cognitive dysfunction*, 2nd ed. Thorofare, N.J.: Slack Inc.

Index

A

Acquisitional frame of reference, 70-73
  functional approach, 72
  human occupation approach, 72-73
  perceptual motor therapy, 72
  perceptual motor training, 72
  skill training approaches, 70-72
Activities of daily living, rating system, 190
Activities of daily living
  clinic activities, 79-81
  enjoyable activities, 81-82
  grading, 78-79
Activity analysis, evaluation, 10-11
Acuity, driver rehabilitation, 123
Adult learner, 82-84
  behavioristic theory, 82-83
  self theory, 83
Albert's Test, 39, 40
  unilateral visual inattention, 157
Allen Cognitive Level Test, 4
Alternating attention, 27, 143-144
  cognitive goals, 176
  Symbol Digit Modalities Test, 147-148
  tests, 145-148
  Trail Making Test, 145-146
  treatment, 176
Apraxia, child, 112
Arousal
  clinical observations, 143
  cognitive goals, 175
  cognitive treatment, 85-86
  description, 23-24
  evaluation, 23-24
    functional implications, 24
  functional observations, 141-143

  guide, 141-143
  treatment, 175
Assessment of Motor and Process Skills, 6
Attention
  alternating attention, 27, 143–144
    Symbol Digit Modalities Test, 147–148
    tests, 145–148
    Trail Making Test, 145–146
  cognitive treatment, 86-88
  description, 24-25
  evaluation, 25-30
  functional implications, 25
  functional observations, 143-144
  guide, 143-148
  selective attention, 27, 143
    tests, 144–145
  sustained attention, 25–27, 143
    Random Letter Test, 144–145
    tests, 144–145
    Visual Vigilance Test, 144
Auditory deficit, cognitive and perceptual evaluation, 19
Avocational Group, 185
Ayres Figure-Ground Test, 45
  visual analysis, 161-162

B

Behavior, 13
Behavioristic theory, adult learner, 82-83
Bilateral integration
  Double Circles Test, 168-169
  treatment, 181-182
Bilateral Simultaneous Stimulation Test, unilateral tactile
  inattention, 167-168
Block arrangement problem, problem solving, 153

Block Design Construction Test, visual construction, 165-166
Body awareness
    description, 50
    evaluation, 50-54
    functional implications, 50
    functional observations, 166-167
    guide, 166-167
    perceptual goals, 181
    tests, 167-172
    treatment, 104-111, 181
Body parts, identification, 108
Body parts identification
    perceptual goals, 182
    treatment, 182
Brain, functional unit, 75-77

C

Cambridge Apraxia Battery, 5
Cancellation task, sustained attention, 144
Caregiver instruction, motor planning, 115. *See also* Adult learner
Case example, 131-137
Chart review, evaluation, 9-10
Chessington Occupational Therapy Neurological Assessment Battery, 5
Child, apraxia, 112
Clinic activities, 79-81
Cognition, driver rehabilitation, 125-127
Cognition evaluation chart, driver rehabilitation, 122
Cognitive and perceptual evaluation. *See also* Specific type
    auditory deficit, 19
    expressive language deficit, 19-20
    factors infuencing, 13-21
    formal testing, 6
    motor function, 20-21
    occupational therapist assessments, 4-6
    overview, 23
    primary senses, 15-19
    psychosocial factors, 13-15
    receptive language deficit, 19
    standardized tests, 4-6
    tactile sensory testing, 18-19
    techniques, 23-58
Cognitive and perceptual treatment techniques, 85-115. *See also* Specific type
Cognitive deficit, driver rehabilitation, treatment, 129-130
Cognitive evaluation, guide, 141-153
Cognitive evaluation techniques, 23-36
Cognitive treatment, 85-95
    arousal, 85-86
    attention, 86-88
    memory, 89-92
    orientation, 88-89
    problem solving, 92-95
    selective attention, 86-88
    sustained attention, 86
    topographical orientation, 89
Computer, unilateral visual inattention, 100-101
Contrast sensitivity, driver rehabilitation, 124
Copying, unilateral visual inattention, 38-39, 156-157

Cross Test, 42
    visual spatial awareness, 158-159
Crossing-out task, unilateral visual inattention, 39-40

D

Developmental frame of reference, 70
    sensorimotor approach, 70
    sensory integrative approach, 70
Digit repetition test, sensory memory, 150
Distant memory, 30
Drawing, unilateral visual inattention, 38-39, 156-157
Driver rehabilitation, 117-130
    acuity, 123
    behind-the-wheel evaluation, 119
    clinical evaluation, 118-119
    cognition, 125-127
    cognition evaluation chart, 122
    cognitive deficit, treatment, 129-130
    contrast sensitivity, 124
    driver training, 119-122
    evaluation, 123-127
    glare recovery, 124
    glare vision, 124
    night vision, 124
    ocular mobility, 124
    perception, 124-125
    perception evaluation chart, 121
    perceptual deficit, treatment, 129
    poor performance, 122-123
    referral, 117-118
    Rehabilitation Institute of Chicago Driver Knowledge Test, 127
    vision evaluation chart, 119, 120
    visual deficit, treatment, 128-129
    visual field, 123-124
Driver training, driver rehabilitation, 119-122

E

Eat group, 184-185
Encoding, 30
Environmental adaptation, 84
Estimation of Time Test, orientation, 149
Evaluation
    activity analysis, 10-11
    arousal, 23-24
        functional implications, 24
    attention, 25-30
    body awareness, 50-54
    chart review, 9-10
    cognitive, 23-36
    driver rehabilitation, 123-127
    formal testing, 11-12
    interview, 10
    memory, 31
    methods, 9-12
    midline orientation, 54
    motor planning, 58
    orientation, 34
    philosophy, 9-12

problem solving, 35-36
purpose, 9
right-left discrimination, 54
tactile discrimination, 53
treatment effectiveness, 67
unilateral tactile inattention, 51
unilateral visual inattention, 37-41
   functional observations, 37-38
visual analysis, 43-50
visual construction, 47-50
visual perception, 36-43
visual spatial awareness, 42-43
visual synthesis, 43-50
Expressive language deficit, cognitive and perceptual
   evaluation, 19-20

F

Face-Hand Test, 168
Figure-ground analysis, 43-44
Figure-Ground Screening Test, visual analysis, 161
Financial problem, problem solving, 152
Finger localization test, tactile discrimination, 169
Frame of reference, 69-73. *See also* Specific type
Functional activities, 77-78
Functional brain unit, 75-77
Functional occupations programs, 187

G

Glare recovery, driver rehabilitation, 124
Glare vision, driver rehabilitation, 124
Goal writing, 175-190
   activities for daily living goals vs. component skill
     goals, 187-190
   group goals, 184
   skill deficit evaluation, 61-67
     functional impact, 62-63
Group treatment, 184-187
GROW (Group Rehabilitation on Ward), 185

H

Hemianopia, 15-16
Hooper Visual Organization Test, 45
   visual synthesis, 162-163
Human occupation approach, acquisitional frame of
   reference, 72-73

I

Intellectual Housework Assessment, 5
Interview, evaluation, 10

J

Judgment of Line Orientation Test, 42
   visual spatial awareness, 159

L

Language, motor-planning deficit, 111-112
Lesion
   location, 73-74
   symptoms, 73-74
Letter Cancellation Task, unilateral visual inattention,
   157-158
Life role, 14
Line bisection test, unilateral visual inattention, 38, 39, 156
Loewenstein Occupational Therapy Cognitive
   Assessment, 4
Long-term memory, 30, 150
   cognitive goals, 177
   treatment, 177

M

Memory
   cognitive treatment, 89-92
   description, 30
   evaluation, 31
   functional implications, 30-31
   functional observations, 149-150
   guide, 149-151
   long-term memory, 30, 150
     cognitive goals, 177
     treatment, 177
   sensory modality classification, 30
   short term memory, 30, 149–150
     cognitive goals, 176–177
     tests, 150–151
     treatment, 176–177
     Visual Memory Test, 150–151
   time classification, 30
Memory acquisition, 30
Memory deficit, treatment, 90-92
Midline orientation
   description, 54
   evaluation, 54
   functional implications, 54
   perceptual goals, 182-183
   tests, 171-172
   treatment, 108-111, 182-183
Mnemonic device, 91
Model of Human Occupation, 13
Motor-Free Visual Perception Test, 4
Motor function, cognitive and perceptual evaluation, 20-21
Motor planning. See also Motor-planning deficit
   caregiver instruction, 115
   conceptualization problems, 112
   description, 54-55
   evaluation, 58
   functional observations, 172-173
   guide, 172-174
   perceptual goals, 183-184
   production problems, 113
   skilled movement sequences, 113-115
   tests, 173-174
   treatment, 111-115, 183-184
Motor-planning deficit
   classification, 55

conceptual system, 55
functional implications, 55-58
language, 111-112
production system, 55
Multisensory stimulation, unilateral visual inattention, 96-97

N

Nervous system
   hard-wired system, 74-75
   soft-wired system, 74-75
Neural plasticity, 75
Neurological function, 73-77
Night vision, driver rehabilitation, 124
Nonstandardized test, 12

O

Occupational therapy cognitive protocol
   formal testing, 6
   literature review, 3-4
Ocular mobility, driver rehabilitation, 124
Ontario Society of Occupational Therapists Perceptual
   Evaluation, 5
Orientation
   cognitive treatment, 88-89
   description, 31-34
   Estimation of Time Test, 149
   evaluation, 34
   functional implications, 32-34
   functional observations, 148
   guide, 148-149
   orientation interview, 148-149
   tests, 148-149
Orientation interview, 148-149

P

Perception, driver rehabilitation, 124-125
Perception evaluation chart, driver rehabilitation, 121
Perceptual deficit, driver rehabilitation, 129
Perceptual evaluation, guide, 155-174
Perceptual motor orientation group, 185-186
Perceptual motor therapy, acquisitional frame of reference,
   72
Perceptual motor training, acquisitional frame of reference,
   72
Primary senses, cognitive and perceptual evaluation, 15-19
Problem solving
   block arrangement problem, 153
   cognitive goals, 177-179
   cognitive treatment, 92-95
   description, 34-35
   evaluation, 35-36
   financial problem, 152
   functional implications, 35
   functional observations, 151-152
   guide, 151-153
   problem-solving simulations, 151
   Rey Complex Figure Test, 151
   tests, 151-153

Three-Dimensional Block Design Test, 151
   treatment, 177-179
Problem-solving simulations, problem solving, 151
Psychosocial factors, cognitive and perceptual evaluation,
   13-15

R

Random Letter Test, sustained attention, 144-145
Reaction Time Measure of Visual Field, unilateral visual
   inattention, 158
Receptive language deficit, cognitive and perceptual
   evaluation, 19
Referral, driver rehabilitation, 117-118
Rehabilitation Institute of Chicago cognitive and perceptual
   evaluation, 3, 6-7
Rehabilitation Institute of Chicago Driver Knowledge Test,
   driver rehabilitation, 127
Rey Complex Figure, 46
Rey Figure Test, problem solving, 151
Right-left discrimination
   description, 53-54
   evaluation, 54
   functional implications, 54
   perceptual goals, 182
   tests, 171
   treatment, 108, 182
Rivermead Perceptual Assessment Battery, 5

S

Saccades, 17-18
Saint Mary's CVA Evaluation, 4
Schenkenberg Line Bisection Test, 38, 39
Selective attention, 27, 143
   cognitive goals, 176
   cognitive treatment, 86-88
   tests, 145
   treatment, 176
Self theory, adult learner, 83
Sensory memory, 30
   digit repetition test, 150
   tests, 150
Sensory registration, treatment, 95
Short-term memory, 30, 149-150
   cognitive goals, 176-177
   tests, 150-151
   treatment, 176-177
   Visual Memory Test, 150-151
Short-term visual memory, 32-33
Skill deficit evaluation
   goal writing, 61-67
      functional impact, 62-63
   treatment planning, 61-67
      functional impact, 62-63
Snellen test, 16
Spatial awareness. See also Visual Spatial Awareness
   perceptual goals, 180
   treatment, 180
Stroke group, 186-187
Stroke re-entry group, 187

Sustained attention, 25-27, 143
cancellation task, 144
cognitive goals, 175-176
cognitive treatment, 86
Random Letter Test, 144-145
tests, 144-145
treatment, 175-176
Visual Vigilance Test, 144
Sustained auditory attention, 26
Symbol Digit Modalities Test, 27, 29
alternating attention, 147-148

T

Tactile discrimination
description, 51-52
evaluation, 53
finger localization test, 169
function implications, 52-53
perceptual goals, 182
Tactile Form Perception Test, 169-170
tests, 169-171
treatment, 106-108, 182
Tactile Form Perception Test, tactile discrimination, 169-170
Tactile sensory loss
perceptual goals, 181
treatment, 104, 181
Tactile sensory testing, cognitive and perceptual evaluation, 18-19
Test of Orientation for Rehabilitation Patients, 4
Three-Dimensional Block Construction Test, visual construction, 166
Three-Dimensional Block Design Test, problem solving, 151
Topographical orientation
cognitive treatment, 89
functional observations, 149
guide, 149
Trail Making Test, 27, 28
alternating attention, 145-146
Treatment approach, 73-82
Treatment effectiveness, evaluation, 67
Treatment planning, skill deficit evaluation, 61-67
functional impact, 62-63

U

Unilateral tactile inattention
Bilateral Simultaneous Stimulation Test, 167-168
description, 51
evaluation, 51
functional implications, 51
tests, 167-169
treatment, 104-105, 181-182
Unilateral visual inattention
Albert's Test, 157
computer, 100-101
copying, 38-39
copying tasks, 156-157
crossing-out task, 39-40

description, 37, 95
drawing, 38-39, 156-157
evaluation, 37-41
functional observations, 37-38
functional implications, 37
functional observations, 155-156
guide, 155-158
high-level speed and complexity tasks, 41
increasing awareness, 96
Letter Cancellation Task, 157-158
line bisection, 38, 39, 156
multisensory stimulation, 96-97
perceptual goals, 179
Reaction Time Measure of Visual Field, 158
tests, 156-158
treatment, 95-105, 179
treatment of severe deficits, 96
vestibular stimulation, 97-98
visual scanning training, 98-99

V

Vestibular stimulation, unilateral visual inattention, 97-98
Vision evaluation chart, driver rehabilitation, 119, 120
Visual acuity, 16-17
Visual analysis
Ayres Figure-Ground Test, 161-162
evaluation, 43-50
Figure-Ground Screening Test, 161
functional observations, 159-160
perceptual goals, 179-180
tests, 160-162
treatment, 101-102, 179-180
Visual Discrimination of Abstract Shapes Test, 160
Visual Form Discrimination Test, 160-161
Visual construction, 46-50
Block Design Construction Test, 165-166
description, 46-47
evaluation, 47-50
functional implications, 47
functional observations, 163
guide, 163-166
perceptual goals, 180
tests, 163-166
Three-Dimensional Block Construction Test, 166
treatment, 102-104, 180
Visual deficit, driver rehabilitation, treatment, 128-129
Visual discrimination, 43
Visual Discrimination of Abstract Shapes Test, visual analysis, 160
Visual Discrimination of Abstract Shapes Screening Form, 43
Visual field, 15-16
driver rehabilitation, 123-124
Visual Form Discrimination Test, 44
visual analysis, 160-161
Visual Memory Test, short-term memory, 150-151
Visual perception
evaluation, 36-43
guide, 155-159
treatment, 95-104
Visual pursuit, 18

Visual range of motion, 17
Visual scanning training, unilateral visual inattention, 98-99
Visual screening, 15
Visual spatial awareness
    clinical observations, 158
    Cross Test, 158-159
    description, 41
    evaluation, 42-43
    functional implications, 41-42
    functional observations, 158
    guide, 158-159
    Judgment of Line Orientation, 159

tests, 158-159
treatment, 101
Visual synthesis
    description, 43, 44
    evaluation, 43-50
    functional implications, 43, 44-46
    Hooper Visual Organization Test, 162-163
    perceptual goals, 179-180
    tests, 162-163
    treatment, 101-102, 179-180
Visual vigilance, 26
Visual Vigilance Test, sustained attention, 144

Teach LE dressing

237

Pt is alert + grasps instructions well
verbal cueing may or may not be helpful
Sensation appeared to be intact on left side.
Tasks may be repeated several times during one
training session,
Backward chaining - can be used to assist the
Pt in learning ADL skills until the last step
of the process is reached. Then the PT performs the
Last ~~task~~ STEP independently, which affords a sense of
completion, when the last step is mastered
the therapist assists until the last two
steps are mastered, then the PT independently
completes these last two steps. The process
continues c the therapist offering less assistance,
PT performs from last step to first independently

Environment should be adequate + safe

Right Affected Side

5C   PUTTING ON SOCKS -
Sit in wheelchair Brakes Locked
with normal ^Left Leg, cross Right (Affected) Leg over
open top of sock with Left hand Thumb and two
fingers, work sock onto the foot and pull
over heel and pull up sock eliminating wrink
The PT would place the unaffected Left Leg
on the affected Leg and follow the same
steps using his Left hand to put on his
Left sock.

PUTTING ON UNDERWEAR or TROUSERS
Sit in chair with Locked wheelchair
position normal Leg in front of midline
of body with knee flexed to 90 degrees.
using A normal hand reach forward and
grasp ankle

Pedretti
P 257